AF180447

Operative Techniques in Liver Surgery

Operative Techniques in Liver Surgery

Edited by Everett Bailey

hayle medical
New York

Hayle Medical,
750 Third Avenue, 9th Floor,
New York, NY 10017, USA

Visit us on the World Wide Web at:
www.haylemedical.com

© Hayle Medical, 2019

This book contains information obtained from authentic and highly regarded sources. Copyright for all individual chapters remain with the respective authors as indicated. All chapters are published with permission under the Creative Commons Attribution License or equivalent. A wide variety of references are listed. Permission and sources are indicated; for detailed attributions, please refer to the permissions page and list of contributors. Reasonable efforts have been made to publish reliable data and information, but the authors, editors and publisher cannot assume any responsibility for the validity of all materials or the consequences of their use.

ISBN: 978-1-63241-638-4

The publisher's policy is to use permanent paper from mills that operate a sustainable forestry policy. Furthermore, the publisher ensures that the text paper and cover boards used have met acceptable environmental accreditation standards.

Trademark Notice: Registered trademark of products or corporate names are used only for explanation and identification without intent to infringe.

Printed in China.

Cataloging-in-Publication Data

Operative techniques in liver surgery / edited by Everett Bailey.
p. cm.
Includes bibliographical references and index.
ISBN 978-1-63241-638-4
1. Liver--Surgery. 2. Surgery, Operative--Technique. 3. Operations, Surgical. I. Bailey, Everett.
RD546 .O64 2019
617.556--dc23

Table of Contents

Preface

This book aims to highlight the current researches and provides a platform to further the scope of innovations in this area. This book is a product of the combined efforts of many researchers and scientists, after going through thorough studies and analysis from different parts of the world. The objective of this book is to provide the readers with the latest information of the field.

A number of surgical procedures are available for the treatment of malignant and benign liver conditions. Many techniques have evolved over the years to make liver surgery more effective, simpler and safer. It is now possible to perform complicated, major and more involved liver surgical procedures within a few hours and without the requirement of blood transfusions. The most common type of liver surgery is liver resection, which involves the complete or partial removal of the liver. It is mostly performed for the purpose of removing a tumor. Liver tumors can also be addressed using minimally invasive, catheter-based procedures and treatments. Surgeries for the treatment of liver lesions such as cysts, hemangiomas and adenomas can be done laparoscopically or in a conventional open surgical procedure, depending on the location of the lesion. The objective of this book is to give a general view of the different operative techniques of liver surgery, and their applications. It strives to provide a fair idea about liver surgery and to help develop a better understanding of the latest advances within this surgical specialization. It will be a vital reference text for hepatologists, gastroenterologists, surgeons and students alike.

I would like to express my sincere thanks to the authors for their dedicated efforts in the completion of this book. I acknowledge the efforts of the publisher for providing constant support. Lastly, I would like to thank my family for their support in all academic endeavors.

Editor

1

Safety of liver resection and effect on quality of life in patients with benign hepatic disease: Single center experience

Carsten Kamphues[1*], Sabine Engel[1], Timm Denecke[2], Roberta Bova[1], Michael Hippler-Benscheidt[1], Gero Puhl[1], Peter Neuhaus[1] and Daniel Seehofer[1]

Abstract

Background: Although liver resection has long been established for selected patients with benign hepatic disease, the success of surgical treatment of these patients cannot be evaluated exclusively through postoperative morbidity and mortality. Therefore, the aim of the study was to prove the safety of liver resection in the treatment of benign liver tumors and to evaluate the effect of surgical treatment on the patients' qauality of life.

Methods: A total of 146 patients who underwent liver resection because of benign liver tumors were included in this study. Postoperative outcome was assessed and patients evaluated their quality of life before surgery and at the present time using the European Organization for Research and Treatment of Cancer Quality of Life Questionnaire Core-30 (QLQ C-30).

Results: The rate of serious (> grade 2) complications was 4.1% with no postoperative death. The quality of life assessment revealed an overall improvement of general health status after resection (0.7 vs. 0.56, $p < 0.001$) and additionally a significant reduction of 6 out of 9 symptoms. Furthermore, compelling benefits in the patients' social and emotional coping could be detected after surgery.

Conclusions: Liver resection for benign liver disease is a safe procedure and leads to a significant improvement of quality of life in selected patients.

Background

In recent years benign liver tumors have been diagnosed in larger numbers due to advantages in diagnostic imaging modalities [1-4]. Most common benign entities are hemangioma, followed by focal nodular hyperplasia (FNH) and adenoma, which together represent more than 80% of all benign liver tumors [3-5]. Rare benign liver diseases include for instance parasitic liver cysts, cystadenoma, caroli's disease and angiomyolipoma. Although data are heterogenous incidence of simple liver cysts is estimated to be approximately 5% [3-5]. Despite widespread availability of imaging modalities the differentiation between benign and malignant liver tumors remains a diagnostic challenge. While the accurate distinction between FNH and adenoma, as well as hepatocellular carcinoma, may be difficult, it is essential with regard to the appropriate treatment strategy [6]. Percutaneous liver biopsy often has limited benefit and must be regarded as contraindicated, especially in hypervascular tumors such as hemangioma [7].

Most benign tumors do not require aggressive treatment and the indication for resection of benign hepatic lesions remains controversial [3,4,8,9]. Today, hepatectomy is an accepted treatment for primary and secondary liver malignancies with low mortality-rates and morbidity of less than 30% [3,4,10,11], but major liver surgery for benign liver disease remains under discussion. Currently accepted indications for surgical resection of a benign liver tumor include suspicion of malignancy and severe or progressive tumor-related symptoms [3,4,11]. Large or growing hepatic adenomas should also be resected based on the risk of malignant degeneration

* Correspondence: carsten.kamphues@charite.de
[1]Department of General, Visceral and Transplantation Surgery, Universitätsklinikum Charité, Campus Virchow Klinikum, Humboldt-Universität, D-13353 Berlin, Germany
Full list of author information is available at the end of the article

and severe bleeding. In patients with parasitic liver cysts (e.g. echinococcus) a resection of the cyst is also recommended.

Postoperative morbidity and mortality as well as recurrence rate are the main factors evaluating the clinical outcome of patients undergoing major liver resection. However, a number of biological, social and clinical parameters that are meaningful for the patient are not reflected by these data, especially after resection of benign liver tumors. Based on the modern concepts of health-related quality of life (QoL) several questionnaires, such as the EORTC-QLQ-C30, have been developed in recent years, measuring the subjective outcome for patients after hepatobiliary surgery [12-15]. Assessment of quality of life, such as disease-free or overall survival, has become an important tool for the assessment of cancer patients [16,17], but no study has so far evaluated the quality of life liver resection has on patients with benign liver tumors.

The aim of the study was therefore to evaluate the postoperative outcome of patients who underwent liver resection due to benign liver disease in a primary hepatobiliary center. Furthermore, this study represents the first evaluation of quality of life after resection of benign hepatic tumors overall.

Methods

Between April 2002 and May 2008 all patients who underwent liver resection for benign liver disease at our center were included in the study. Patients were excluded in case of occurrence of any malignant disease during the follow-up period.

For all patients eligible for the study the following data were collected in a prospective database: demographics, indication, details of surgical procedure, postoperative complications according to the score by Dindo et al. [18], follow up, including recurrence rate and survival, as well as quality of life before surgery and at the present time.

Indications for surgery were suspicion of malignancy, severe or progressive symptoms, diagnosis of parasitic liver cysts as well as diagnosis or suspicion of adenoma. Surgical procedures for benign liver tumors included: left and right hemihepatectomy, extended left and right hemihepatectomy, unisegmentectomy, plurisegmentectomy, atypical resection and combinations of these techniques. Patients undergoing laparoscopic fenestrations of liver cysts were excluded from the present analysis; however, patients who underwent formal liver resection for liver cysts or cystic liver tumors were included.

Quality of life

Quality of life before and after surgery was assessed by sending a quality of life questionnaire to all patients included in this study after recovery from surgery. The patients were asked to evaluate their quality of life before surgery and at present time. Since there is no specific questionnaire for benign liver tumors available, the European Organization for Research and Treatment of Cancer Quality of Life Questionnaire Core-30 (QLQ C-30, Version 3.0) was used. This questionnaire is normally used in clinical cancer trials, but also adequate for assessing quality of life in patients with benign liver tumors, whose symptoms and discomfort are often similar to cancer patients. The questionnaire consists of 30 items incorporating 5 functional scales (physical, role, social, emotional, cognitive), 9 symptom scales (fatigue, nausea/vomiting, pain, dyspnoea, insomnia, loss of appetite, constipation, diarrhea, financial difficulties) and a global health scale [19]. Beyond the questionnaire all patients were asked if they would undergo liver resection for a benign hepatic lesion again, based on their present quality of life.

Ethics

For this study ethical approval was obtained from the institutional ethical committee (EA2/047/09, Ethical committee of the Charité, University Clinic, Berlin) and all patients gave informed consent prior to the enrolment in the study.

Statistics

Statistical analysis was performed using PASW Statistics 18.0 (SPSS Inc., Chicago, IL) and the R statistical software (Version 2.8.1, GNU/Linux). All quantitative data were expressed as median and range, unless otherwise indicated. Differences between quality of life parameters were tested using the Wilcoxon-test for paired samples. A p-value of less than 0.05 was regarded as statistically significant.

Results

The study population consisted of 146 patients who had undergone liver resection due to benign liver disease at our center. There was an expected majority of female patients in the study population and preoperative blood samples did not reveal limited liver function in any of the patients. Relevant demographic and preoperative parameters of the entire cohort as well as the quality of life subpopulation are summarized in Table 1.

Diagnosis and indication

Main diagnosis in the study population was FNH in 45 patients (30.8%), followed by hemangioma in 28 patients (19.2%) and echinococcus cyst in 21 patients (14.4%). Table 2 categorizes the diagnoses for liver resection in this study.

Table 1 Demographics and preoperative liver values of all patients and the Quality of Life subpopulation.

	All patients (n = 146)	QoL group (n = 81)
Age [years]	44 (13 - 74)	46 (16-74)
Gender ratio (male : female)	37 (25.3%) : 109 (74.7%)	16 (19.8%) : 65 (80.2%)
Tumor size [mm]	65 (10 - 230)	70 (8 - 230)
Preoperative bilirubine level [mg/dl]	0.5 (0.2 - 6.2)	0.5 (0.2 - 3.0)
Preoperative AST [U/l]	24 (6 - 259)	24 (8 - 259)
Preoperative ALT [U/l]	26 (4 - 775)	25 (5 - 775)
Preoperative Quick value [%]	97 (27 - 130)	98 (27 - 130)

Values are median (range).

The leading indications for liver resection were severe or progressive symptoms in 77 patients (52.7%), 48 patients (32.9%) underwent liver resection because malignancy could not be completely ruled out through preoperative measures. The remaining 21 patients (14.4%) were resected because of echinococcus cysts.

In 115 patients (78.8%) postoperative histopathological findings could confirm the most likely preoperative diagnosis, whereas in 31 patients (21.2%) the preoperative diagnosis turned out to be misleading.

Operative procedures

The most frequently performed operative procedure was right hemihepatectomy in 39 cases (26.7%), followed by atypical resection (27 patients, 18.5%) and plurisegmentectomy (25 patients, 17.1%). Unisegmentectomy was performed in 17 patients (11.6%) whereas 16 patients (10.9%) underwent left hemihepatectomy. Extended hemihepatectomy was required in 15 patients (10.3%) on the right and in 7 patients (4.8%) on the left side.

The median operative time was 200 (77-517) minutes. In 32 patients (21.9%) a pringle maneuver was performed intraoperatively. 13 patients (8.8%) required blood transfusions during liver resection. The median stay on intensive care unit was 1 (0-10) day and patients were able to leave hospital after a median stay of 9 (2-55) days.

Postoperative complications and follow up

There were a total of 25 postoperative complications (17.1%) and no postoperative death in the entire cohort. 10 patients had sterile fluid collections, of which 3 (2.0%) required percutaneous drainage. 2 patients (1.3%) suffered from postoperative bile leakage and required reoperation on the first postoperative day. Infectious complications (e.g. wound infection, cholangitis) occurred in 12 (8.6%) patients, while one patient suffered a middle cerebral artery stroke despite sufficient anticoagulation. This patient recovered well and was sent to a neurological rehabilitation 16 days after surgery. The rate of serious (≥ grade 3) complications was 4.1% (6 patients) in the study population.

During the follow-up period recurrent disease was observed in 13 out of 146 patients, representing a recurrence rate of 9% for the entire cohort. 6 out of these 13 patients developed liver cysts again, leading to a disease recurrence rate of 40% in this subpopulation, while 5 patients with FNH (11.1% of the FNH population) and one patient each with adenoma (11.1% of the adenoma population) and hemangioma (3.6% of the hemangioma population) had recurrence of their liver disease. However, none of these cases were recurrences in the common sense but patients rather developed growth of preexisting small lesions in the remnant liver based on the fact that all of these conditions can be of multifocal nature. After a median follow-up of 50 months (3-95 months) all patients are still alive.

Table 2 Diagnosis and type of liver resection of the entire cohort and the Quality of Life (QoL) subpopulation.

		All patients (n = 146)	QoL group (n = 81)
Diagnosis			
	FNH	45 (30.8%)	27 (33.3%)
	Hemangioma	28 (19.1%)	14 (17.3%)
	Adenoma	9 (6.2%)	6 (7.4%)
	liver cyst	15 (10.3%)	9 (11.1%)
	echinococcus cyst	21 (14.4%)	9 (11.1%)
	caroli's disease	13 (8.9%)	7 (8.6%)
	others*	15 (10.3%)	9 (11.1%)
Type of liver resection			
	hemi- or extended hemihepatectomy	77 (52.7%)	44 (54.3%)
	parenchyma-sparing resection	69 (47.3%)	37 (45.7%)

others*: liver abscess (6 patients), cystadenoma (5 patients), angiomyolipoma (4 patients)

Quality of life

A total of 81 patients (55.5% of the entire cohort) who had returned a completed questionnaire were included in the quality of life assessment. Details on demographic data as well as diagnosis and type of liver resection are summarized in Table 1 and Table 2. The main indications for surgery were the occurrence of severe symptoms in 44 patients (50.6%) and suspicion of malignancy in 19 patients (19.8%). Postoperative morbidity rate was 17.2% (14 patients) and therefore in total not significantly different from the entire cohort. However, this subpopulation included 5 out of 6 patients with severe complications (6.2%). After a median follow-up of 56 months (17-76 months), 9 patients (11%) had recurrent disease, mainly after resection of benign liver cysts (4 patients = 40% of the liver cyst population). Likewise, all demographic as well as diagnostic and operative details of the quality of life subpopulation revealed no significant differences compared to the parameters of the entire cohort (data not shown). Therefore the quality of life assessment may be regarded as representative for the entire cohort.

Table 3 Results of EORTC QLQ C30 questionnaire before surgery and at present time.

	before Surgery		at present time		p
	mean	SD	mean	SD	
Global health status	0.56	0.30	0.70	0.22	**0.000**
Functional scales					
Physical functioning	0.83	0.22	0.85	0.17	0.16
Role functioning	0.73	0.34	0.77	0.31	0.23
Emotional functioning	0.57	0.29	0.66	0.26	**0.007**
Cognitive functioning	0.80	0.25	0.78	0.27	0.30
Social functioning	0.66	0.36	0.75	0.29	**0.03**
Symptom scales					
Fatigue	0.41	0.33	0.30	0.31	**0.004**
Nausea and vomiting	0.18	0.29	0.12	0.23	0.068
Pain	0.37	0.38	0.24	0.28	**0.001**
Dyspnoea	0.24	0.32	0.21	0.31	0.29
Insomnia	0.40	0.35	0.31	0.34	**0.027**
Appetite loss	0.19	0.32	0.11	0.23	**0.033**
Constipation	0.22	0.30	0.14	0.27	**0.027**
Diarrhoea	0.16	0.27	0.21	0.32	**0.039**
Financial difficulties	0.17	0.33	0.18	0.30	0.98

p< 0.05 is considered significant and in bold.
SD: Standard deviation

Quality of life assessment

Statistical analysis revealed a highly significant improved global health status after resection of benign liver tumor in our population (0.7 vs. 0.56, $p < 0.001$).

The Wilcoxon test for paired samples also showed a remarkable benefit in social ($p = 0.03$) and emotional functioning ($p = 0.007$) after surgery, whereas no impact on physical wellbeing and cognitive functioning was detected.

A reduction of symptoms after operative therapy of benign liver disease was observed in 6 out of 9 symptom scales. Especially for the symptoms pain (0.24 vs. 0.37, $p = 0.001$) and fatigue (0.3 vs. 0.41, $p = 0.004$) the postoperative improvement was highly significant. A detailed analysis of the EORTC QLQ C-30 questionnaire is summarized in Table 3.

At the end of the follow-up period, 78 of 81 patients (96.3%) would again undergo liver resection due to benign liver disease from their present point of view.

Discussion

Despite controversial discussion about the practice of liver surgery in benign liver disease, nowadays liver resection is well-established as treatment of selected patients. Despite ongoing advantages in imaging modalities in recent years, there still is a considerable proportion of patients with an incorrect preoperative diagnosis. In a study by Charny et al. only 42 out of 62 preoperative diagnoses (67.7%) could be confirmed postoperatively by histopathological examination [11]. In the present study the percentage of patients with correct preoperative diagnosis increased to 78.8%, largely due to improved preoperative diagnostics. However, in a relevant number of patients the differentiation between benign and malignant hepatic lesions remains challenging.

In the largest series in literature Feng et al. reported on 827 liver resections for benign hepatic tumors with a postoperative complication rate of 13.5%, showing that liver resection can be regarded as a safe procedure [20]. Similar results were published by Charny et al. [11], who reported on 155 patients undergoing liver resection due to benign hepatic disease with a postoperative morbidity of 21% and no postoperative death. These results can be emphasized by the present study showing an overall complication rate of 17.1% with a mortality of 0%. In this series a total of only 4.1% of the patients had serious complications (≥ grade 3) which required further intervention but all of them recovered well during the follow-up period; however the majority of postoperative complications can be regarded as minor. Comparable data have recently been published by Lordan et al. [21]. In a series of 79 liver resections the rate of serious complications was 1.3% and no postoperative death occurred. This leads to the conclusion that even major hepatic resections of benign liver tumors can be safely performed in specialized hepatobiliary centers. This fact might influence the decision-finding process in these patients.

Furthermore the present study underlines that the recurrence rate of benign liver disease after liver resection is low. In our study 9% of the patients had recurrent disease and none of them required re-intervention. This strengthens the hypothesis that according to the standard parameters, morbidity and tumor recurrence, hepatic resection reaches good results in the treatment of benign liver disease. However, there are some important aspects concerning the patients' subjective feelings, which are not reflected by these parameters. Different health-related quality of life tools like the EORTC QLQ-C30 or the short-form 36 (SF 36) have been developed during the last 15 years in order to measure the effect of different therapeutic strategies on patients life, mainly in oncological patients [22-24]. These days, quality of life tools have also been established in the evaluation of subjective outcome of common hepatobiliary procedures and are therefore incorporated into the decisions of clinicians and patients [12-14]. In a prospective longitudinal study Poon et al. showed a significant enhancement of quality of life in patients with hepatocellular carcinoma after hepatectomy [12]. Similar results were presented in another study by Martin et al. who revealed a significant improvement in long-term quality of life after major hepatectomy in patients with primary or metastatic liver cancer [13]. It is widely accepted that quality of life represents a parameter which is as important as disease-free survival or overall survival in cancer patients [15]. Nevertheless there is hardly any data about quality of life in patients with benign disease so far.

Although, particularly for those patients, for whom morbidity and mortality are not sufficient in evaluating the therapeutic success, this study is, to our knowledge, the first in literature that evaluates the impact of hepatic resection on the quality of life of patients with benign liver tumors. In several other studies it has been shown that 80-89% of all patients with preoperative complaints due to benign liver disease were asymptomatic after liver resection [8,11,21,25], but these studies only focused on a selection of all patients and often referred to a single symptom. In the present study it could be elucidated that hepatic resection leads to a significant improvement of global health status in the entire group of patients with benign liver disease. Beside a reduction of 6 out of 9 analyzed symptoms, a significant impact of liver resection on social and emotional functioning in these patients could be detected. The fact, that 96.3% of the patients would undergo liver resection again from their present point of view stresses the positive effect of liver surgery on patients' everyday lives. Although the interpretation of this study might be limited due to its retrospective character these results give a strong impression of the patients' subjective outcome after resection of benign liver tumors and underline the benefit of surgical treatment from the patients' point of view. The immanent bias of the return rate of the questionnaires in retrospective studies cannot be avoided in the present study as well. However, the Quality of Life subpopulation can be regarded as representative for the entire cohort and therefore all conclusions can be drawn for all the patients in this study.

Conclusions

In conclusion, this study demonstrates that liver resection due to benign liver tumor can be performed safely in a specialized hepatobiliary center. Furthermore, this study is the first in literature to show that surgical treatment of benign liver lesions might lead to an improvement in quality of life by reducing symptoms and improving emotional and social functioning. Further prospective studies are crucial in order to support these results and thus might affect the decision-finding processes in patients with benign liver tumors.

Non-financial competing interests

- Are there any non-financial competing interests (political, personal, religious, ideological, academic, intellectual, commercial or any other) to declare in relation to this manuscript? If so, please specify. - No.
- The authors declare that they have no competing interests.

Acknowledgements and funding
None

Author details
[1]Department of General, Visceral and Transplantation Surgery, Universitätsklinikum Charité, Campus Virchow Klinikum, Humboldt-Universität, D-13353 Berlin, Germany. [2]Department of Radiology, Universitätsklinikum Charité, Campus Virchow Klinikum, Humboldt-Universität, D-13353 Berlin, Germany.

Authors' contributions
CK had full access to all the data in the study and takes responsibility for the integrity of the data and accuracy of analysis. CK, SE, DS and PN were responsible for the study concept and design. The acquisition of data was performed by CK, SE, RB, TD and GP. CK, SE, TD, MHB, DS and GP were involved in the analysis and interpretation of data. The manuscript was written by CK, SE, RB, TD and MHB and critically revised by DS, GP and PN. All authors approved the final version of the manuscript.

Competing interests
Financial competing interests
- In the past five years have you received reimbursements, fees, funding, or salary from an organization that may in any way gain or lose financially from the publication of this manuscript, either now or in the future? Is such an organization financing this manuscript (including the article-processing charge)? If so, please specify. - No.
- Do you hold any stocks or shares in an organization that may in any way gain or lose financially from the publication of this manuscript, either now or in the future? If so, please specify. - No.
- Do you hold or are you currently applying for any patents relating to the content of the manuscript? Have you received reimbursements, fees,

funding, or salary f om an organization that holds or has applied for patents relating to the con:ent of the manuscript? If so, please specify. - No.
• Do you have any other financial competing interests? If so, please specify. - No.

References

1. Choi BY, Nguyen MH: **The diagnosis and management of benign hepatic tumors.** *J Clin Gastroenterol* 2005, **39**:401-12.
2. Federle MP, Brancatelli G: **Imaging of benign hepatic masses.** *Semin Liver Dis* 2001, **5**:17-42.
3. Kammula US, Buell JF, Labow DM, Rosen S, Millis JM, Posner MC: **Surgical management of benign tumors of the liver.** *Int J Gastrointestinal Cancer* 2001, **30**:141-146.
4. Ibrahim S, Chen CL, Wang SH, Lin CC, Yang CH, Yong CC, Jawan B, Cheng YF: **Liver resection for benign liver tumors: indications and outcome.** *Am J Surg* 2007, **193**:5-9.
5. Nichols FC, van Heerden JA, Weiland LH: **Benign liver tumors.** *Surg Clin North Am* 1989, **69(2)**:297-314.
6. DeCarlis L, Pirotta V, Rondinara GF, Sansalone CV, Colella G, Maione G, Slim AO, Rampoldi A, Cazzulani A, Belli L, Forti D: **Hepatic adenoma and focal nodular hyperplasia: diagnosis and criteria for treatment.** *Liver Transpl Surg* 1997, **3**:160-165.
7. Taavitsainen M Airaksinen T, Kreula J, Paivansalo M: **Fine-needle aspiration biopsy of liver hemangioma.** *Acta Radiol* 1990, **31**:69-71.
8. Terkivatan T, de Wilt JH, de Man RA, van Rijn RR, Zondervan PE, Tilanus HW, IJzermans JN: **Indications and long-term outcome of treatment of benign hepatic tumors. A critical appraisal.** *Arch Surg* 2001, **136**:1033-1038.
9. Farges O, Daradkeh S, Bismuth H: **Cavernous hemangiomas of the liver: Are there any indications for resection?** *World J Surg* 1995, **19**:19-24.
10. Jarnagin WR, Gonen M, Fong Y, DeMatteo RP, Ben-Porat L, Little S, Corvera C, Weber S, Blumgart LH: **Improvement in perioperative outcome after hepatic resection: Analysis of 1803 consecutive cases over the past decade.** *Ann Surg* 2002, **236**:397-407.
11. Charny CK, Jarnagin WR, Schwartz LR, Frommeyer HS, DeMatteo RP, Fong Y, Blumgart LH: **Management of 155 patients with benign liver tumours.** *Br J Surg* 2001, **88**:808-813.
12. Poon RT, Fan ST, Yu WC, Lam BK, Chan FY, Wong J: **A prospective longitudinalstudy of quality of life after resection of hepatocellular carcinoma.** *Arch Surg* 2001, **136**:693-699.
13. Martin RC, Eid S, Scoggins CR, McMasters KM: **Health-related quality of life: Return to baseline after major and minor liver resection.** *Surgery* 2007, **142**:676-684.
14. Sajid MS, Iftikhar M, Rimple J, Baig MK: **Use of health-related quality of life tools in hepatobiliary surgery.** *Hepatobiliary Pancreat Dis Int* 2008, **7**:135-137.
15. Banz VM, Inderbitzin D, Fankhauser R, Studer P, Candinas D: **Long-term Quality of Life after hepatic resection: Health is not simply the absence of disease.** *World J Surg* 2009, **33**:1473-1480.
16. Mayer RJ: **Summary of the second international conference on biology, prevention and treatment of gastrointestinal malignancies.** *Ann Oncol* 1995, **6**:645-9.
17. Slevin ML: **Quality of life: philosophical question or clinical reality.** *BMJ* 1992, **305**:466-469.
18. Dindo A, Demartines N, Clavien PA: **Classification of surgical complications.** *Ann Surg* 2004, **240**:205-213.
19. Aaronson NK, Ahmedzai S, Bergman B, Bullinger M, Cull A, Duez NJ, Filiberti A, Flechtner H, Fleishman SB, de Haes JC: **The European Organization for Research and Treatment of Cancer QLQ-C30: a quality-of-life instrument for use in international clinical trials in oncology.** *J Natl Cancer Inst* 1993, **85**:365-376.
20. Feng ZQ, Huang ZQ, Xu LN, Liu R, Zhang AQ, Huang XQ, Zhang WZ, Dong JH: **Liver resection for benign hepatic lesions: A retrospective analysis of 827 consecutive cases.** *World J Gastroenterol* 2008, **14(47)**:7247-7251.
21. Lordan JT, Worthington TR, Quirney N, Fawcett W, Karanjia ND: **Early postoperative outcomes following hepatic resection for benign liver disease in 79 consecutive patients.** *HPB* 2009, **11**:321-325.
22. Sloan JA, Loprinzi CL, Kuross SA, Miser AW, O'Fallon JR, Mahoney MR, Heid IM, Bretscher ME, Vaught NL: **Randomized comparison of four tools measuring overall quality of life in patients with advanced cancer.** *J Clin Oncol* 1998, **16**:3662-3673.
23. Kemmler G, Holzner B, Kopp M, Dünser M, Margreiter R, Greil R, Sperner-Unterweger B: **Comparison of two quality-of-life instruments for cancer patients: the Functional Assessment of Cancer Therapy-General and the European Organization for Research and Treatment of Cancer Quality of Life Questionnaire-C30.** *J Clin Oncol* 1999, **17**:2932-2940.
24. Camilleri-Brennan J, Steele RJ: **Quality of life after treatment for rectal cancer.** *Br J Surg* 1998, **85**:1036-43.
25. Fioole B, Kokke M, van Hillegersberg R, Rinkes IH: **Adequate symptom relief justifies hepatic resection for benign disease.** *BMC Surgery* 2005, **5**:7-11.

Vascular coil erosion into hepaticojejunostomy following hepatic arterial embolisation

Soondoos Raashed[1], Manju D Chandrasegaram[1,2], Khaled Alsaleh[1], Glen Schlaphoff[3] and Neil D Merrett[1,2*]

Abstract

Background: Right hepatic arterial injury (RHAI) is the most common vascular injury sustained during laparoscopic cholecystectomy, occurring in up to 7% of cholecystectomies. RHAI is also the most common vascular injury associated with a bile duct injury (BDI) and is reported to occur in up to 41 – 61% of cases when routine angiography is employed following a BDI.

We present an unusual case of erosion of vascular coils from a previously embolised right hepatic artery into bilio-enteric anastomoses causing biliary obstruction. This is on a background of biliary reconstruction following a major BDI.

Case presentation: A 37-year old man underwent a bile duct reconstruction following a major BDI (Strasberg-Bismuth E4 injury) sustained at laparoscopic cholecystectomy. He had two separate bilio-enteric anastomoses of the right and left hepatic ducts and had a modified Terblanche Roux-en-Y access limb formed.

Approximately three weeks later he was admitted for significant gastrointestinal bleeding and was hypotensive and anaemic. Selective computed tomography angiography revealed a 2 x 2 centimetre right hepatic artery pseudoaneurysm, which was urgently embolised with radiological coils.

Two months later he developed intermittent fevers, rigors, jaundice, and right upper quadrant pain with evidence of intrahepatic biliary dilatation on magnetic resonance cholangiopancreatography. The degree of intrahepatic biliary dilatation progressively increased on subsequent imaging over several months, suggesting stricturing of the bilio-enteric anastomoses. Several attempts to traverse these strictures with a percutaneous transhepatic approach had failed. Then, approximately ten months after the initial BDI repair, choledochoscopy through the Terblanche access limb revealed multiple radiological coils within the bilio-enteric anastomoses, which had eroded from the previously embolised right hepatic artery. A laparotomy was performed to remove the coils, take down the existing obstructed bilio-enteric anastomoses and revise this. Following this the patient recovered uneventfully.

Conclusion: Obstructive jaundice and cholangitis secondary to erosion of angiographically placed embolisation coils is a rarely described complication. In view of the relative frequency of arterial injury and complications following major bile duct injury, we suggest that these patients be formally assessed for associated arterial injury following a major BDI.

Background

Bile duct injury (BDI) associated with laparoscopic cholecystectomy (LC) occurs in 0.3 – 0.6% of cases [1]. Right hepatic arterial injury (RHAI) is the most common vascular injury during LC, occurring in up to 7% of cholecystectomies [2-4]. RHAI is also the commonest vascular injury associated with major BDI, with centers employing routine angiography following a BDI reporting RHAI rates of up to 41 – 61% [1,2,5], presumably secondary to the anatomical proximity of the right hepatic artery (RHA) to the bile duct (BD) [3,6]. Interestingly, where an associated biliary injury exists, arterial occlusions are far more common than pseudoaneurysms, however, where there is no biliary injury, reports of pseudoaneurysms are more common [3]. We present an unusual case of BDI repair complicated by RHA pseudoaneurysm requiring radiological coil embolisation, with a delayed complication of biliary obstruction secondary to erosion of coils into the hepato-enteric anastomosis.

* Correspondence: n.merrett@uws.edu.au
[1]Upper Gastrointestinal Unit, Bankstown Hospital, Sydney, Australia
[2]Division of Surgery, School of Medicine, University of Western Sydney, Sydney, Australia
Full list of author information is available at the end of the article

Case presentation

A previously healthy 37-year old man was transferred to our service with high volume bilious drainage immediately following an elective LC for gallstone pancreatitis. An endoscopic retrograde cholangiopancreatography (ERCP) showed no flow above the mid common bile duct (CBD). Laparotomy found that the CBD was divided at the level of the cystic duct with segmental resection of the common hepatic duct involving the confluence of the hepatic ducts with separation of the right and left hepatic ducts (Strasberg-Bismuth E4 injury). A bile duct reconstruction was performed, bringing together the separated adjacent walls of the right and left hepatic ducts together and suturing them to form a common wall. The bilio-enteric anastomoses were then performed over separate externalised stents via a modified Terblanche Roux-en-Y limb [7]. The anastomoses on subsequent imaging gave the appearance of a preserved confluence, because of the sutured common adjoining walls of the right and left separated ducts. There was an uneventful recovery and he was discharged 10 days post-operatively with the biliary stents in situ.

One week after discharge, the patient experienced a gastrointestinal bleed and presented with melaena to a nearby hospital. He was found to have a haemoglobin level of 90 g/L (Reference range: 130 – 180 g/L) and was transfused with two units of packed red blood cells. He underwent a gastroscopy and colonoscopy to investigate this. No obvious cause for his bleeding was found, and one colonic pedunculated polyp was removed. His bleeding settled and he was discharged three days after admission. Our unit was not notified of this admission.

Two days following this discharge, the patient had an episode of haematochezia associated with collapse at home. He was taken to the emergency department of our hospital where he was hypotensive (blood pressure 92/63 mmHg) and tachycardic (heart rate 115 beats/min). His abdomen was soft and non-tender, and digital rectal examination revealed dark red blood. His haemoglobin level was 111 g/L. He was initially resuscitated with crystalloids, but had further episodes of fresh rectal bleeding. Repeat haemoglobin was 58 g/L, and packed red blood cell transfusion was commenced. Urgent selective computed tomography angiography was performed revealing a 2 × 2 centimetre aneurysm arising from the RHA/cystic artery adjacent to surgical clips. The aneurysm was embolised with platinum and stainless steel radiological coils (Figure 1, Figure 2). A tubogram through the biliary stents after the procedure showed no evidence of leakage or stricture of the biliary anastomoses. He had no further bleeding and was discharged three days later. Four weeks later, the stents were removed in the outpatient rooms.

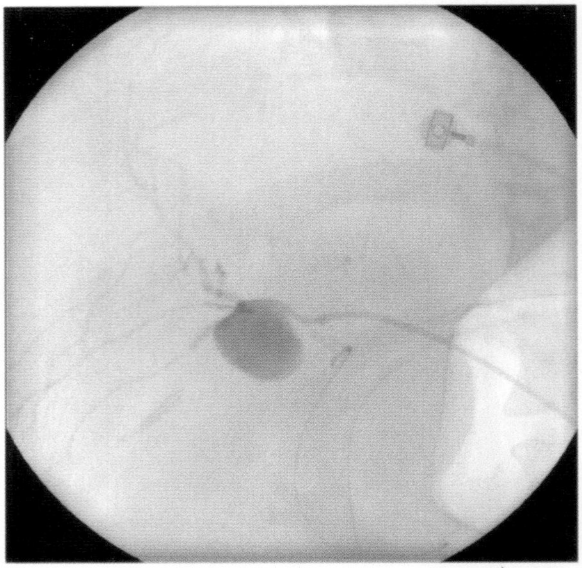

Figure 1 Pseudoaneurysm of the right hepatic artery on angiogram.

Two months later the patient developed intermittent fevers, rigors, jaundice and right upper quadrant pain. His liver function tests revealed a cholestatic picture with an elevated bilirubin of 59 μmol/L (Reference range: 0 – 17 μmol/L), ALP 473 U/L (Reference range: 30 – 115 U/L) and GGT 721 U/L (Reference range: < 66 U/L).

A magnetic resonance cholangiopancreatography (MRCP) was performed, showing slight prominence of the intrahepatic biliary radicles above the level of the right and left main hepatic ducts, with preservation of

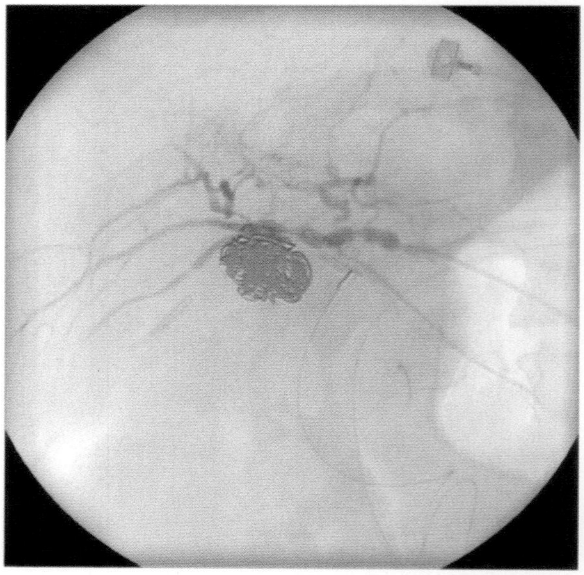

Figure 2 Coil embolisation of right hepatic arterial pseudoaneurysm.

the contour of the biliary ducts without evidence of irregularity or stenosis. A hepatobiliary iminodiacetic acid (HIDA) scan to assess biliary excretion showed mild retention of tracer in left hepatic lobe inferiorly in pre- and post-cholecystokinin images but no evidence to suggest biliary stenosis. It also suggested poor emptying from the Roux loop and it was felt that associated bacterial overgrowth within the Roux loop may have been responsible for his symptoms and he was kept on low dose oral antibiotics with improvement of his liver function tests at six weeks (bilirubin 9 U/L, ALP 361 U/L and GGT 504). Progress MRCP two months later revealed increasing intrahepatic biliary dilatation with the left main hepatic duct increasing in diameter from 6.6 mm on the previous MRCP to 9.8 mm, suggesting a significant bilio-enteric anastomotic stricture.

Thus, approximately 10 months after his BD reconstruction, he was admitted electively for percutaneous transhepatic cholangiography (PTC) and balloon dilatation of this bilio-enteric anastomosis. After confirmation of the stricture by PTC, a 4 French catheter was inserted into his left ductal system and an 8.5 French pigtail catheter was placed into his right ductal system but neither could be advanced into the enteric limb (Figure 3). Two further attempts were made at PTC balloon dilatation, but both failed. It was decided to attempt to visualise the anastomosis through the Terblanche access limb. Choledochoscopy through the modified Terblanche access limb showed multiple radiological coils from the previous embolisation of the RHA pseudoaneurysm at the site of the anastomoses, causing a mechanical obstruction (Figure 4, Figure 5). Laparotomy was performed and the bilio-enteric anastomoses were taken down to remove the coils. The right and left ductal systems were evaluated with intraoperative cholangiogram and the bilio-enteric anastomoses were revised using the existing Roux limb around 10 French infant feeding catheters, which were externalised again through the modified Terblanche limb.

Post-operative recovery was uneventful. A cholangiography through the catheters showed good drainage of contrast through the bilio-enteric anastomoses. The

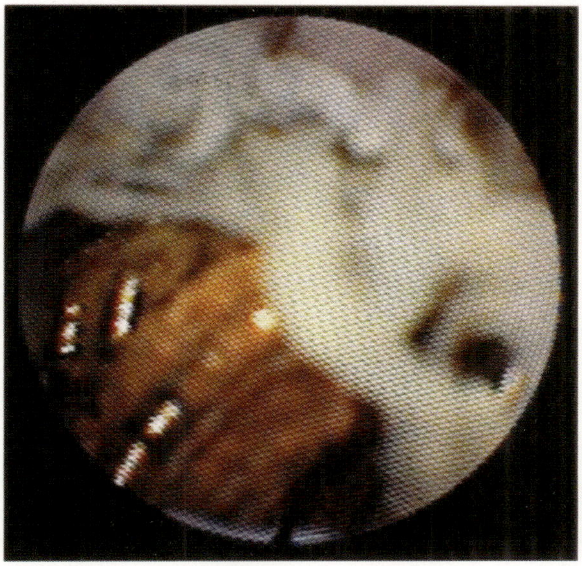

Figure 4 Coils seen around hepaticojejunostomy from within Roux limb on choledochoscopy.

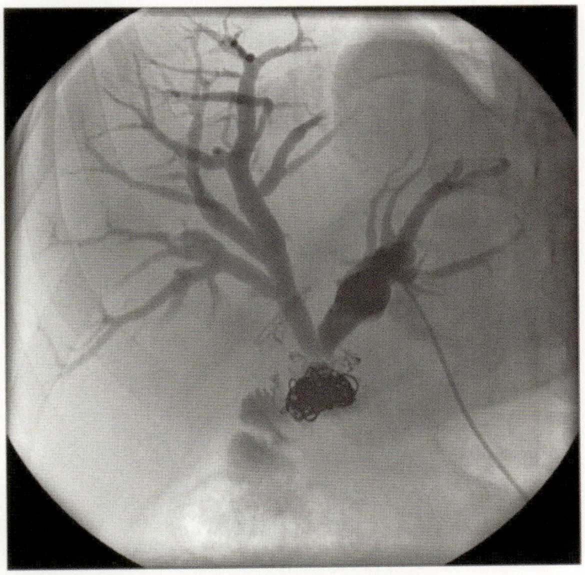

Figure 3 Biliary catheter in left hepatic ductal system.

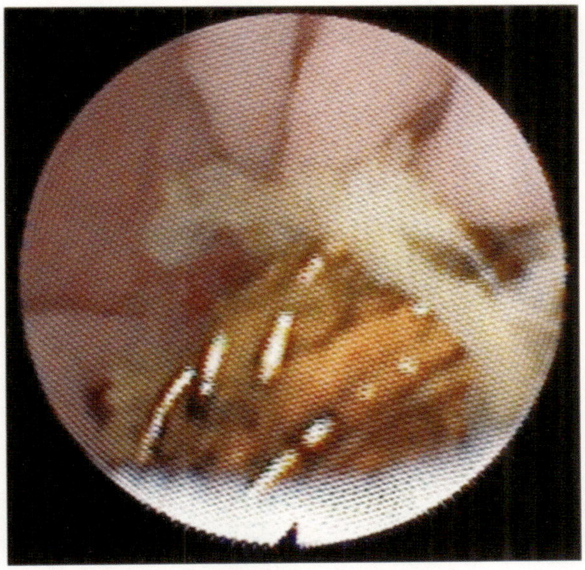

Figure 5 Coils seen around hepaticojejunostomy from within Roux limb on choledochoscopy.

Table 1 Vascular coil migration from right hepatic artery to common bile duct

Author	Age/ sex	Primary operation	Timing of RHApA bleed post-primary operation	Management of bleed	Time after which vascular coils migrated to CBD	Presenting symptom	Management
Current study	38 M	Bile Duct Reconstruction after BDI following cholecystectomy	1 week	Required one attempt at coil embolisation "packing technique" with flow maintained within the artery.	10 months	Obstructive jaundice and Cholangitis	3 attempts with PTC to traverse biliary obstruction failed, bilateral biliary catheter drainage, and re-operation to revise hepaticojejunostomy
Van Steenbergen et al. [22]	72 M	Liver transplantation for primary biliary cirrhosis	10 weeks	Coil embolisation "packing technique" with flow maintained within the artery. Bleeding recurred with revascularization of aneurysm. ePTFE covered coronary stent placed to exclude pseudoaneurysm	5 years	Stone and coils in bile duct, described as "biliary colic"	ERCP (failed removal), coils and stone removed with PTC
AlGhamdi et al. [23]	55 F	Liver transplant for Hepatitis C cirrhosis and hepatocellular carcinoma	13 weeks post-transplant, (had 2 balloon angioplasties of hepatic artery jump graft 10 weeks post-transplant for stenosis)	Embolisation of bleeding aneurysm, and balloon covered stent used to treat hepatic artery stenosis. Further small pseudoaneurysm at junction of hepatic artery and jump graft managed with coil packing and further covered stent to exclude pseudoaneurysm.	3 months	Coil migration identified at time of biliary stent replacement for biliary stricture.	Coils and stones removed at ERCP with further balloon dilatation of stricture.
Turaga et al. [27]	65 M	Difficult cholecystectomy for gangrenous GB with T-tube choledochotomy after failed CBD stone retrieval	3 weeks	Required one attempt at embolisation	1 year	Obstructive jaundice and Cholangitis	ERCP (failed removal) → required open bile duct exploration, removal of coils and insertion of T-tube. Artery and pseudoaneurysm ligated
Kao et al. [28]	65 F	Cholecystectomy and T-tube choledochostomy	Not reported	Coil embolisation	8 years	Obstructive jaundice	PTC performed for biliary drainage followed by ERCP for removal of coils and stone from CBD
Ozkan et al. [14]	58 M	Subtotal Cholecystectomy for cholecystitis	4 weeks, Required 2 attempts at embolisation	Coil embolisation, "packing technique" with flow maintained within the artery. Required further embolisation 3 days later for rebleed, and growth of neck of pseudoaneurysm	2 years	Pancreatitis	ERCP identified coils → required open bile duct exploration, removal of coils and stones, and drainage of pseudocyst with cystojejunostomy

M: Male, F: Female, RHApA: RHA pseudoaneurysm, PTC: Percutaneous transhepatic cholangiography, ERCP: Endoscopic retrograde cholangiopancreatography.

patient was discharged 10 days after his operation, with total resolution of his jaundice and improvement in eating, drinking and general daily function. The stents were removed at six weeks and six years later the patient remained well with normal liver function tests and no further episodes of cholangitis.

Discussion

From cadaveric studies, RHAI occurs in up to 7% of cholecystectomies. RHAI without concomitant BDI or portal vein injury rarely causes clinically significant liver or biliary ischaemia [2-4]. This may be due to the ability of the hilar marginal arteries to shunt blood from the left hepatic arterial system across to the remaining distal divided RHA system. It has been suggested that RHAI combined with biliary injuries can lead to ischaemic stricturing which may not become stable for several months following the injury and may be responsible for anastomotic stricturing after early repair [3]. Review of the vascularity of the BD has suggested that high anastomoses are to be preferred to low anastomoses [8]. Interestingly, there is disagreement as to whether a RHAI actually worsens biliary injury, which may relate to referral patterns and timing of repair [1]. Schmidt et al. found on univariate and mutivariate analyses that associated arterial injury and repair in the presence of active peritonitis were associated with increased complications after BDI [9]. However the delayed repair view is not universal, with many authors supporting early repairs [1,10,11]. A recent paper has emphasised that early repair by a specialist Hepatobiliary surgeon is associated with equivalent stricture rates to delayed repair but improved quality of life, return to normal activities and lower cost [12].

Hepatic artery pseudoaneurysm following LC has a reported incidence of 0.5 – 0.8% and can present four weeks post-operatively but may occur up to 13 months post-operatively [13-16]. Radiographic embolisation has been used successfully in the management of post-cholecystectomy pseudoaneurysms [13,15-18]. A variety of embolic agents have been described, including coils, Gelfoam, tissue adhesives, thrombin, detachable balloons and autologous clot [15]. Tulsyan et al. reported technical success in endovascular treatment of 11 hepatic artery pseudoaneurysms using coils, N-butylcyanoacrylate (N-BCA) glue or a combination of both depending on the desired rate of polymerisation [19]. The ideal placement of coils is a point of contention, with some authors advocating packing of the pseudoaneurysm itself and others suggesting "sandwich packing" (i.e. distal and proximal coil packing) to avoid rupturing the pseudoaneurysm [17], as well as to avoid coil migration [20,21]. In the elective setting, combination of stenting with a covered stent to maintain arterial flow and the packing and exclusion technique have been proposed, but no large series of this technique have yet been described and it may be problematic in the emergency setting [22-24].

Aneurysm coil migration from all sites into the gastrointestinal tract has been reported in at least twelve cases [25,26]. Coil migration into the CBD from the RHA has been reported in five cases (Table 1) [27,28]. Coil erosion into the BD or bilio-enteric anastomoses causing biliary obstruction is exceedingly rare, and we were only able to find three other reports of this in the literature [14,27,28].

Conclusion

Obstructive jaundice and cholangitis secondary to erosion of angiographically placed embolisation coils is a rarely described complication following treatment of arterial injury subsequent to iatrogenic BDI. In view of the relative frequency of arterial injury and complications following major BDI, we would suggest that these patients be formally assessed for associated arterial injury.

Competing interests

The authors declare that they have no competing interests.

Authors' contributions

SR, MC, KA, GS and NM were involved in the conception and design of the case report and ongoing critical revisions of the manuscript. All authors gave final approval of the version to be published.

Acknowledgement

We have no sources of funding to declare.

Author details

[1]Upper Gastrointestinal Unit, Bankstown Hospital, Sydney, Australia. [2]Division of Surgery, School of Medicine, University of Western Sydney, Sydney, Australia. [3]Interventional and Diagnostic Radiology, Liverpool Hospital, Sydney, Australia.

References

1. Pekolj J, Alvarez F, Palavecino M, Clariá R, Mazza O, De Santibañes E. Intraoperative management and repair of bile duct injuries sustained during 10,123 laparoscopic cholecystectomies in a high-volume referral center. J Am Coll Surg. 2013;216(5):894–901.
2. Alves A, Farges O, Nicolet J, Watrin T, Sauvanet A, Belghiti J. Incidence and consequence of an hepatic artery injury in patients with postcholecystectomy bile duct strictures. Ann Surg. 2003;238(1):93–6.
3. Strasberg S, Helton W. An analytical review of vasculobiliary injury in laparoscopic and open cholecystectomy. HPB (Oxford). 2011;13(1):1–14.
4. Halasz N. Cholecystectomy and hepatic artery injuries. Arch Surg. 1991;126(2):137–8.
5. Koffron A, Ferrario M, Parsons W, Nemcek A, Saker M, Abecassis M. Failed primary management of iatrogenic biliary injury: incidence and significance of concomitant hepatic arterial disruption. Surgery. 2001;130(4):722–8.

6. Stewart L, Robinson T, Lee C, Liu K, Whang K, Way L. Right hepatic artery injury associated with laparoscopic bile duct injury: incidence, mechanism, and consequences. J Gastrointest Surg. 2004;8(5):523–30.
7. Krige J, Bornman P, Harries-Jones E, Terblanche J. Modified hepaticojejunostomy for permanent biliary access. Br J Surg. 1987;74(7):612–3.
8. Terblanche J, Worthley C, Spence R, Krige J. High or low hepaticojejunostomy for bile duct strictures? Surgery. 1990;108(5):828–34.
9. Schmidt S, Settmacher U, Langrehr J, Neuhaus P. Management and outcome of patients with combined bile duct and hepatic arterial injuries after laparoscopic cholecystectomy. Surgery. 2004;135(6):613–8.
10. Stewart L. Iatrogenic biliary injuries: identification, classification, and management. Surg Clin North Am. 2014;94(2):297–310.
11. Perera M, Silva M, Hegab B, Muralidharan V, Bramhall S, Mayer A, et al. Specialist early and immediate repair of post-laparoscopic cholecystectomy bile duct injuries is associated with an improved long-term outcome. Ann Surg. 2011;253(3):553–60.
12. Dageforde L, Landman M, Feurer I, Poulose B, Pinson C, Moore D. A cost-effectiveness analysis of early vs late reconstruction of iatrogenic bile duct injuries. J Am Coll Surg. 2012;214(6):919–27.
13. Ozkan OS, Walser EM, Akinci D, Nealon W, Goodacre B. Guglielmi detachable coil erosion into the common bile duct after embolization of iatrogenic hepatic artery pseudoaneurysm. J Vasc Interv Radiol. 2002;13(9 Pt 1):935–8.
14. Rivitz S, Waltman A, Kelsey P. Embolization of an hepatic artery pseudoaneurysm following laparoscopic cholecystectomy. Cardiovasc Intervent Radiol. 1996;19(1):43–6.
15. Sansonna F, Boati S, Sguinzi R, Migliorisi C, Pugliese F, Pugliese R. Severe hemobilia from hepatic artery pseudoaneurysm. Case Rep Gastrointest Med. 2011;2011:1–5.
16. Milburn J, Hussey J, Bachoo P, Gunn I. Right hepatic artery pseudoaneurysm thirteen months following laparoscopic cholecystectomy. EJVES Extra. 2007;13(1):1–3.
17. Nicholson T, Travis S, Ettles D, Dyet J, Sedman P, Wedgewood K, et al. Hepatic artery angiography and embolization for hemobilia following laparoscopic cholecystectomy. Cardiovasc Intervent Radiol. 1999;22(1):20–4.
18. Johnson SR, Koehler A, PL K, Hanto DW. Long-term results of surgical repair of bile duct injuries following laparoscopic cholecystectomy. Surgery. 2000;128(4):668–77.
19. Tulsyan N, Kashyap VS, Greenberg RK, Sarac TP, Clair DG, Pierce G, et al. The endovascular management of visceral artery aneurysms and pseudoaneurysms. J Vasc Surg. 2007;45(2):276–83.
20. Takahashi T, Shimada K, Kobayashi N, Kakita A. Migration of steel-wire coils into the stomach after transcatheter arterial embolization for a bleeding splenic artery pseudoaneurysm: report of a case. Surg Today. 2001;31(5):458–62.
21. Shah NA, Akingboye A, Haldipur N, Mackinlay JY, Jacob G. Embolization coils migrating and being passed per rectum after embolization of a splenic artery pseudoaneurysm, "The Migrating Coil": a case report. Cardiovasc Intervent Radiol. 2007;30(6):1259–62.
22. Van Steenbergen W, Lecluyse K, Maleux G, Pirenne J. Successful percutaneous cholangioscopic extraction of vascular coils that had eroded into the bile duct after liver transplantation. Endoscopy. 2007;39 Suppl 1:E210–1.
23. AlGhamdi HS, Saeed MA, AlTamimi AR, O'Hali WA, Khankan AA, AlTraif IH. Endoscopic extraction of vascular embolization coils that have migrated into the biliary tract in a liver transplant recipient. Dig Endoscopy. 2012;24(6):462–5.
24. DeFreitas D, Phade S, Stoner M, Bogey W, Powell C, Parker F. Endovascular stent exclusion of a hepatic artery pseudoaneurysm. Vasc Endovascular Surg. 2007;41(2):161–4.
25. Tekola BD, Arner DM, Behm BW. Coil migration after transarterial coil embolization of a splenic artery pseudoaneurysm. Case Rep Gastroenterol. 2013;7(3):487–9.
26. Han YM, Lee JY, Choi IJ, Kim CG, Cho S-J, Lee JH, et al. Endoscopic removal of a migrated coil after embolization of a splenic pseudoaneurysm: a case report. Clin Endosc. 2014;47(2):183–7.
27. Turaga KK, Amirlak B, Davis RE, Yousef K, Richards A, Fitzgibbons RJJ. Cholangitis after coil embolization of an iatrogenic hepatic artery pseudoaneurysm: an unusual case report. Surg Laparosc Endosc Percutan Tech. 2006;16(1):36–8.
28. Kao W, Chiou Y, Chen T. Coil migration into the common bile duct after embolization of a hepatic artery pseudoaneurysm. Endoscopy. 2011;43:E364–5.

3

Clinical symptoms and sonographic follow-up after surgical treatment of nonparasitic liver cysts

Hubert Scheuerlein*, Falk Rauchfuss, Julia Franke, Karin Jandt, Yves Dittmar, Gudrun Trebing and Utz Settmacher

Abstract

Background: The optimal treatment of nonparasitic liver cysts is still a topic of debate. Only symptomatic cysts are being considered as requiring treatment. Aim of this study is to evaluate our experience with this disease over the past ten years with a structured follow-up program.

Methods: From January 2000 to August 2010, 56 consecutive patients with nonparasitic liver cysts were treated at our institution. We assessed morbidity, recurrence and complication rates, quality of life as well as pre- and post-operative sonographic status of the cysts and course of clinical symptoms.

Results: In 84% of the patients surgery was started as a laparoscopic procedure. Conversion rate was 6.4%. Average diameter of deroofed cysts was 12 cm. Overall complication rate was 16% and overall recurrence rate 28.3% (8.7% recurrences at the surgical site, 19.6% new or enlarged cysts). One half of the patients were symptom-free after surgery and the other half had at least one persisting symptom post-operatively. In one half of these patients with persisting symptoms, symptoms were ameliorated by surgery. In the other half of patients the number of symptoms increased after surgery. Two thirds of the overall patients reported their post-operative health as being good or very good.

Conclusions: Surgical deroofing is the most effective treatment option for symptomatic liver cysts. Half of our patient population retained at least one symptom from a group of more than ten abdominal symptoms.
Only the minority of these cases may be attributed to true recurrence, de-novo cysts or growing pre-existing cysts. The analysis of our cases suggests that the persistent symptoms in our patients may in part be due to the fact that the association between clinical complaints and the liver cysts was not sufficiently established. A more rigid patient selection should be implemented in order to achieve better results from the treatment of cysts. Because even large cysts are frequently asymptomatic, patient selection should not primarily be based on the cyst size only. The decision should be based strictly on the correlation between cyst / cyst location and symptoms / clinical complaints. In our opinion, further diagnostic procedures may be necessary in individual cases to clarify such a correlation.

Background

Nonparasitic liver cysts occur in up to 5% of the population [1,2]. There are simple (single or multiple) cysts (simple liver cyst, SLC) as opposed to polycystic liver disease (PCLD). There is currently a general agreement that only symptomatic cysts should be treated. 10%-16% of patients with liver cysts develop symptoms at some stage in life [3]. Symptoms develop at an advanced age and are non-specific. Women are more frequently affected [4,5]. As the recurrence rate of percutaneous drainage alone is up to 100%, this procedure cannot be accepted as the only treatment [6]. For sclerotherapy very heterogeneous success rates between 0% and 100% are being reported with a low complication rate and short hospital stay [7]. In a recent prospective sclerotherapy study in 20 patients with 20% saline the cysts had completely disappeared after 2 years follow-up in 40% of the patients [8]. There are no larger or randomized comparative studies. Thus, sclerotherapy cannot be evaluated sufficiently with respect to its definitive value as yet. Laparoscopic cyst deroofing is the gold standard for treatment if this is feasible with respect to the location and configuration of the cysts [9,10]. Its value, too, has not been definitively assessed, but there are data

* Correspondence: Hubert.Scheuerlein@med.uni-jena.de
Department of General, Visceral and Vascular Surgery, University Hospital Jena, Erlanger Allee 101, 07747 Jena, Germany

that the short-term outcomes of laparoscopic fenestration were superior to the open approach [11]. Very heterogeneous success rates between 43% and 96% are being reported [2]. Irrespective of the surgical methods, true recurrence and growing remnant cysts are frequently reported in the literature. There is no definitive correlation with clinical symptoms. Studies with a larger sample size (> 50) and/or specific pre- and post-operative comparison of symptoms are scarce [2,11]. The value of this present study lies in its systematic sonografic and clinical follow-up after surgical cyst deroofing with a large patient population and long follow-up period.

Methods

Between January 2000 and August 2008, 56 consecutive patients with symptomatic nonparasitic hepatic cysts were evaluated and treated at our institution.

The decision for surgery was generally based on a minimum cyst size of 5 cm and abdominal pain, dyspnea and/or vegetative symptoms caused by adjacent organ compression or increased abdominal pressure and, therefore, causing gastrointestinal transport impairments, resulting in nausea, vomiting, oesophageal reflux, loss of appetite and/or early satiety. Mainly cysts located on the liver margin or underneath the surface within the parenchyma of the segments II, III, IVb, V and VI were selected for laparoscopic surgery.

There were 49 women and 7 men, with a mean age of 59 years (range 39 to 81 years). 4 patients had PCLD. All patients underwent pre-operative sonography. The echinococcus serology was negative in all cases.

These were the criteria for sonographic evaluation as benign / non-parasitic liver cyst: smooth margins, no septum, watery / clear cyst fluid, no contrast enhancement and calcifications. Further diagnostic procedures were initiated in cases of even the slightest suspicion of parasitic or neoplastic cyst.

All operations were performed as deroofing. The decision for open or laparoscopic surgery was made by the respective surgeon depending on his/her experience, cyst location and relevant co-morbidities (e.g. vena cava thrombosis being a contra-indication against the laparoscopic technique). The decision whether to perform an omentoplasty was also made exclusively by the operating surgeon. For open surgery, access was gained via a J incision. Laparoscopic surgery was performed via a 3-trocar-technique in the region of the right hypochondrium (in individual cases, another trocar was used as auxiliary trocar). For deroofing, we attempted to remove a maximum of the cyst roof ("wide deroofing"). The operating surgeon decided on the dissection method and in most cases, ultrasonic dissection was performed (Ultracision harmonic scalpel, Ethicon Endo Surgery, Norderstedt, Germany).

A specific questionnaire with regard to medical history (including a detailed history of the medication, paying special attention to female sexual hormones), symptoms and quality of life was developed. The patients were interviewed post-operatively and were asked to compare their current clinical complaints with the pre-operative complaints. All patients had additionally been invited for a sonographic and clinical follow-up examination. The pre- and post-operative sonographic examination was standardized on the basis of the Couinaud segment classification. Statistics were performed with SPSS 18 (chi-square test, Kruskal-Wallis test, paired t-test, Wilcoxon test). Patients were analysed regarding demographics, cyst morphology, symptoms and complaints, therapeutic procedures, postoperative complications according to Clavien-Dindo classification and longterm results (synopsis of relevant demographic and clinical characteristics in Table 1).

An approval of the local ethic's committee was not needed in this design, since all patients give their consent to follow-up investigations and further use of their data when entering our department. Furthermore, the study design was non-invasive.

Results

General aspects

For pre-operative work-up, 77% of patients had computed tomography in addition to sonography and 5% had an MRI.

Complete follow-up (sonography, clinical examination and complete questionnaire) was achieved in 46/51 patients (90%). The average follow-up period was 43 months (3–119 months). Four patients had died during follow-up (the cause of death was not related to the liver cyst or

Table 1 Demographic and clinical characteristics

Male : Female	7:49
Simple liver cysts : Polycystic liver disease	52:4
Age, years (range)	59 (39–81)
BMI, kg/m^2 (range)	27 (19–41)
ASA I, n (%)	9 (16)
ASA II, n (%)	42 (75)
ASA III, n (%)	5 (9)
Diameter of dominant cyst, cm (range)	12 (6–20)
Laparoscopic/open deroofing, n (%)	47 (84)/9 (16)
Conversion rate (%)	6.4
Simultaneous cholecystectomy, n (%)	16 (29)*
Postoperative complication rate (%)	16**
Recurrence rate (%)	8.7

*8/47 (17%) laparoscopic, 8/9 (89%) open; **13% laparoscopic, 33% open, not significant.
Abbreviations: BMI Body Mass Index, *ASA* American Society of Anesthesiologists.

surgery for liver cysts) and one patient with PCLD had a liver transplantation.

The cysts had been known for 40 months on average (0–360 months). The average BMI was 27 kg/m^2 (19–41 kg/m^2). 46/49 women (94%) had given birth. Use of female sexual hormones postmenopausal or for contraception was recorded in 22% and 67% of patients, there was no significant association with symptoms or cyst size. All surgical samples were examined by the pathologist and there was no malignancy. 41/56 (73%) did have prior abdominal surgery and 24/49 (49%) female patients did have prior gynaecological surgery. 18/56 (32%) patients did have other concomitant diseases of the gastrointestinal tract (Table 2). As for non-abdominal co-morbidities, these were mainly cardiac/circulatory (43%) and metabolic (32%). 16/56 (29%) patients had a simultaneous cholecystectomy (6× gall stones, 9× close proximity to the cyst, 1 both factors). 7/56 (13%) patients underwent previous treatment for their cysts elsewhere (5 percutaneous drainages, 1 laparoscopic and 1 open cyst fenestration). 9/56 (16%) patients were ASA class I, 42/56 (75%) were ASA class II and 5/56 (9%) were ASA class III. There was no surgical mortality.

Pre-operative symptoms

The distribution of pre-operative symptoms is shown in Table 3 (multiple answers possible, minimum number of symptoms 1, maximum number of symptoms 7).

Cyst status

17/52 (33%) patients with SLC had single and 35/52 (67%) had multiple cysts. Of the 4 patients with PCLD 2 had Gigot stage I and 2 had Gigot stage III. Only the left or the right liver lobe was affected in 7 (13%) and 11 (20%) cases, respectively. In the remaining 38 patients, both lobes were affected. There was a cyst related hepatomegaly in 41% of the patients. The average diameter of the deroofed cysts was 12 cm (6–20 cm). In one third of the patients, the segments IVa, VII and VIII were affected (these are considered as being difficult to access via the laparoscopic approach).

Table 2 Concurrent diseases of the gastrointestinal tract (multiple answers permitted)

Disease	n
Gallstones	8
Diverticulosis of the sigmoid colon	4
Steatosis hepatis	3
GERD	3
Gastritis	3
Peptic ulcer	1
Exocrine pancreatic insufficiency	1

GERD – Gastroesophageal reflux disease.

Table 3 Pre-operative symptoms (multiple answers permitted)

Symptom	n	%
Upper abdominal pain	33	58.9
Feeling of pressure	32	57,1
Fullness	8	14,3
Nausea	8	14,3
Weight loss	3	5,4
Vomiting	3	5,4
Dyspnoea	3	5,4
Early satiety	2	3,6
Loss of appetite	2	3,6

Laparoscopic surgery

In 47/56 (84%) patients surgery was started as a laparoscopic procedure. In 3 patients, there was a conversion to open surgery (conversion rate 6.4%). The reasons for conversion were hemorrhage (2 cases) and an incidental finding of a peritoneal metastasis from breast cancer (1 case). The average surgical duration was 80 min (16–230 min). In cases of simultaneous cholecystectomy (8 cases) the surgical duration was significantly prolonged, on average by 20 min ($p = 0.014$). A mean number of 2 cysts (1–9 cysts) were deroofed. In 5 patients, omentoplasty was performed. The average post-operative hospital stay was 6 days (4–13 days) following deroofing and cholecystectomy and 5.2 days (2–19 days) after deroofing only, respectively. The difference was not significant ($p = 0.291$).

Laparotomy

9/56 patients (including 2/4 patients with PCLD, both stage Gigot I) have had a primary laparotomy. The reasons for primary laparotomy included: cyst-related inferior vena cava thrombosis (2 cases), massive cystic liver (1 case), recurrence (1 case), previous Billroth-II resection (1 case), abscess (1 case) and position or morphology of the cysts deemed unfavourable (3 cases). The mean surgical duration was 106 min (44–173 min). An average of 2 cysts (1–3 cysts) have been fenestrated. Omentoplasty was performed in 3 cases. A simultaneous cholecystectomy was performed in 8 patients. When compared to the laparoscopic procedure, the post-operative hospital stay was significantly longer (mean 8.3 days, range 6–21 days; $p = 0.004$).

Complications

Intraoperative complications

There were 8 intra-operative complications in the laparoscopic group. These were injuries to the liver parenchyma (4 cases), one injury to the left hepatic vein, one hemorrhage during omentoplasty, one bile leak and one injury to the adrenal gland. The injury to the hepatic vein and one parenchymal hemorrhage led to conversion, all others were managed laparoscopically. There were no complications in the laparotomy group. Thus, the total intra-operative complication rate was 14% (8/56; laparoscopy group 8/47 (17%), laparotomy group 0/9 (0%)). The intra-operative complication rate was not significantly different ($p = 0.361$).

Postoperative complications

The total post-operative complication rate was 16% (9/56; laparoscopy group 6/47 (13%), laparotomy group 3/9 (33%)). There was a total of 14 complications, including 10 complications according to the Clavien-Dindo classification I (5 pleural effusions; ascites, impaired wound healing, partial respiratory insufficiency, dyspnoea, fever, one case each), one Clavien-Dindo classification II (urinary tract infection) and 3 cases of Clavien-Dindo classification IIIa (biloma / bile leak). There was a significant difference between the two surgical techniques ($p = 0.031$).

Follow-up

Immediate post-operative sonography

In 50/56 (89%) patients, a sonographic examination was performed immediately after surgery. In 29/50 (58%) patients, there were no more cysts, in 21/50 (42%) patients, remaining cysts have been observed. The total cysts volume had been reduced on average by 47% (6%-85%) through surgery in patients with remnant cysts.

Sonographic follow-up examination

The mean follow-up period was 43 months (3–119 months). 46/56 (82%) patients had a sonographic follow-up examination. Only 2/46 (4%) patients had no sonographic evidence of cysts. 11/46 (24%) patients had single and 33/46 (72%) patients had multiple cysts (including 3 patients with PCLD). There was cyst-related hepatomegaly in 15/46 (33%) patients. Only 3 patients with remaining cysts did not have any clinical complaints. In 8 patients, the size of the cysts had increased as compared to the immediate post-operative examination.

Symptoms and recurrence rate during follow-up

23/46 (50%) patients were completely symptom-free and 23/46 (50%) patients had persisting symptoms. 3/23 (13%) patients with persisting symptoms had no symptom change in the pre-/post-operative comparison, whereas 12/23 (52%) patients had increasing and 8/23 (35%) patients decreasing symptoms (Table 4). The post-operative symptoms included feeling of pressure (33%), upper abdominal pain (24%), fullness (15%), dyspnoea (15%), nausea (13%), early satiety (11%) and weight loss (2%; multiple answers possible). In 3/8 (38%) of the patients with decreased symptoms there was probably an association with a new cyst (5 cm, 7 cm and 11 cm, respectively). In 7/12 (58%) of the patients with increased symptoms relevant cysts have been observed (5–20 cm, average cyst size 9 cm). In one of these patients the increasing clinical complaints were most likely caused by a symptomatic incisional hernia. In the 3 patients with identical symptoms pre- and post-operatively, there might have been an association with a new cyst of 5 cm in size and in one case this was probable for a cyst of 15.5 cm. Therefore in altogether 12/23 (52%) patients with persisting or increasing symptoms this may generally be explained by a new cyst (8 of these 12 patients with a new cyst had a cyst size of at least 6 cm). Recurrences developed in 13/46 (28.3%) patients. 4 of those (4/46, 8.7%) have been "true surgical" recurrences at the former surgical site. All recurrences occurred after laparoscopic fenestration. There was, however, no significant association between recurrence and surgical technique ($p = 0.562$). 3 patients did have further surgery for liver cysts during the follow-up period. There was one open surgical revision (adhesions/stenosis of the gastroduodenal junction) and 2 laparoscopic re-operations. The

Table 4 Symptom change in patients with persisting symptoms

Symptom change	Number of symptoms Pre-operative → Post-operative	Δ (Difference)
No change (n = 3)	2 → 2	0
	1 → 1	0
	1 → 1	0
Symptom increase (n = 12)	2 → 6	4
	4 → 7	3
	1 → 4	3
	1 → 3	2
	1 → 3	2
	1 → 3	2
	1 → 3	2
	2 → 3	1
	2 → 3	1
	1 → 2	1
	1 → 2	1
	1 → 2	1
Symptom decrease (n = 8)	5 → 1	4
	4 → 2	2
	6 → 5	1
	3 → 2	1
	2 → 1	1
	2 → 1	1
	2 → 1	1
	2 → 1	1

Kruskal-Wallis test did not show any difference between the surgical techniques with respect to the number of reported clinical complaints. The decrease of the number of symptoms post-operatively as compared to pre-operatively was significant after laparoscopic surgery ($p = 0.004$) but did not improve after open or conversion surgery ($p = 0.667$ and $p = 1.000$, respectively).

Symptoms and description of the quality of life

7/46 (15%) patients reported their current health condition as being very good while 24/46 (52%) patients reported it as being good. 15/46 (33%) reported their current health condition as constricted, 13 of these 15 patients felt impaired in their daily lives by the reported symptoms. On a scale from 0–10, 33/46 (72%) patients did not report any impairment (0). 6/46 (13%) patients reported minor impairment (grade 1–3) and 7/46 (15%) patients reported moderate to major impairment (grade 4–8). 13/33 (39%) patients with an impairment degree of 0 in their daily lives did report at least 1 symptom in their history of clinical complaints.

Discussion

For SLCs cyst deroofing (laparoscopic wherever possible) is considered as being the therapeutic gold standard. The symptoms in patients with liver cysts are non-specific. Die Zystengröße allein scheint eine untergeordnete Rolle zu spielen, da selbst bei großen kongenitalen Leberzysten asymtpmatische Verläufe keine Seltenheit sind [3]. It is certain that other factors play a role, in particular the location of the cysts. So far, in the literature, there are hardly any considerations of psychosomatic factors that may play a role in a certain patient proportion which may be difficult to identify; these factors are complex and difficult to measure.

For reasons of clarity of the terminology and because of the fact that too small a fenestration may favour recurrence, the term complete cyst *deroofing* should be used in order to emphasize this aspect [3,12].

The value of the current study is in its rather concise follow-up (clinical examination, sonography, questionnaire) in a sufficiently large patient population and long follow-up period. Our patient population is comparable to those of other groups on the topic with respect to age, gender distribution, cyst size, symptoms and complication rate [2,10,13]. Studies with more than 50 patients and a specific follow-up are scarce [2,10,11,13,14]. A sufficiently long follow-up period is of critical importance in patients with liver cysts because there is evidence that a relatively large patient proportion (5-50% according to the literature) develops recurrent clinical symptoms from cysts within 3–5 years [2]. The mean follow-up period in this current study is 43 months. This duration was reached or surpassed in only half of the studies published so far [2]. There are only scarce exact comparisons of pre- and post-operative symptoms in the literature [2,11].

Our altogether recurrence rate is as high as 28.3%. For principal reasons in our opinion the type of recurrence (i.e. a "true surgical recurrence" at the former surgical site vs. a "recurrence of the disease" in terms of completely new or enlarged pre-existing cysts) should be considered as different entities in an analysis of surgical outcome. This discrimination can only be made by an accurate imaging during the follow-up and will not be done in the daily routine. Split like this our surgical recurrence rate was 8.7% and recurrent disease occurred in 19.6%, both rates being independent of the surgical approach.

Our study includes 4 patients with PCLD. Cyst deroofing (possibly laparoscopically) in Gigot stage I may provide a long lasting improvement. The recurrence rate in PCLD is generally higher, and more frequently liver resection is the treatment of choice [2]. Thus, there is a fundamental difference between SLC/PCLD stage I and PCLD stage II/III. In cases of diffuse disease, reduced nutritional status, extreme hepatomegaly and ascites, liver transplantation may be considered (in cases of GFR < 40 ml/min with simultaneous kidney transplantation) [15].

As in selected patients with PCLD the decision for resection or deroofing may be made, these cases were primarily included in the analysis. However, numerous reports in the literature suggest that patients with PCLD should be analyzed separately. Even though our 4 patients with PCLD should not have falsified our results significantly, we would strictly separate these two entities in future studies.

In all studies, females predominate (1:3 – 1:9) [2,10,12,13]. The age peak is around 60 years, as it is in our patient population. Between the age of 30 and 60 years, there is a progressive growth of cysts for reasons that are not known so far [16]. Several authors have linked this to the influence of estrogens [17]. In our patient population, we did not observe a significant association between female sexual hormones and symptoms or cyst size.

16/56 (29%) of our patients underwent simultaneous cholecystectomy for concomitant cholecystolithiasis or immediate proximity of the gallbladder to the cyst (8 open, 8 laparoscopically; 6 concomitant cholecystolithiasis, 9 immediate proximity, 1 concomitant cholecystolithiasis and immediate proximity).

The decision for surgery was based on the liver cyst even though it is not possible to clarify definitively if in case of concomitant gall stones the reported symptoms may be attributed to these (none of these patients did show typical signs of gall stone related disease, such as relevant elevated laboratory parameters, sonographic criteria or typical symptoms in the medical history). In case of gall stones, we generally perform a cholecystectomy simultaneously at our institution, except in cases where the patients decides otherwise.

In 84% of the patients, the cyst deroofing was started as a laparoscopic procedure, the conversion rate was 6.4%. There was previous abdominal or gynaecological surgery in 73% and 49%, respectively, while only in one case the previous abdominal surgery (Billroth-II resection) was the reason for a primary open procedure. In a total of 9 cases, the surgical procedure was primarily open (3 unfavorable cyst locations, 2 vena cava thromboses, 1 PCLD, 1 recurrence, 1 abscess, 1 Billroth-II resection). As reported in the literature, this approach was reserved for particular situations. In both cases of a concomitant vena cava thrombosis, successful thrombectomy was performed.

Three fourths of the patients were ASA stage II and almost one tenth were stage III. This explains the comparatively long hospital stay of 6 and 8 days, respectively (laparoscopic and open group, respectively).

In the literature, there are occasional reports about predominant affection of the right or left lobe. We could not confirm that observation in our patient population. In one third of our patients with laparoscopic surgery, segments IVa, VII and VIII were affected; access to these is considered to be difficult. This is as such not a contraindication against the laparoscopic approach, neither did it affect the conversion rate in a negative way. We believe that this confirms the experience of other authors, that this problem is met by an on-going learning curve on one hand and by specific patient positioning (modified left sided position) as required on the other hand.

In the laparoscopy group, the intra-operative complication rate was 17% (possibly related to the learning curve) while it was 0% in the laparotomy group (difference not significant). Those were mainly bleeding complications which led to conversion in 2 cases. The post-operative complication rate of 16% was within the data reported in the literature. 3 cases (Clavien-Dindo grade IIIa) required intervention for bile leakage (sonographically guided drainage and/or ERC). The difference in the post-operative complication rate (laparoscopy vs. laparotomy 13% vs. 33%) was significant but does reflect in general the selection of "more difficult" patients for open surgery.

The use of omentoplasty is being discussed controversially in the literature. We have employed it in 14% of our patient population (8/56; 5 laparoscopically, 3 open). None of our patients with omentoplasty developed a recurrence. However, in one case, there was intra-operative bleeding from the omentum majus during laparoscopic omentoplasty; this did not necessitate conversion. Because of the few cases of omentoplasty in our patient population, we cannot make a definitive statement. There are reports about recurrence in the literature despite omentoplasty [10,18]. Furthermore, there is evidence that omentoplasty may cause additional complications or favour recurrence [10,19]. The data in the literature are controversial and there as many proponents as opponents of omentoplasty [2,9,10,18-21] while in more recent publications the value of omentoplasty is being viewed critically [10,18,19,21]. Currently, a falciform ligament pedicle graft is being proposed as an alternative prophylaxis against recurrence, but there are no long-term data available so far [22].

Half of our patient population (23/46, 50%) were completely symptom-free after cyst deroofing. The other half reported persisting symptoms. Only in some of these patients a new cyst is the explanation for the reported complaints.

This high rate may be explained by the design of the interview. 11 symptoms, possibly related to liver cysts, have been included in the interview. As soon as even only one of the 11 possible symptoms was reported in the post-operative interview, this was declared as persistent clinical complaints. In retrospect, this interview design is unspecific. Finally, the liberal decision for surgery may be an explanation as symptoms which may have had other causes may have not been decisively clarified and may have been falsely attributed to liver cysts. It may be beneficial to assess the psychosomatic aspects separately in order to relate them to the respective somatic complaints.

Our work also suggests that un-specific symptoms may have been judged too un-critically as being the cause of clinical complaints and, thus, have been judged to be relevant for the decision making (Table 3). The association between cyst location and the specific complaints should possibly have been established more precisely and only a very obvious association should lead to surgery (e.g. a relatively large cyst exerts pressure on the gastro-duodenal junction). We will, thus, perform more intensive diagnostics (in particular endoscopically) of the vicinity in the future in order to rule out concomitant disease. Furthermore, we consider the introduction of the cyst aspiration test in the future for better patient selection.

Irrespective of the accuracy of the follow-up, a recurrence rate of approximately 5% and an associated reoperation rate of less than 10% may be assumed [2,23,24]. As opposed to earlier reports in the literature [3,25], our data and numerous other studies show, that the laparoscopic procedure as such is no longer a risk factor for a higher probability of recurrence [2,11,13]. Carrying a low rate of complications and conversions, it is, thus, to be considered the treatment of choice for the vast majority of cases. In our study, we have mainly used the ultrasound dissector in the laparoscopically treated patients. Several authors see a potential association of the recurrence rate with the dissection technique. However, the development of recurrence is supposedly more affected by the extent of the fenestration/deroofing (and, thus, only indirectly by the dissection technique) [10,26].

Several groups report the avoidance of cyst recurrence after an ablation of the cyst lining in the residual fenestrated cystic cavity with argon beam coagulation [25,27]. We have used this technique so far only for liver resections. The results with argon beam coagulation to the cyst lining in the literature appear to be promising so that we will use it in the future in order to avoid cyst recurrence.

Conclusions

In conclusion, our results, in context with the data from the literature may be summed up as follows: only symptomatic cysts should be operated. True/symptomatic recurrence develops in 5% to maximally 10% of patients. Recurrences will become most probably symptomatic again. In approximately one fifth of patients new cysts develop or existing cysts grow. It is currently not clear under which circumstances such conditions become symptomatic. In our study in one half of the patients the symptoms continued at varying degrees. In order to address this point appropriately, a more extensive diagnostic work-up and a meticulous patient selection are necessary in our hands. With respect to QoL, our results provide only very general information. Two thirds of the overall patients reported their post-operative health as being good or very good.

So far, the literature does not distinguish strictly between true recurrence (i.e. a new cyst exactly at the location where surgery was performed) and remaining cysts that grow in due course or de-novo symptomatic cysts. For the sake of better comparability of study results, a standardized follow-up (including sonography on a regular basis) as well as a sufficiently long follow-up period of at least 3 years are required. In adequately selected patients, laparoscopic (or open) deroofing is nevertheless the most effective treatment option for symptomatic patients. Our data may be limited by the retrospective character of our analysis. The above mentioned questions and particularities require further scientific evaluation.

Competing interests

The authors declare that they have no competing interests.

Authors' contributions

HS collected the data, analysed the data and wrote the manuscript; FR analysed the data and wrote the manuscript; JF collected the data, analysed the data and wrote the manuscript; KJ analysed the data and wrote the manuscript; YD analysed the data and wrote the manuscript; GT performed the ultrasound investigations, collected the data and wrote the manuscript; US analysed the data and wrote and revised the manuscript. All authors read and approved the final manuscript.

References

1. Caremani M, Vincenti A, Benci A, *et al*: **Ecographic epidemiology of non-parasitic hepatic cysts.** *J Clin Ultrasound* 1993, **21**:115–118.
2. Loehe F, Globke B, Marnoto R, *et al*: **Long-term results after surgical treatment of nonparasitic hepatic cysts.** *Am J Surg* 2010, **200**:23–31.
3. Gigot JF, Legrand M, Hubens G, *et al*: **Laparoscopic treatment of nonparasitic liver cysts: adequate selection of patients and surgical technique.** *World J Surg* 1996, **20**:556–561.
4. Gaines PA, Sampson MA: **The prevalence and characterization of simple hepatic cysts by ultrasound examination.** *Br J Radiol* 1989, **62**:335–337.
5. Cowles RA, Mulholland MW: **Solitary hepatic cysts.** *J Am Coll Surg* 2000, **191**:311–321.
6. Tocchi A, Mazzoni G, Costa G, *et al*: **Symptomatic nonparasitic hepatic cysts: options for and results of surgical management.** *Arch Surg* 2002, **137**:154–158.
7. Moorthy K, Mihssin N, Houghton PW: **The management of simple hepatic cysts: sclerotherapy or laparoscopic fenestration.** *Ann R Coll Surg Engl* 2001, **83**:409–414.
8. Jusufovic R, Zerem E: **Percutaneous treatment of symptomatic non-parasitic benign liver cysts with 20% NaCl solution.** *Med Arh* 2011, **65**:35–37.
9. Palanivelu C, Jani K, Malladi V: **Laparoscopic management of benign nonparasitic hepatic cysts: a prospective nonrandomized study.** *South Med J* 2006, **99**:1063–1067.
10. Treckmann JW, Paul A, Sgourakis G, *et al*: **Surgical treatment of nonparasitic cysts of the liver: open versus laparoscopic treatment.** *Am J Surg* 2010, **199**:776–781.
11. Qiu Jg WH, Jiang JW, *et al*: **Laparoscopic fenestration vs open fenestration in patients with congenital hepatic cysts: a meta-analysis.** *World J Gastroenterol* 2011, **17**:3359–3365.
12. Sendt W, Weber T, Retschke S, *et al*: **Symptomatic non-parasitic liver cysts: early and long-term results of surgical management.** *Zentralbl Chir* 2009, **134**:149–154.
13. Mazza OM, Fernandez DL, Pekolj J, *et al*: **Management of nonparasitic hepatic cysts.** *J Am Coll Surg* 2009, **209**:733–739.
14. Koperna T, Vogl S, Satzinger U, *et al*: **Nonparasitic cysts of the liver: results and options of surgical treatment.** *World J Surg* 1997, **21**:850–854.
15. Aussilhou B, Douflé G, Hubert C, *et al*: **Extended liver resection for polycystic liver disease can challenge liver transplantation.** *Ann Surg* 2010, **252**:735–743.
16. el Mouaasouy A, Naruhn M, Lauchart W, *et al*: **Treatment of symptomatic non-parasitic liver cysts using percutaneous drainage and irrigation with hypertonic saline solution.** *Chirurg* 1991, **62**:810–813.
17. Duca S, Cazacu M, Vlad L, *et al*: **Nonparasitic abdominal serous cysts. A multiple case report.** *Acta Chir Belg* 1993, **93**:18–24.
18. Wahba R, Kleinert R, Prenzel K, *et al*: **Laparoscopic deroofing of nonparasitic liver cysts with or without greater omentum flap.** *Surg Laparosc Endosc Percutan Tech* 2011, **21**:54–58.
19. Tagaya N, Nemoto T, Kubota K: **Long-term results of laparoscopic unroofing of symptomatic solitary nonparasitic hepatic cysts.** *Surg Laparosc Endosc Percutan Tech* 2003, **13**:76–79.
20. Emmermann A, Zornig C, Lloyd DM, *et al*: **Laparoscopic treatment of nonparasitic cysts of the liver with omental transposition flap.** *Surg Endosc* 1997, **11**:734–736.
21. Civello IM, Matera D, Maria G, *et al*: **Laparoscopic fenestration of symptomatic non-parasitic cysts of the liver.** *Hepatogastroenterology* 2005, **52**:849–851.
22. Faulds JM, Scudamore CH: **Technical report of a novel surgical technique: laparoscopic cyst fenestration and falciform ligament pedicle graft for treatment of symptomatic simple hepatic cysts.** *J Laparoendosc Adv Surg Tech A* 2010, **20**:857–861.
23. Morino M, De Giuli M, Festa V, *et al*: **Laparoscopic management of symptomatic nonparasitic cysts of the liver. Indications and results.** *Ann Surg* 1994, **219**:157–164.
24. Tan YM, Chung A, Mack P, *et al*: **Role of fenestration and resection for symptomatic solitary liver cysts.** *ANZ J Surg* 2005, **75**:577–580.
25. Gigot JF, Metairie S, Etienne J, *et al*: **The surgical management of congenital liver cysts.** *Surg Endosc* 2001, **15**:357–363.
26. Petri A, Höhn J, Makula E, *et al*: **Experience with different methods of treatment of nonparasitic liver cysts.** *Langenbecks Arch Surg* 2002, **387**:229–233.

4

Minimal invasive surgery in treatment of liver metastases from colorectal carcinomas: case studies and survival rates

Domenico Loffredo[1], Alberto Marvaso[1], Sandro Ceraso[2], Nicola Angelo Cinelli[3], Aldo Rocca[4], Mario Vitale[5], Michele Rossi[6], Eugenio Annibale Genovese[7], Bruno Amato[4], Mariapia Cinelli[8*]

From 26th National Congress of the Italian Society of Geriatric Surgery
Naples, Italy

Abstract

Background: Liver represents the main organ subject to metastases from colorectal tumors. Resections of liver metastases from colorectal cancer have a well-considered therapeutic role underlined by survival of 5 years by approximately 50-60% of surgical cases as is deduced from an analysis of the most recent literature. The objective of surgery is to eradicate the metastases present and obtain a margin free from neoplastic impact of amplitude of approximately 1 cm with residual liver quantity at the end of the intervention that allows the patient to survive. Currently the dimensions and the number of colorectal liver metastases (CRLM) do not limit the hepatectomy. Purpose of this work is to evaluate the survival, according to our case studies of patients treated only with the wedge resection (atypical resection) approximately 1 cm from the margins of metastases.

Methods: In *"A. Rizzoli" Lacco Ameno Hospital (Ischia)*, from 2005 to 2010, 12 liver resections were performed for metastases from colorectal carcinoma with atypical resection. Synchronous surgical treatment with resection of the colorectal carcinoma and metastases was performed in 6 patients, 2 female and 4 male (Group 1). Surgical liver metastasectomy post-colectomy was performed on 6 patients, 3 female and 3 male (Group 2).

Results: No patient was treated with chemotherapy. The mortality rate of intraoperative and perioperative infection was in both cases of 0%. Survival:11 patients treated surgically from 2005-2010 with synchronous surgery resection (Group 1) and liver metastasectomy (Group 2) are currently living. One 77-years-old patient died three years after surgery for BPCO.

Conclusions: This result was able to be obtained due to the wedge resection technique routinely used in our Hospital, associated with the indispensable use of intraoperatory ultrasound (IOUS). Significant differences between the synchronous and non-synchronous intervention emerged only regarding the number of days of hospital stay, higher in the first case.

Introduction

Colorectal cancer is third in incidence in the western countries, only preceded of prostate and lung cancer in men and breast and lung cancer in women. The combination of molecular events that lead to colorectal adenocarcinoma is very varied and includes genetic and epigenetic anomalies. Were described at least two different genetic pathways. These are the APC/beta catenine pathway associated with WNT and the classic adenoma-carcinoma sequence (which represents up to 80% of sporadic colon tumors); and the pathway of the micro satellite instability, associated with defects in the system for repairing the DNA mismatch. There is, then, a third group of colon tumors presenting an increase in the methylation of the CpG island without micro satellite instability; many of these tumors hide Kras mutations.

* Correspondence: mariapia.cinelli@unina.it
[8]Department of Public Health, University of Naples "Federico II" Naples, Naples, Italy
Full list of author information is available at the end of the article

Many causes work together to determine the colorectal tumor; among them were identified some associated with lifestyle, others genetic and others of non-hereditary type. Lifestyle and family history have long been identified as factors increasing the risk of occurrence of these lesions: nutritional factors (diet with a large amount of animal fats and refined sugars and low in fiber), obesity, low physical activity, smoking and excess alcohol [1]. There are many hereditary pathologies, such as genetic factors, that predispose onset of colorectal carcinoma, among these the syndromes characterized by the occurrence of polyps (most of the colorectal carcinomas, approximately 80%, originated from precancerous lesions such as adenomatous polyps with dysplastic component), familial adenomatous polyps (FAP), Polyps Associated with MYH gene (MAP), Gardner's syndrome, Turcot's syndrome; and those without polyps such as Lynch's syndrome or Hereditary Non Polyposis Colorectal Carsinosis (HNPCC)[2-4]. The probability that a polyp of the colon may evolve toward an invasive form of cancer depends on the dimensions of the polyp itself: is low (less than 2%) for dimensions lower than 1.5 cm; intermediate (2% - 10%) for dimensions between 1.5 - 2.5 cm; significant (more than 10%) for lesions of dimensions greater than 2.5 cm.[5]. Additional risk conditions that are included among non-hereditary factors consist of chronic inflammatory intestinal illnesses such as Crohn's disease and ulcerous rectal colitis [6]. Age also is among the risk factors; the occurrence is 10 times higher among people between the ages of 60 and 65 compared to those from 40 to 45. Colorectal tumor is located, in half of the cases, in the sigma and in the rectum; in one case in four (25%) of patients, the ascending colon is affected, while the location of the illness in the transverse and descending colon is verified in approximately one case in five (20%). Most frequent istotype of large intestine tumor is represented by adenocarcinoma, in 90-95% of all colon tumors. Metastasis at the hepatic level represents one of the most frequent forms of neoplastic progressions the large intestine, followed by lungs, encephalon and skeleton [7]. It is estimated that the 25% of patients with colorectal carcinoma presenting liver metastases have already been diagnosed with this. Surgical resection of colorectal liver metastases (CRLM) is currently the only therapeutic option able to significantly improve long-term survival, offering possibility of potential cure. The 5-year survival rate in patients treated surgically exceeds 58%, while 10 years of survival exceeds 25% [8]. In contrast, patients who are not candidates for hepatectomy present average survival lower than 12 months and at 5 years the survival rate is equal to 0.9% [9]. In this article, we wish to emphasize the aspect of the average survival of the patients undergoing resection of liver metastases, presenting case studies for patients operated on in our center between the years 2005-2010 and thus demonstrate the major role of surgery in liver metastases from colorectal cancer. First we must identify criteria indicating surgical resection. Our objective surgery is to eradicate all liver metastases and create the conditions for at least a centimeter of healthy tissue is left around the lesion removed according to the "wedge resection" approach. In reality, these limits were discussed by Cady and Kokudo, who in their studies affirm the possibility of holding the margins of resection in healthy tissue also at less than 1 cm, when technically not avoidable, without modifying survival and radicalism of the operation[10]. Current approach indicates that the resection may be performed, as long there remains a sufficient amount of liver that allows to patient survive during regeneration phase [11]. It is seen, from literature, that after the resection, at least two contiguous liver segments must be present. The remaining segments must present a branch of portal vein, a branch of the hepatic artery, and a bile duct. Furthermore, liver remaining must represent 20-25% of total functioning hepatic volume [12]. This hepatic volume is calculated based on preoperatory axial imaging and is called a future liver remnant, FLR, and must be without illnesses as cirrhosis, steatosis and steatopathy associated with chemotherapy (CASH). In the past patients with more than three metastases or with extrahepatic diseases, were not eligible for surgery, today introduction of preoperatory chemotherapy and new chemotherapy drugs as well as the progress of modern surgical technique, amplified the outcome of eligible patients. Currently size and number of liver metastases from colorectal carcinoma (CRLM) do not limit hepatectomy, thus making possible the removal of all metastases present with negative margins, maintaining adequate functionality of remaining liver. As an example we can report a case treated by us in 2009, included in group 2, of a female patient of about 60 years subject to surgical treatment to remove seven liver metastases from colorectal carcinoma. The patient, is in good health, is regularly subject to monitoring and has not presented relapse. The presence of extrahepatic disease does not automatically exclude the patient from surgery. Cases of long-term survival have been reported in a significant number of patients who underwent a complete resection of extrahepatic lesions, especially in the case of pulmonary metastases. Decision-making in these cases is strictly related to the experience of the medical and surgical team, the prognostic clinical factors (performance status, synchronous and metachronous metastases, time to appearance, serological tumour marker levels) and the patient's life expectancy [13]. The optimal surgical strategy for patients with synchronous colorectal liver metastases is not yet well-considered. Traditionally, the standard therapy for most patients with colorectal cancer and synchronous colorectal liver metastases consists of colorectal resection first to prevent bleeding, perforation or obstruction, followed 6 weeks later by staged liver resection [14]. Alternatively patients may be subject simultaneously to colorectal and liver resection. A further therapeutic option for patients with synchronous colorectal liver metastases (CLM) consists of the "liver-first approach"- firstly starting with chemotherapy, secondly doing the liver surgery and lastly, performing the colorectal resection. The rationale of this approach is the reflection that, in patients with advanced or technically doubtful resectable synchronous liver metastases from colorectal cancer, CLM might progress during treatment of the primary, precluding curative treatment in a second stage. Since the curability of liver metastases in this situation but not the primary tumor decides the prognosis of the patient, resection of the primary should be postponed. Initial chemotherapy would control and would reduce the dimensions of liver metastases and would be contextual to radiotherapy for the primary tumor [15]. In our experience, the optimal surgical strategy for the patients that present metastases and primary tumors is the synchronous removal of the primitive tumor and liver metastases. Patients, therefore, may undergo simultaneous colorectal and liver resection. In patients with inoperable liver metastases, neoadjuvant chemotherapy may reduce their capacity, resizing them and thus making the patient a candidate for surgical intervention. According to the literature, the use of Folfox (5-fluorouracil infusion + oxaliplatin), Folfiri (5-fluorouracil, leucovorin, irinotecan) or Folfirinox (oxaliplatino, irinotecan, 5-fluorouracil and leucovorin) combined with biological agents such as cetuximab (better prognosis in the cases of mCRC with Kras wild type), may improve the rates of response and make the 20% of patients considered inoperable, possible candidates for surgical treatment [16]. Standard chemotherapies have systemic toxicities and different efficacy [17-19]. Conversely, there is no hint of a remodeling of the Ca^{2+} toolkit, that has been observed in other malignancies, including renal cellular carcinoma [20,21], and prostate cancer[22], and has been put forward as alternative target for selective molecular therapies [19]. In this cancer main consequences of neoadjuvant chemotherapy, however, may be: liver toxicity, steatosis, complications of the biliary tract and susceptibility to infection. To minimize the complications, surgical intervention should be performed approximately one month after the end of chemotherapy.

Materials and methods

Purpose of this work is to evaluate survival, regarding our case studies of all patients under our observation and treated only with the surgical technique of wedge resection (atypical resection) in order to obtain a margin of at least 1 cm free from metastatic involvement. This includes evaluating mortality differences and in peri- and post-operatory complications among the patients undergoing synchronous and non-synchronous resection interventions. Liver resection is considered typical when it is conducted on an anatomic fissure plan architecturally distinct in the vascular structures, especially based on the portal system. In contrast, liver resection is considered atypical, the extension of the pathological process is considered rather than the vascular architecture of the liver.

In "A. Rizzoli" Lacco Ameno Hospital (Ischia), from 2005 to 2010, 12 liver resections were performed for colorectal carcinoma metastases with atypical resection. Patients were retrospectively divided in two groups:

Group 1: six patients, two female and four male, subject to synchronous surgical treatment with resection of the colorectal carcinoma and metastases;

Group 2: six patients, three female and three male, subject to surgical treatment of post-colectomy liver metastasectomy.

An interesting fact is that none of the patients in our study was subjected to preoperative or postoperative chemotherapy. The average age of the patients was 60 years (range 43 - 77), with prevalence for men (7 cases compared with 5), but this is considering the fact that the colorectal neoplasias are most frequent in these latter. Selection criteria for our patients were the following:

1. General operability of the patient in consideration of concomitant diseases;
2. Adequate FLR (future liver remnant);
3. At least two remaining contiguous hepatic sectors after the resection that present adequate blood flow [23]. The clinical risk score (CRS) was useful to select eligible patients and estimate an initial prognostic preoperatory value. It assigns one point to each of the following criteria:

1. Lymph nodes condition;
2. Disease-free interval from the primary to discovery of the liver metastases of < 12 months;
3. Number of tumors > 1;
4. Preoperative carcinoembryonic antigen (CEA) level > 200 ng/ml;
5. Size of the largest tumor > 5 cm.

The 5 year survival rate for patients with 0 points was 60%, whereas that for patients with 5 points

was 14%. Fong et al. concluded that patients with a CRS of 0, 1, 2, have a highly favorable outcome and surgical resection is undoubtedly rational therapy for such patients. Patients with CRS of 3 or 4 have worst prognosis and they should be preventively treated with adjuvant therapy [24].

Liver anatomy

Liver anatomy was not widely understood until the middle twentieth century. In the most anatomical textbooks, the liver appears little more than a box into which vessels enter and leave but without any internal anatomy.

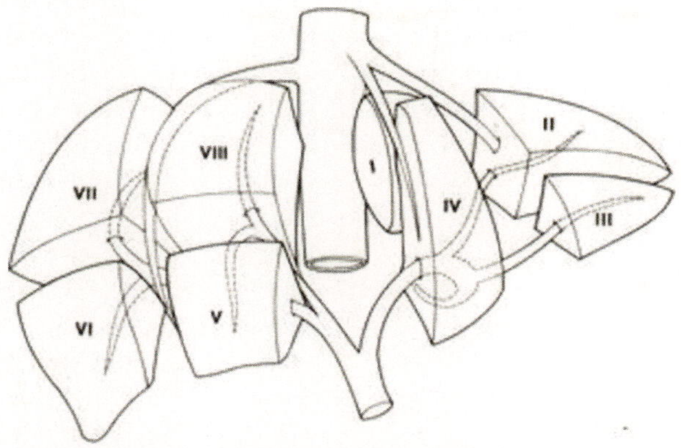

Figure 1 Segmentazione epatica by Couinaud.

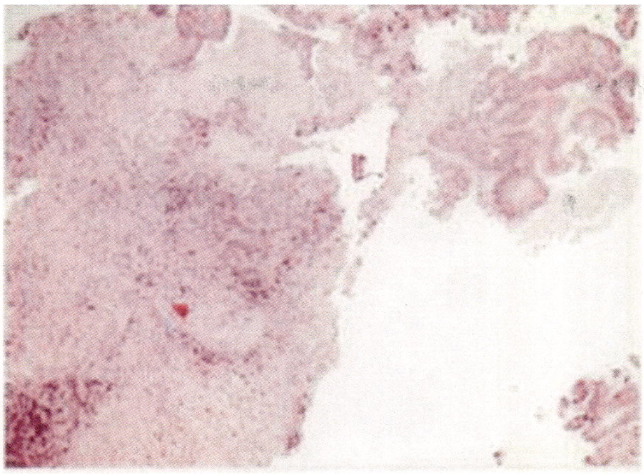

Figure 2 Biopsy of the case with a diagnosis of hepatic infiltration colonic adenocarcinoma.

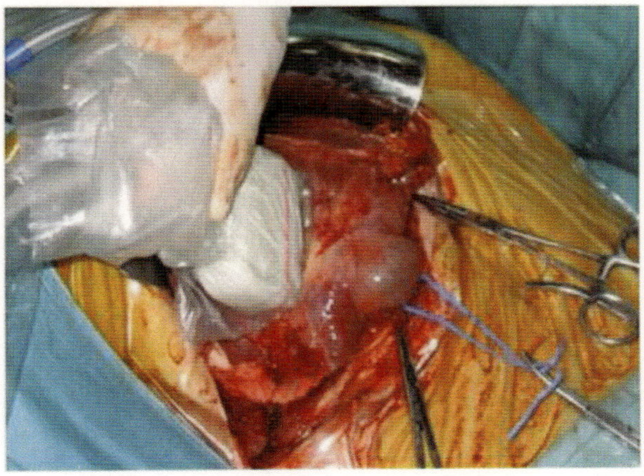

Figure 3 *Intraoperatory ultrasound*: the intraoperatory high resolution ultrasound may identify very small liver lesions (including the marginal ones) that are often unrecognized preoperatory with other imaging methods.

Claude Couinaud et al in France first described the segmental anatomy of the liver, which is essential to modern liver surgery. In substance the liver has 4 sectors and 8 segments. Every segment has a portal vein, hepatic artery, and bile duct and hepatic vein branches. This means they can all be resected separately leaving for the most part the other segments of the liver uncompromised [25]. Even today liver segmentation is inspired by Couinaud and divides the liver into 8 segments, each independent regarding the arterial and venous contribution as well as the vein flow (Figure 1). Main fissure demarcates the line between the gallbladder and lower caval vein and the plane of the medial-suprahepatic vein. Spigelian caudate lobe is placed dorsally and represents segment I; Left lobe is divided into segments II, III, IV; Right lobe in the segments V, VI, VII, VIII. Suprahepatic veins delimit the internal segments of the liver:Right suprahepatic veins separates the VI and the VII segment from V and from VIII; Medial suprahepatic veins separates the V and the VIII segment from IV.

Preoperative assessment

Medical history conducted in patients with neoplastic disease showed weight loss, low-grade fever and pain. Laboratory exams showed leukopenia, increased transaminases, alkaline phosphatase, as well as hyperbilirubinemia and hypoalbuminemia. Instrumental methods used were the ultrasound, MRI, CT scan with cytology and sometimes angiography. Furthermore, in all patients was observed an increase in some tumoral markers, including CEA, alpha-fetoprotein and TPA.

Surgical procedure

Now we illustrate the main points of the phases of surgical resection of liver metastases in a patient of 52 years, treated in our hospital in 2006 (Group 2) (Figure 2 and 3). In 2004, Sahani et al. reported advantages of the IOUS hepatospecific regarding the MRI with contrast media. The sensitivity of IOUS and MRI was respectively 94.3% and 86.7% [26].

Multiple liver metastases (Group2)

Other interesting element emerged evaluating the patient 60 years already described, belonging to group 2, wich were removed well seven liver metastases. The important aspect is determined by the mini-invasive surgical treatment of hepatic metastasis because the resection was performed with margins from 0.5 cm to 1 cm., under strict control intraoperative ultrasound and documented in various phases (Figure 4). The patient is alive today and has no metastatic relapse in routine follow-up.

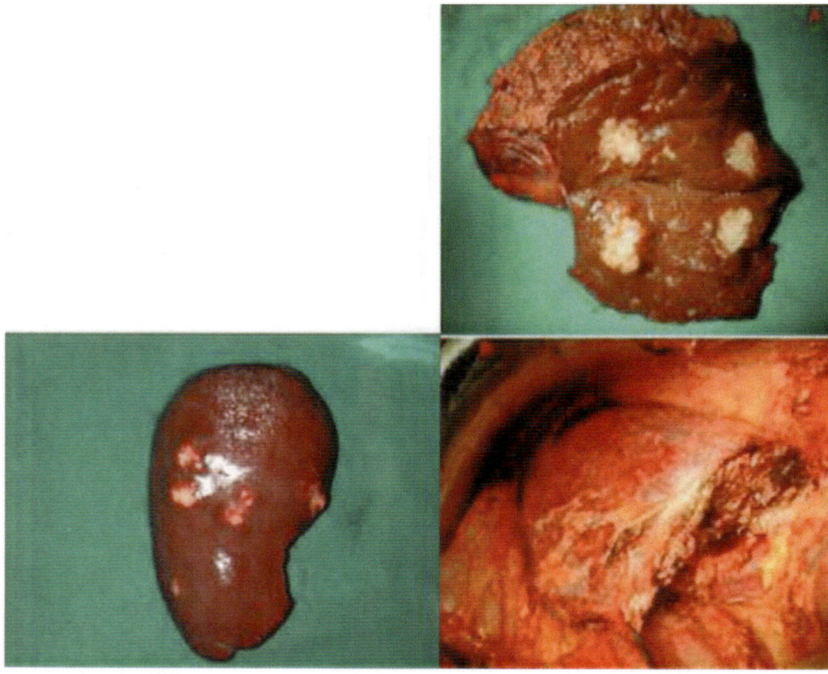

Figure 4 Resection margins of seven hepatic metastases < 1 cm from the lesion (Group 2).

Liver metastasis and colorectal carcinoma (synchronous surgery resection) (Group1)

We illustrate the case of a patient of 67 years operated in our hospital in 2005, belonging to group1, submitted to surgical treatment of simultaneous resection of adenocarcinoma of the ascending colon and liver metastasis. The patient is currently undergoing periodic monitoring (Figure 5). Finally we examine the case of another patient 71 years of age treated by us in 2007, which is also subjected to surgical treatment of synchronous resection of adenocarcinoma of the left colon and liver metastastasi two large 6x4 and 7x5 cm. (Group1) (Figure 6).

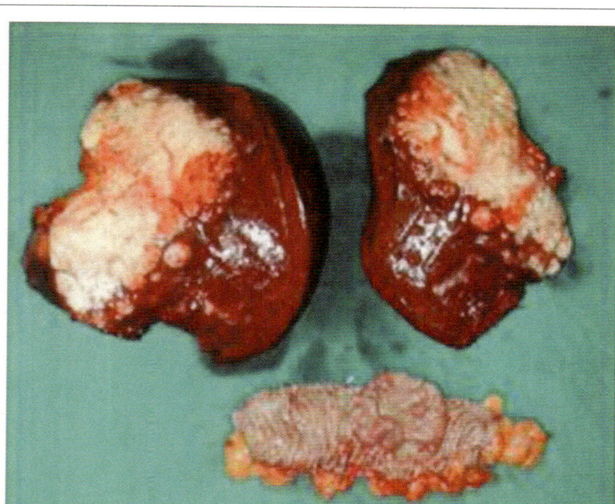

Figure 5 Surgical sample of liver metastasis and colon carcinoma (synchronous surgery resection) Group1.

Results

Twelve patients affected by colorectal carcinoma and liver metastasis were treated surgically at the Hospital in Ischia through:

1) Synchronous surgical treatment with resection of colorectal carcinoma and metastasis, performed in 6 patients, 2 female and 4 male (Group 1).

2) Surgical treatment of liver metastasectomy post-colectomy performed in 6 patients, of which 3 female and 3 male (Group 2).

Mortality

The mortality rate of intraoperative and perioperative infection was in both cases of 0%. ***Postoperatory complications***

A patient treated in our hospital of liver metastasis (Group 2), with a broncopnemopatia chronic obstructive (BPCO) history, reported a right pleural effusion after six days, he was quickly treated. This 77 years-old patient died three years after intervention for BPCO. Another female patient, 65 years of age with metastasis in the liver segments VII and VIII infiltrating the diaphragm, pneumothorax reported in the sixth day, treated with aspiration and medication (Group 2).

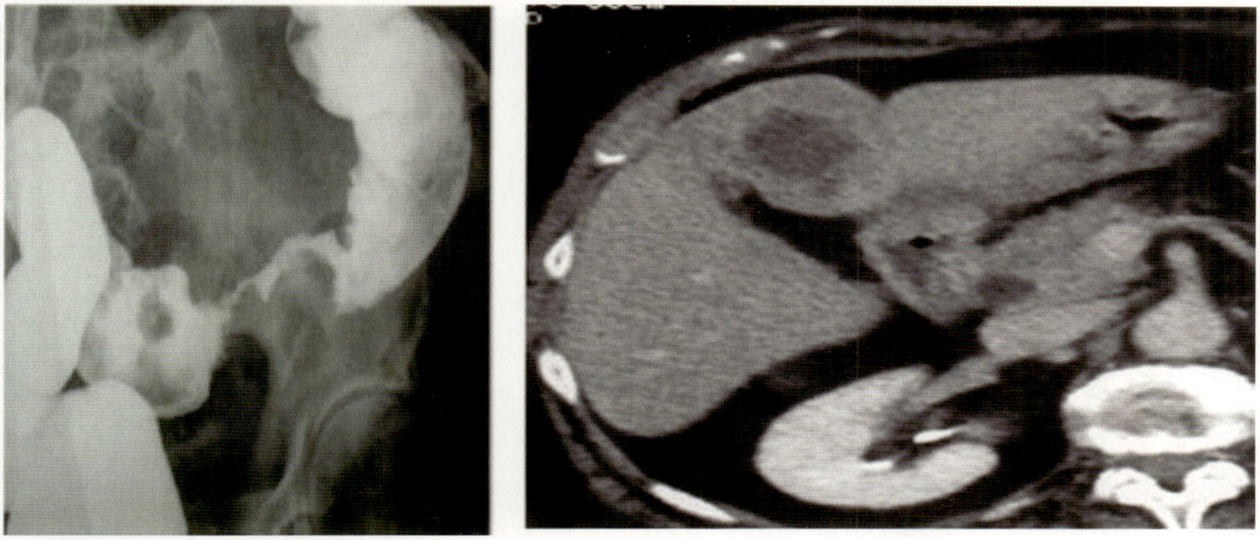

Figure 6 Hemicolectomy sin + metastasis of 6x4 and 7x5 cm (Group1).

Hospital stay

The average hospital stay is of 15 days after the synchronous surgical treatment of colorectal carcinoma and liver metastasis (Group 1), while the average stay is 9 days after the liver metastasis (Group 2) (Figure 7).

Survival

Eleven patients treated surgically from 2005-2010 with synchronous surgery resection (Group 1) and liver metastasectomy (Group 2) are currently living. One 77-years-old patient died three years after surgery for BPCO.

Monitoring hemostasis

In no case was it necessary to perform transfusions on the surgically-treated patients.

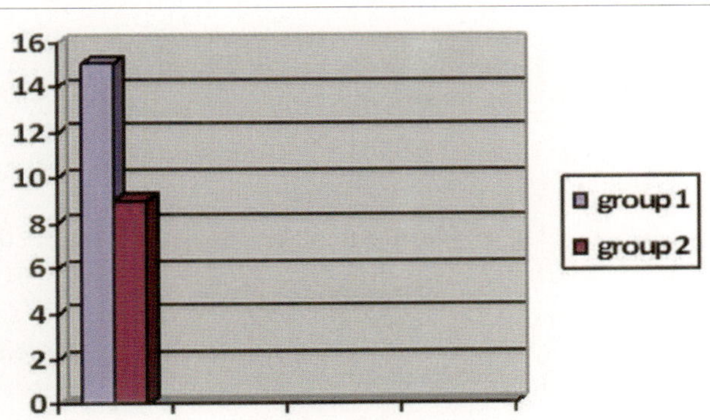

Figure 7 Average hospital stay. Synchronous resection of colorectal liver metastases, 15 days (Group 1). Resection of liver metastases, 9 days (Group 2).

Conclusion

Cancer and other chronic disease have an increased incidence in old age induced by oxidative stress mechanisms [27,28]. Oxidant overproduction occurs in response to several stressors like drugs, chemicals, hypercaloric diet and physical exercise [29]. Colorectal cancer is third in incidence in the western countries and median age of occurrence is in the sixth and seventh decades. Surgery for colorectal liver metastasis is now well established, it has produced very significant benefits for patients. According to our experience, it is useful to surgically treat all patients with liver metastasis removables and you need to resect as much as possible metastases as long as you manage to get a free margin of at least 1 cm without neoplastic disease. Outcome was obtained in 11 patients treated with the exception of female patient, 60 years of Group 2, who had seven liver metastasis removed, leaving, however, a free margin from the lesion equal to 0.5 cm of free tissue. This result was able to be obtained, in our opinion, due to the wedge resection technique routinely used in our center, associated with the indispensable use of intraoperatory ultrasound (IOUS). The confirmation of the resectionability of the secondary effects on the liver and the safety of the surgical strategy to adopt, including the delimitation of the resection margin, only takes place on the operating table after bimanual palpation and intraoperatory ultrasound. This may in fact indicate foci of the disease smaller than 3 mm not shown in the investigations, evaluate the anatomic relationship between the tumor and the vascular peduncle and guide the excision of lesions. The occurrence of operatory mortality and infection was equal to 0% for both groups. No significant difference emerged in mortality between patients subject to synchronous and non-synchronous resection; The times of stay regarding synchronous intervention were higher compared with metastasectomy. Since 2011 we have surgically treated other cases that we do not include in our work for brief follow-up.

Competing interests
The authors declare that they have no competing interests.

Authors' contributions
DL: conceived the study, carried out the surgical procedures, analyzed and interpreted the data. AM: conceived the study, carried out the surgical procedures, analyzed and interpreted the data. SC: critically revised the manuscript. NAC: performed statistical analysis. AR: analyzed and interpreted the data. MV: critically revised the manuscript. MR: perfomed image diagnostic procedures, critically revised the manuscript. EAG: perfomed image diagnostic procedures, critically revised the manuscript. BA: analyzed and interpreted the data, critically revised the drafted manuscript. MPC: conceived the study, analyzed and interpreted the data, drafted the manuscript. All authors read and approved the final manuscript.

Authors' information
DL: Staff Surgeon at *Lacco Ameno Hospital (Ischia)*
AM: Head Surgeon at *Lacco Ameno Hospital (Ischia)*
SC: Vascular Perfusionist
NAC: Economist for Health
AR: Student at University of Naples "Federico II"
MV: Associate Professor of Endocrinology at University of Salerno
MR: Associate Professor of Radiology at University of Rome "Sapienza"
EAG: Associate Professor of Radiology at University of Cagliari
BA: Associate Professor of Surgery, University of Naples "Federico"
MPC: Assistant Professor of Anatomy, University of Naples "Federico"

Declarations
Publication charges for this article were covered by research funds of the project Bando Faro 2012 - Finanziamenti per l'Avvio di Ricerche Originali, cofounded by the Compagnia di San Paolo and by the Polo per le Scienze e le Tecnologie per la Vita of the University Federico II in Naples.
This article has been published as part of *BMC Surgery* Volume 13 Supplement 2, 2013: Proceedings from the 26th National Congress of the Italian Society of Geriatric Surgery. The full contents of the supplement are available online at http://www.biomedcentral.com/bmcsurg/supplements/13/S2

Authors' details
[1]Asl Na 2-Hospital A. Rizzoli of Lacco Ameno (Ischia), Naples, Italy. [2]Perfusion Science, University of Naples "Federico II", Naples, Italy. [3]Bioethics, Catholic University "Sacred Heart", Rome, Italy. [4]Department of Clinical Medicine and Surgery, University of Naples "Federico II" Naples, Naples, Italy. [5]Department of Medicine and Surgery, University of Salerno, Baronissi (SA), Italy. [6]Department of Radiology, Sant'Andrea Hospital, University of Rome "Sapienza", Rome, Italy. [7]Department of Radiology, University of Cagliari, Cagliari, Italy. [8]Department of Public Health, University of Naples "Federico II" Naples, Naples, Italy

References
1. Chan AT, Giovannucci EL: **Primary prevention of colorectal cancer.** *Gastroenterology* 2010, **138**:2029-43.
2. Jasperson KW, Tuohy TM, Neklason DW, *et al*: **Hereditary and familial colon cancer.** *Castroenterology* 2010, **138**:2044-58.
3. Truta B, Allen BA, Conrad PG, Weinberg V, Miller GA, Pomponio R, Lipton LR, Guerra G, Tomlinson IP, Sleisenger MH, Kim YS, Terdiman JP: **A comparison of the phenotype and genotype in adenomatous polyposis patients with and without a family history.** *Fam Cancer* 2005, **4(2)**:127-33.
4. Thirlwell C, Howarth KM, Segditsas S, Guerra G, Phillips RK, Talbot IC, Gorman M, Novelli MR, Sieber OM, Tomlinson IP: **Investigation of pathogenic mechanisms in multiple colorectal adenoma patients without germline APC or MYH/MUTYH mutations.** *Br J Cancer* 2007, **96(11)**:1729-34.
5. Park DH, Kim HS, *et al*: **Clinicopathologic characteristics and malignant potential of colorectal flat neoplasia compared with that of polypoid neoplasia.** *Dis Colon Rectum* 2008, **51**:43-49.
6. Freeman HJ: **Colorectal cancer risk in Crohn disease.** *World J Gastroenterol* 2008, **14**:1810-11.
7. Biasco G, Derenzini E, Grazi GL, Ercolani G, Ravaioli M, Pantaleo MA, Brandi G: **Treatment of liver metastases from colorectal cancer: Many doubts, some certainties.** *Cancer Treatment Reviews* 2006, **32**:214-228.
8. Yang AD, Brouquet A, Vauthey JN: **Extending limits of resection for metastatic colorectal cancer: risk benefit ratio.** *J Surg Oncol* 2010, **102**:996-1001).
9. Van den Eynde M, Hendlisz A: **Treatment of colorectal liver metastases: a review.** *Rev Recent Clin Trials* 2009, **4(1)**:56-62.
10. Chandrakanth Are, Mithat Gonen, Kathleen Zazzali, Ronald PDeMatteo, William RJamagin, Yuman Fong, Leslie HBlumgart, Michael D'Angelica: **The Impact of Margins on Outcome After Hepatic Resection for Colorectal Metastasis.** *Annals of Surgery August* 2007, **246(2)**:295-301.
11. Adam R, Whicherts DA, de Haas RJ, Ciacio O, Levi F, Paule B, Ducreux M, Azoulay D, Bismuth H, Castaind D: **Patients with initially unresectable colorectal liver metastases: is there possibility of cure.** *J Clin Oncol* 2009, **27**:1829-1835.
12. Hemming AW, Reed AI, Howard RJ, Fujita S, Hochwald SN, Caridi JG, Hawkins IF, Vauthey JN: **Preoperative portal vein embolization for extended hepatectomy.** *Ann Surg* 2003, **237**:686-691, discussion 691-3.
13. Elias D, Sideris L, Pocard M, *et al*: **Results of R0 resection for colorectal liver metastases associated with extraliver disease.** *Ann Surg Oncol* 2004, **11(3)**:274-80.
14. Hopt UT, Drognitz O, Neeff H: **Timing of resection in patients with colorectal carcinoma and synchronous liver metastases.** *Zentralbl Chir* 2009, **134**:425-429.
15. Mentha G, Roth AD, Terraz S, Giostra E, Gervaz P, Andres A, Morel P, Rubbia-Brandt L, Majno PE: **'Liver first' approach in the treatment of colorectal cancer with synchronous liver metastases.** *Dig Surg* 2008, **25**:430-435.
16. Adam R, Hoti E, Bredt LC: **Evolution of neoadjuvant therapy for extended liver metastases-have we reached our [non-resectable] limit.** *J Surg Oncol 2010* **102**:922-931.
17. Moccia F, Bonetti E, Dragoni S, Fontana J, Lodola F, Berra Romani R, Laforenza U, Rosti V, Tanzi F: **Hematopoietic progenitor and stem cells circulate by surfing on intracellular Ca2+ waves: A novel target for cell-based therapy and anti-cancer treatment?** *Curr Signal Transd T* 2012, **7(7)**:161-176.
18. Moccia F, Dragoni S, Lodola F, Bonetti E, Bottino C, Guerra G, Laforenza U, Rosti V, Tanzi F: **Store-dependent Ca(2+) entry in endothelial progenitor cells as a perspective tool to enhance cell-based therapy and adverse tumour vascularization.** *Curr Med Chem* 2012, **19(34)**:5802-5818.
19. Dragoni S, Laforenza U, Bonetti E, Lodola F, Bottino C, Guerra G, Borghesi A, Stronati M, Rosti V, Tanzi F, Moccia F: **Canonical Transient Receptor Potential 3 channel triggers VEGF-induced intracellular ca2+ oscillations in endothelial progenitor cells isolated from umbilical cord blood.** *Stem Cells and Development* 2013, **22(19)**:2561-2580.
20. Lodola F, Laforenza U, Bonetti E, Lim D, Dragoni S, Bottino C, Ong HL, Guerra G, Ganini C, Massa M, *et al*: **Store-operated Ca2+ entry is remodelled and controls in vitro angiogenesis in endothelial progenitor cells isolated from tumoral patients.** *PLoS One* 2012, **7(9)**:e42541.
21. Sanchez-Hernandez Y, Laforenza U, Bonetti E, Fontana J, Dragoni S, Russo M, Avelino-Cruz JE, Schinelli S, Testa D, Guerra G, *et al*: **Store-operated Ca(2+) entry is expressed in human endothelial progenitor cells.** *Stem Cells Dev* 2010, **19(12)**:1967-1981.
22. Shapovalov G, Skryma R, Prevarskaya N: **Calcium channels and prostate cancer.** *Recent Pat Anticancer Drug Discov* 2013, **8(1)**:18-26.
23. Reinhart TGrundmann: *World J Gastrointest Surg* 2011, **3**:183-186.
24. Nordlinger B, Guiguet M, Vaillant JC, Balladur P, Boudjema K, Bachellier P, *et al*: **Surgical resection of colorectal carcinoma metastases to the liver. A prognostic scoring system to improve case selection, based on 1,568 patients.** *Association Francaise de Chirurgie Cancer* 1996, **77**:1254-1262.
25. Couinaud C, Delmas A, Patel J: **La foie: etudes anatomiques et chirurgicales.** Masson Paris; 1957.
26. Sahani DV, Kalva SP, Tanabe KK, *et al*: **Intraoperative US in patients undergoing surgery for liver neoplasms: comparison with MR imaging.** *Radiology* 2004, **232**:810-4.

5

Diffuse large B-cell lymphoma of the colon with synchronous liver metastasis: a rare case report mimicking metastatic colorectal adenocarcinoma

Domenico Risio[1*], Rossana Percario[1], Margherita Legnini[1], Francesco Caldaralo[1], Domenico Angelucci[2], Camilla Marinelli[2], Alberto D'Aulerio[1], Roberto Cotellese[1], Luca Napolitano[1] and Paolo Innocenti[1]

Abstract

Background: Primary colorectal lymphoma represents a rare minority among the colonic neoplasms. Early diagnosis is often difficult because of unspecific symptoms, with subsequent delays in diagnosis and management. We describe a rare case of colonic lymphoma presenting with synchronous liver metastasis.

Case presentation: A 70-year-old male with a 6-mo history of vague abdominal pain, constipation and melena was referred to our hospital. Computed tomography scan of abdomen revealed the presence of a mass along the proximal ascending colon. Colonoscopy biopsy showed external compression of the cecum with two ulcerations of mucosa, but it was not consistent for a definitive diagnosis. Because the difficulties in the preoperative pathological diagnosis, the high risk of bowel obstruction and the correlated hemorrhagic risk, the patient underwent a right hemicolectomy associated with locoregional lymphadenectomy and liver resection.
The surgically resected right colon and liver tumors were all immunohistochemically diagnosed as diffuse large B-cell lymphomas (DLBCL). The patient refused any other antineoplastic treatment; he is alive and free of disease at 3 years after initial diagnosis.

Conclusions: Primary colonic lymphomas represent a rare minority among the colonic neoplasms. Their correct pre-operative identification is crucial for the design of treatment. This case highlights the difficulty in diagnosing of primary colonic lymphoma. To our knowledge, this is the first report of a colonic lymphoma presenting with a colonic mass and a synchronous liver metastasis.

Keywords: Diffuse large B-cell lymphoma (DLBCL), Liver metastasis, Mantle cell lymphoma (MCL), Multiple lymphomatous polyposis (MLP), Primary colonic lymphoma (PCLs)

Background

Primary colonic lymphoma (PCLs) is rare comprising 10–20% of all gastrointestinal lymphomas and less than 1% of large bowel malignancies. It is the third most common large bowel malignancy after adenocarcinoma and carcinoid [1]. Patients often present with vague and non-specific symptoms that subsequently lead to delay in diagnosis which often occurs after laparotomy and surgical resection. It is often associated with inflammatory bowel disease and immunosupression. Males are predominantly affected with highest incidence at the age of 50–70 years. Most PCLs have a B-cell lineage and are classified as diffuse large B-cell lymphomas (DLBCL) [2]. The optimal treatment for PCL is controversial. Here, we present an unusual case of diffuse large B-cell lymphomas of the cecum with synchronous liver metastasis.

* Correspondence: domenicorisio@virgilio.it
[1]Unit of General and Laparoscopic Surgery, "G. d'Annunzio" University, Via dei Vestini 31, 66100 Chieti, Italy
Full list of author information is available at the end of the article

Case presentation

A 70-year-old male presented with a 6-mo history of vague abdominal pain. The patient also complained of constipation, fatigue, weight loss and melena.

The patient's history included repaired right sided inguinal hernia, pulmonary fibrosis, hypertension and angina pectoris which was treated using coronary stents 5 months ago and dual antiplatelet therapy. He underwent a colonoscopy 6 years before, and the result was negative for colorectal diseases. The abdomen was soft, tender to palpation over the right and lower quadrant. Clinical examination on admission revealed the existence of a palpable mass in the right iliac fossa. Laboratory data, including tumor markers and leucocitary formula, were all within the normal limits, except for the hemoglobin level (hgb 8.8 g/dl). A colonoscopy revealed external compression of the cecum and mucosa appears edematous with two hemorrhagic ulcerations (Figure 1). Biopsies obtained during the colonoscopy were not diagnostic.

Abdominal computed tomography (CT) with intravenous contrast showed a ulcerated mass at the proximal ascending right colon, with associated adenopathy of the ileo-colic pedicle and in the retroperitoneum (Figure 2). Hypovascular heterogeneous single lesion with diameters of 3.5 cm suggestive for metastases from colorectal adenocarcinoma was detected during the portal venous phase of liver enhancement in segment 6 based on Couinaud's classification (Figure 3). The single liver lesion appears round and no radiological signs suggestive of vascular infiltration were present.

Computed tomography guided tru-cut biopsy of the liver nodule was not performed because of the rapid deterioration of the overall health status of patient. We didn't have repeat a new colonoscopy because of the patient's refusal.

During hospital stay, the patient presented a new episode of rectal bleeding and signs of hypovolemia such as tachycardia, hypotension, and low urine output. So blood transfusions were performed to replace blood lost.

Both the rapid health deterioration of patient and the high hemorragic risk associated with the risk of bowel obstruction prompted us to perform a right hemicolectomy associated with loco-regional lymphadenectomy.

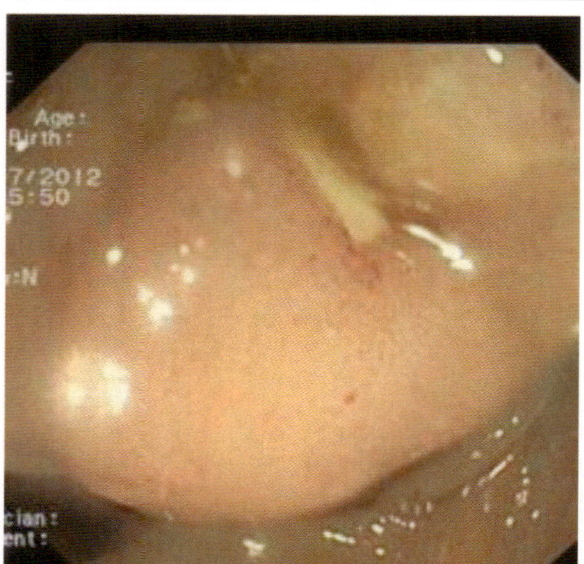

Figure 1 Colonscopy showed external compression of the cecum and mucosa appears edematous with hemorrhagic ulcerations.

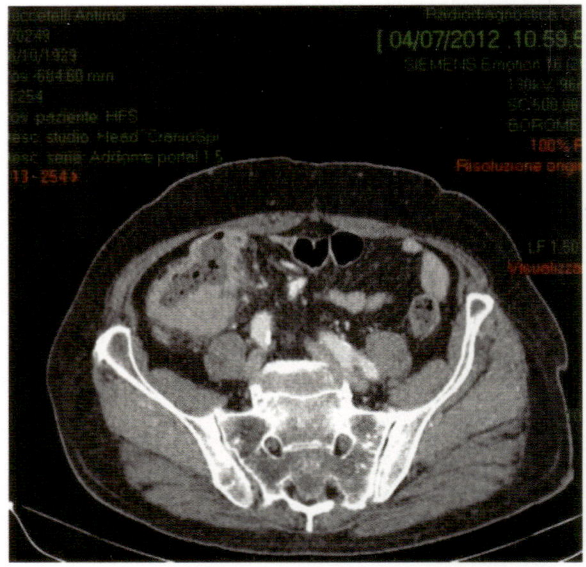

Figure 2 Abdominal computed tomography (CT) with intravenous contrast detected a ulcerated massat the proximal ascending right colon, with associated adenopathy of the ileo-colic pedicle.

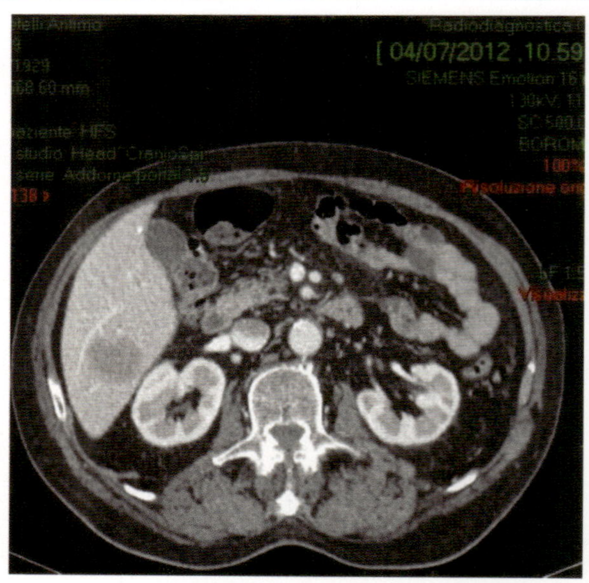

Figure 3 Hypovascular lesion with diameters of 3.5 cm suggestive for metastases from colorectal adenocarcinoma was detected in the liver segment 6 based on Couinaud's classification.

Under Pringle's maneuver a limited anatomic resection of segment 6 was performed.

Gross examination of the resected specimen showed a distinct lesion in the cecum. Microscopic examination revealed diffuse large B cell lymphoma of the cecum and portions of colonic tissue infiltrated by the neoplasm.

The cells were monotonous with irregular nuclear membranes and prominent nucleoli with easily found mitotic activity. Immunohistochemical staining was also performed and revealed the tumor to be CD10+, CD3+, CD79+ (Figure 4) and negative for BCL6 and MUM1.

The liver resected specimen revealed a metastasis of non-Hodgkin's lymphoma with central necrosis. Morphologic and immunohistochemical results confirmed the diagnosis of synchronous presentation of diffuse large B-cell lymphomas with mesenteric lymph nodes and a single liver metastasis. He was discharged home 12 days after his operation.

Four weeks after surgery, the patient underwent bone marrow biopsy for a further evaluation of the disease. Bone biopsy was negative for neoplastic involvement.

At 3-year follow-up, patient is alive and free of disease.

Discussion

The colon is an uncommon site of involvement of Non-Hodgkin's lymphoma (NHL). The most frequently involved colonic site at diagnosis is the ileocaecal region (approximately half of the cases), followed by the caecum, the sigmoid and the rectum. Clinical presentation of colonic lymphoma is quite vague and variable. The most common symptoms of colonic lymphoma are abdominal pain and weight loss with a palpable mass identified on physical examination. Primary colonic lymphomas usually occurs between the fourth and seventh decade of life.

The etiology of DLBCL is unknown, but some risk factors and predisposing conditions have been identified such as immunodeficienty and inflammatory bowel diseases [3]. Despite the severe luminal narrowing, lymphoma is less likely to cause obstruction because it does not elicit a desmoplastic response and submucosal lymphoid infiltration weakens the muscularis propria of the wall. However, its appearance may resemble that of other disease processes involving the cecum. The correctly diagnosis is often challenging and usually based on histological findings after operative colonic resection.

In general, the diagnosis of colonic lymphoma could be based on the CT appearance of extensive abdominal and/or pelvic lymphadenopathy. Even in the absence of lymphadenopathy, characteristic images such as location at the cecum, demarcation from the peri-colonic fat with no invasion of surrounding viscera and the presence of perforation in the absence of desmoplastic reaction should raise the suspicion of a lymphoma. Fisher et al. suggest that without the presence of enlarged lymph nodes it is difficult to distinguish this type of tumor from primary adenocarcinoma [4]. Radiologic examination of large bowel and colonoscopy with biopsy could not sufficient for definitive diagnosis of colonic lymphoma, but US and/or CT are invaluable for the staging of the disease. Malignant lymphoma of the colon has been reported in association with a variety of other entities, especially those of altered immune status and associations with chronic ulcerative colitis, Crohn's disease, and celiac disease. Sciaudone et al. reported the presence of non-Hodgkin mantle cell lymphoma (MCL) with multiple lymphomatous polyposis (MLP) in a patient with a history of recurrent abdominal pain, diarrhea and rectal bleeding. They showed the importance of considering multiple lymphomatous polyposis in differential diagnosis of patients affected by atypical inflammatory bowel disease, because, although the clinical, radiological, endoscopic, and histological presentation of gastrointestinal MCL is very informative, it should be kept in mind that morphological features alone may not be sufficient to diagnose of colonic non-Hodgkin lymphoma [5].

Wang et al. showed that the morphology of primary colonic lymphoma (PCL) is variable, resulting in a wide range of endoscopic features, including mass lesions, narrowing of the lumen, ulceration, mucosal irregularities, and aphthous lesions [6]. Wyatt revealed that

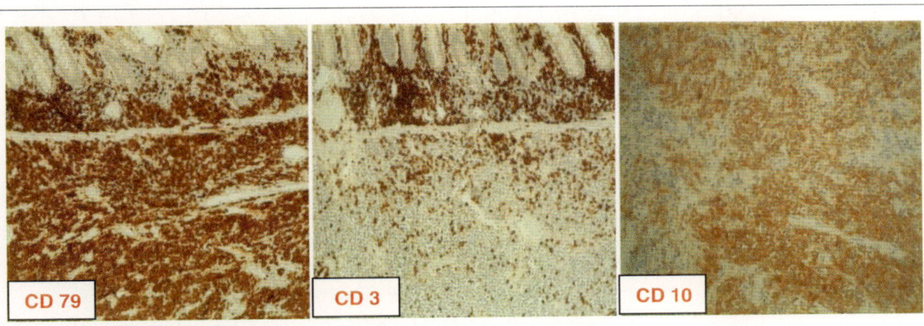

Figure 4 Immunohistochemical profile of diffuse large B cell lymphoma of the cecum. Diffuse large B-cell lymphoma cells were diffusely positive for CD 79, CD 3 and strongly positive for CD 10.

endoscopic findings of colonic lymphoma are classified by ulceration, infiltration, and the presence of a mass [7].

Furthermore for B-cell lymphomas, fungating mass is the most common endoscopic type (54.0%) [8].

The different presentations of colonic lymphoma could be better revealed by the use of double contrast barium enema technique. The radiologic changes may be similar to those found in Crohn's disease, amoebiasis or pseudomembranous colitis [9]; they can be divided into five groups: mucosal nodularity, endo-exoenteric mass, intraluminal mass, mural infiltration and mesenteric invasion [10].

The diagnosis of primary colonic lymphomas (PCL) was initially established in 1961 and included the following diagnostic five criteria [11]:

1. No palpable superficial lymphadenopathy;
2. No enlargement of the mediastinal lymph nodes on chest X-ray;
3. Normal white blood cell count;
4. Predominance of the bowel lesion, and adjacent lymph nodes affected at laparotomy;
5. Absence of any tumor in the liver or spleen at laparotomy.

Our patient's disease met all these criteria preoperatively, except for the liver lesion detected by abdominal CT scan, but the radiologic characteristics of this lesion were similar to those of liver metastases from colorectal cancer. Abdominal computed tomography (CT) images revealed one hypovascular space-occupying lesions with diameters of 3 5 cm with internal heterogeneity due to a relative lack of effect of the contrast medium in the liver (Figure 3). This suggested the presence of metastasis releated to colon cancer. Furthermore it revealed enlarged lymph nodes around the stomach.

The most common histological subtype of colorectal lymphoma is diffuse large B-cell lymphoma (DLBCL), as our case reported [12]. Other histologies include follicular lymphoma, Burkitt lymphoma and Mantle cell lymphoma [13].

Colonic biopsies performed by our endoscopist were non-diagnostic and the diagnosis was made postoperatively after colonic resection. For definitive diagnosis is crucial to define morphology and immunophenotyping. Diffuse large B-cell lymphoma cells generally express pan B cell markers such as CD20, CD19, CD22, CD45 and CD79a; seventy percent of tumor cells express BCL-6 protein; CD10 is expressed in 30 to 60% of cases [14]. In our case, the tumour cells were strongly positive for CD10+ and CD3+. CD10 is considered to be a marker of follicular centre B-cell differentiation. Ohshima et al. reported that CD10 expression was closely associated with improved survival in patients with diffuse large B-cell lymphomas. So they concluded that that CD10 expression may be useful, in combination with clinical parameters, for determining the prognosis of DLBC [15].

In our case, the lymphoma presented as a colonic mass on colonoscopy, but it was not obvious on CT examination. We didn't perform double contrast barium enema because of the patient's refuseal. Some authors have reported rare cases of emphysematous colitis [16] as the first clinical manifestation, and also masquerading Crohn's disease [17]. A multidisciplinary tumor board should manage all aspects of care of patients with colonic lymphoma.

Future advancements in molecular genetics, tumor analysis, and immunohistochemistry could led to most effective management strategies for patients with colonic lymphoma.

Accurate staging of bone marrow status is crucial to optimize the therapeutic strategy. Bone marrow biopsy (BMB) remains the gold standard to determine bone marrow involvement (BMI) but has poor sensitivity because the sample size may be small or the BMI focal [18].

Treatment of colorectal lymphoma usually involves chemotherapy, radiation, surgery or a combination of these. Quayle et al. reported that radiation therapy might not be the preferred option for the treatment of colonic lymphoma, because of a high risk of complications involving the small and large bowels [19]. Nowadays, due to the introduction of new active drugs as monoclonal antibodies like rituximab as part of chemotherapy treatment, the role of surgery is debatable. Some authors propose that surgery could be beneficial to prevent perforation or bleeding; on the other hand others suggest that early diagnosis and chemotherapy might avoid a surgical procedure. In our opinion, surgery may be beneficial in those patients at risk of complications such as hemorrhage, obstruction and perforation, but it should be associated with postoperative chemotherapy. Moreover, surgery alone with or without radiotherapy must be reserved for selected cases, as localized low-grade lymphomas, because the vast amount of lymphomas, moderate and high grade B cell lymphoma, generally extends beyond local fields. In these cases, chemotherapy, with or without surgical excision remains the basis of the treatment.

Conclusion

This case is the first report of colonic lymphoma arising from the cecum with synchronous liver metastasis. It was impossible to achieve a correct preoperative diagnosis and the indication for surgery was supported by the high hemorrhagic risk associated with the risk of bowel obstruction and by rapid deterioration of the overall health status. In our case, both tomography and colonscopy showed findings mimicking colonic adenocarcinoma.

Colonic lymphoma is extremely rare and the variable imaging tests are non-specific; the diagnosis is rarely made before surgery and usually confirmed by histopathological investigation after surgery. This kind of tumour should be considered in the differential diagnoses of colon mass with with enlarged lymph nodes in the abdomen or pelvis and synchronous liver nodules when the biopsies obtained during the colonoscopy were not diagnostic.

Competing interests
The authors declare that no conflict of interest to declare.

Authors' contributions
PI and ML performed the surgery and has given final approval of the version to be published; DR participated to surgery and wrote the manuscript; RP conducted a literature search and contributed to drafting the manuscript; AD, and FC participated in the acquisition and interpretation of radiological data; DA and CM carried out the histological and bio-molecular studies; LN and RC supervised the draft and cared the patien's follow-up. All authors read and approved the final manuscript.

Acknowledgements
We thank Dr. Daniela Tella for reviewing English language.

Author details
[1]Unit of General and Laparoscopic Surgery, "G. d'Annunzio" University, Via dei Vestini 31, 66100 Chieti, Italy. [2]Unit of Pathology, "G. d'Annunzio" University, Chieti, Italy.

References

1. Mahfoud T, Tanz R, Khmamouche MR, Regragui A, Ichou M, Errihani H: **Primary non-Hodgkin's lymphoma of the colon: a case report and literature review.** *J Gastrointest Cancer* 2012, **43**(4):619–621.
2. Daum S, Ullrich R, Heise W, Dederke B, Foss HD, Stein H, Thiel E, Zeitz M, Riecken EO: **Intestinal non-Hodgkin's lymphoma: a multicenter prospective clinical study from the German Study Group on Intestinal non-Hodgkin's Lymphoma.** *J Clin Oncol* 2003, **21**(14):2740–2746.
3. Doolabh N, Anthony T, Simmang C, Bieligk S, Lee E, Huber P, Hughes R, Turnage R: **Primary colonic lymphoma.** *J Surg Oncol* 2000, **74**:257–262.
4. Fisher RI, Oken MM: **Clinical practice guidelines: non-Hodgkin's lymphomas.** *Cleve Clin J Med* 1995, **62**(Suppl 1):SI6e42. quiz SI43e45.
5. Sciaudone G, Pellino G, Selvaggi F: **Diagnostic pitfalls: cancerization in IBD versus mantle cell lymphoma presenting with multiple lymphomatous polyposis.** *Inflamm Bowel Dis* 2011, **17**(6):E28–E30.
6. Wang MH, Wong JM, Lien HC, Lin CW, Wang CY: **Colonoscopic manifestations of primary colorectal lymphoma.** *Endoscopy* 2001, **33**(7):605–609.
7. Wyatt SH, Fishman EK, Jones B: **Primary lymphoma of the colon and rectum: CT and barium enema correlation.** *Abdom Imaging* 1993, **18**(4):376–380.
8. Myung SJ, Joo KR, Yang SK, Jung HY, Chang HS, Lee HJ, Hong WS, Kim JH, Min YI, Kim HC, Yu CS, Kim JC, Kim JS: **Clinicopathologic features of ileocolonic malignant lymphoma: analysis according to colonoscopic classification.** *Gastrointest Endosc* 2003, **57**(3):343–347.
9. Bruneton JN, Thyss A, Bourry J, Bidoli R, Schneider M: **Colonic and rectal lymphomas: a report of six cases and review of the literature.** *Rofo* 1983, **138**(3):283–287.
10. O'Connell DJ, Thompson AJ: **Lymphoma of the colon: the spectrum of radiologic changes.** *Gastrointest Radiol* 1978, **2**:377–385.
11. Dawson IM, Cornes JS, Morson BC: **Primary malignant lymphoid tumours of the intestinal tract: report of 37 cases with a study of factors influencing prognosis.** *Br J Surg* 1961, **49**:80–89.
12. Bairey O, Ruchlemer R, Shpilberg O: **Non- Hodgkin's lymphomas of the colon.** *Isr Med Assoc J* 2006, **8**:832–835.
13. Wong MT, Eu KW: **Primary colorectal lymphomas.** *Colorectal Dis* 2006, **8**:586–591.
14. Stein H, Lennert K, Feller AC, Mason DY: **Immunohistological analysis of human lymphoma: correlation histological andimmunological categories.** *Adv Cancer Res* 1984, **42**:67–147.
15. Ohshima K, Kawasaki C, Muta H, Muta K, Deyev V, Haraoka S, Suzumiya J, Podack ER, Kikuchi M: **CD10 and Bcl10 expression in diffuse large B-cell lymphoma: CD10 is a marker of improved prognosis.** *Histopathology* 2001, **39**(2):156–162.
16. Chou YH, Hsu HL, Lee JC, Lin BR, Liu KL: **Emphysematous colitis of ascending colon with portal venous air caused by diffuse large Bcell lymphoma.** *J Clin Oncol* 2010, **28**(28):496–497.
17. Kashi MR, Belayev L, Parker A: **Primary extranodal Hodgkin lymphoma of the colon masquerading as new diagnosis of Crohn's disease.** *Clin Gastroenterol Hepatol* 2010, **8**:A20.
18. The International Non-Hodgkin's Lymphoma Prognostic Factors Project, Shipp MA, Harrington DP, Anderson JR, Armitage JO, Bonadonna G, Brittinger G, Cabanillas F, Canellos GP, Coiffier B, Connors JM, Cowan RA, Crowther D, Dahlberg S, Engelhard M, Fisher RI, Gisselbrecht C, Horning SJ, Lepage E, Lister TA, Meerwaldt JH, Montserrat E, Nissen NI, Oken MM, Peterson BA, Tondini C, Velasquez WA, Yeap BY: **A predictive model for aggressive non-Hodgkin's lymphoma.** *N Engl J Med* 1993, **329**:987–994.
19. Quayle FJ, Lowney JK: **Colorectal lymphoma.** *Clin Colon Rectal Surg* 2006, **19**(2):49–53.

6

Clamp-Crushing versus stapler hepatectomy for transection of the parenchyma in elective hepatic resection (CRUNSH)

Nuh N Rahbar[1†], Heike Elbers[1†], Moritz Koch[1], Thomas Bruckner[2], Patrick Vogler[1], Fabian Striebel[1], Peter Schemmer[1], Arianeb Mehrabi[1], Markus W Büchler[1] and Jürgen Weitz[1*]

Abstract

Background: Hepatic resection is still associated with significant morbidity. Although the period of parenchymal transection presents a crucial step during the operation, uncertainty persists regarding the optimal technique of transection. It was the aim of the present randomized controlled trial to evaluate the efficacy and safety of hepatic resection using the technique of stapler hepatectomy compared to the simple clamp-crushing technique.

Methods/Design: The CRUNSH Trial is a prospective randomized controlled single-center trial with a two-group parallel design. Patients scheduled for elective hepatic resection without extrahepatic resection at the Department of General-, Visceral- and Transplantation Surgery, University of Heidelberg are enrolled into the trial and randomized intraoperatively to hepatic resection by the clamp-crushing technique and stapler hepatectomy, respectively. The primary endpoint is total intraoperative blood loss. A set of general and surgical variables are documented as secondary endpoints. Patients and outcome-assessors are blinded for the treatment intervention.

Discussion: The CRUNSH Trial is the first randomized controlled trial to evaluate efficacy and safety of stapler hepatectomy compared to the clamp-crushing technique for parenchymal transection during elective hepatic resection.

Background

Hepatic resection forms the cornerstone of therapy for a variety of benign and malignant diseases of the liver [1]. While advances in patient selection, surgical technique, perioperative management and imaging tools reduced mortality substantially, morbidity of patients undergoing hepatic resection remains as high as 30-60% even at high-volume centers [2-7]. Due to the risk of intraoperative hemorrhage as well as postoperative morbidity (e.g. bile leakage, posthepatectomy hemorrhage), the period of actual transection of the liver parenchyma represents a crucial step during hepatic resection. Various studies could indeed demonstrate intraoperative hemorrhage as predictor of poor perioperative outcome in patients undergoing hepatic resection [1,8]. Although various devices have been developed to facilitate parenchymal transection with the ultimate aim to reduce intraoperative blood loss [9], a recent systematic review and meta-analysis failed to show a benefit of these tools compared to the simple clamp-crushing technique [10]. However, to the present there is no randomized controlled trial (RCT) evaluating the technique of stapler hepatectomy. Based on the well-established role of stapling devices in various surgical fields and their common use for division of hepatic veins and portal branches [11-13], vascular staplers may facilitate rapid division of the liver parenchyma with immediate sealing of vascular and biliary structures. In theory, these features enable hepatic resection to be being carried out with less intraoperative blood loss as well as lower operation time.

* Correspondence: juergen.weitz@med.uni-heidelberg.de
† Contributed equally
[1]Department of General, Visceral and Transplant Surgery, University of Heidelberg, Germany
Full list of author information is available at the end of the article

Existing evidence and need for the trial

Several recent systematic review articles including a Cochrane review on transection techniques showed that there is a lack of high-level evidence, i.e. randomized controlled trials, on the use of stapling devices for parenchymal transection in elective hepatic resection [9,10,14,15]. While there are several articles on the technique of stapler hepatectomy as well as retrospective non-controlled studies [16-18], there is currently no RCT evaluating efficacy and safety of stapler hepatectomy compared to standard technique of parenchymal transection. The largest single-center experience on stapler hepatectomy has been reported from the Department of Surgery, University of Heidelberg. This analysis comprised 300 patients who underwent hepatic resection using the technique of stapler hepatectomy for transection of the parenchyma [19]. Even though this report and others suggests stapler hepatectomy to be rapidly feasible as well as effective and safe in controlling intraoperative blood loss [14,20], it's retrospective, non-randomized study design does not justify general recommendations.

Aim of this trial

There is clinical uncertainty and ongoing discussion among liver surgeons regarding the optimal method of parenchymal transection in patients undergoing elective hepatic resection. While the clamp-crushing technique still represents the reference technique for routine liver resections [10], transection of liver parenchyma using vascular staplers may offer a new and safe technique potentially reducing intraoperative blood loss, operation time as well as peri-operative morbidity. As morbidity of patients undergoing hepatic resection remains high, approaches to reduce peri-operative complications are urgently required. Due to the lack of evidence it has to be evaluated, if the technique of stapler hepatectomy decreases intraoperative blood loss as a known predictor of peri-operative morbidity compared to the clamp-crushing technique. In case of comparable or more favorable secondary outcomes such as peri-operative mortality, transection time and need for re-interventions, this advantages would favor stapler hepatectomy as a routine technique for elective liver resections. As RCTs are generally considered to generate the most valid scientific evidence on a treatment's effects, the efficacy and safety of stapler hepatectomy needs to be evaluated in a randomized fashion.

Methods/Design

Trial population and patient recruitment

Patients scheduled for elective hepatic resection at the Department of General-, Visceral- and Transplantation Surgery, University of Heidelberg will be screened for enrollment into the trial. Patients meeting the eligibility criteria will be enrolled into the study. Informed consent is obtained at least on the day before surgery.

Subject Inclusion Criteria

Subjects matching the following criteria are eligible for inclusion into the clinical trial:

- Patients scheduled for elective hepatic resection
- Stapler hepatectomy and clamp-crushing feasible based on preoperative imaging
- Age equal or greater than 18 years
- Informed consent

Subject Exclusion Criteria

Subjects matching any of the following criteria must not be included into the clinical trial:

- Concomitant extraheptic resection planned
- Participation in concurrent intervention trials
- Expected lack of compliance
- Impaired mental state or language problems

Study objectives and endpoints

The primary objective of this trial is to show that intraoperative blood loss during elective hepatic resection can be reduced by stapler hepatectomy as compared to the clamp-crushing technique.

The primary efficacy endpoint of the CRUNSH Trial is total intraoperative blood loss [ml], which is defined as blood loss from skin incision until closure of the skin. Intraoperative blood loss is measured according to the blood collected in the suction containers. Spilling water and ascites is subtracted. Furthermore, swabs are squeezed and their content will also be sucked and added to the fluid collected in the suction containers. To obtain a more precise estimate for the individual patient patient's individual transection area will be considered as a continuous covariate multivariate analysis. The transection area will be assessed using an imprint of the resected specimen on a paper sheet with a known density of 80 mg/m^2.

To further evaluate efficacy and safety of stapler hepatectomy compared to the clamp-crushing technique, a set of general as well as surgical variables are documented as secondary endpoints [21]. The secondary endpoints of the trial are summarized together with their definition in Table 1.

Standardisation of treatments

Patients' intra- and perioperative care will be standardized and kept identical except for the technique of hepatic transection.

Patients receive combined neuraxial and general anaesthesia. However, general anesthesia alone may be

Table 1 Secondary endpoints of the CRUNSH Trial

Secondary endpoint	Definition and assessment of outcomes
Blood loss during liver transection [mL]	Blood loss from beginning of parenchymal transection until minor oozing is stopped. To assess blood loss during liver transection the suction device will be connected to a new suction container for the period of actual hepatic transection.
Blood transfusion:	Administration of blood transfusions is documented for the intraoperative and postoperative period until 48 hours postoperatively. Documentation includes number of patients who received blood transfusions as well as amount of transfused packed red blood cells (PRBC) [units].
Operation time [min]:	Time from skin incision to placement of last skin staple/suture.
Liver transection time [min]:	Time from beginning to end of liver transection.
Duration of postoperative hospital stay [days]:	Time from day of operation to day of discharge.
Duration of ICU stay [days]:	Time on the Intensive Care Unit (ICU). Patients' stay in the recovery room and Intermediate Care (IMC) unit exceeding 24 hours is considered as ICU stay.
Morbidity:	The following predefined complications are documented within the CRUNSH Trial: Posthepatectomy hemorrhage [23]: Drop of hemoglobin level > 3 g/dl after the end of surgery compared to postoperative baseline level and/or any postoperative transfusion of PRBCs for a falling hemoglobin and/or the need for invasive re-intervention (e.g. embolization or re-laparotomy). Postoperative biliary leakage [24]: Presence of bile fluid (bilirubin level more than three times the serum level) in the abdominal cavity or drains on or after postoperative day or the need for reintervention (i.e. interventional drainage and/or relaparotomy due to bile fluid collections or biliary peritonitis). Further biliary complications: Biliary complications such as postoperative biliary stricture detected via ERCP and/or MRCP Intraabdominal fluid collection/abscess: Intraabdominal fluid collection detected on any imaging modality (e.g. ultrasound, CT scan) associated with abdominal discomfort/pain and/or elevation of infectious parameters. Posthepatectomy liver failure [25]: Increased INR or need of coagulation products (FFP, coagulation factors) to normalize the INR and increased serum bilirubin on or after postoperative day five. Pneumonia: Pulmonary infection with evidence of increased infection parameters (CRP > 2 mg/dl and/or leukocytes > 10 0000/ml) which are unlikely to be caused by a different pathologic process and evidence of pulmonary infiltrates on chest x-ray, requiring antibiotic therapy.
In-hospital mortality:	Death due to any reason within the patient's initial hospital stay.
Liver biochemical tests:	Serum levels of Alanine-Aminotransferase (ALT), Aspartate-Aminotransferase (AST), Gamma-glutamyl transferase (GGT), Quick's time/INR, Total Bilirubin, Albumin on postoperative day 1, 3 and 5.
Need for portal triad clamping:	Need for clamping of the hepatic pedicle to control intraoperative hemorrhage.
Resection margins	The proportion of patients with malignant tumors who have a positive resection margin will be documented.
Need for invasive re-interventions:	Invasive re-interventions such as placement of interventional drains, ERCP with stent placement and re-laparotomy within 30 days after the index operation or during patients' initial hospital stay.

chosen, if neuraxial anesthesia is not considered safe by the executing anesthesiologist and lack of patient consent.

Following laparotomy via an extended right subcostal incision, a bilateral subcostal incision (with or without vertical midline extension or a reversed L-shaped incision from xiphoid to the tip of the twelfth right rib the abdomen is initially explored for extrahepatic disease. Intraoperative ultrasound of the liver is carried out regularly to exclude previously undetected lesions. Transection of the hepatic parenchyma is carried out under low central venous pressure (< 5 cmH_2O). Central venous pressure (CVP) is lowered via fluid restriction and clamping of the inferior vena cava (IVC) [22]. If these prove insufficient to lower CVP to a level < 5 cmH_2O, the Trendelenburg position and administration of nitrocompounds may be used in addition. Resections are carried out without use of hepatic inflow control (i.e. portal triad clamping). However, inflow control may be used by the surgeon, if considered necessary and will be documented as a secondary endpoint. Transfusion of PRBC within the CRUNSH Trial is standardized accoriding to the standards of care at the Department of General-, Visceral- and Transplantation and the Department of Anesthesiology, University of Heidelberg (Table 2).

Argon beam coagulation is applied to stop minor oozing once resection is completed and sealants may be used, if deemed necessary by the executing surgeon. After hemostasis is considered secure, easy-flow drains are placed in the subphrenic and subhepatic space and the abdomen is closed in a standardized manner.

Trial interventions

Group A: Clamp-crushing technique

The transectional line is marked and the liver capsule is cauterized. The liver parenchyma is then crushed stepwise using a regular Pèan clamp. Vessels of less than 2 mm in diameter are coagulated with the irrigated bipolar forceps. The remaining vessels are clipped or ligated. The hepatic veins and the portal triad are divided using sutures or the Autosuture Endo Gia™ Universal Stapler

Table 2 Transfusion triggers within the CRUNSH Trial

Risk profile	Minimum hemoglobin (conversion factor 0.621)
< 40 years **no** additional risk factors **no** organ function impairment	< 5.5 g/dl or 3.4 mmol/l
≥ 40 years **no** additional risk factors **no** organ function impairment	< 6 g/dl or 3.7 mmol/l
organ function impairment	< 7 g/dl or 4.3 mmol/l
coronary artery disease with no ischemia carotid artery stenosis with no ischemia history of transient ischemic attack	< 8 g/dl or 5.0 mmol/l
coronary artery disease with ischemia e.g. troponin elevation carotid artery stenosis with ischemia history of stroke	< 10 g/dl or 6.2 mmol/l

and Endo Gia™ Universal Angulating 45 mm loading units with 2.5 mm staples (Covidien).

Group B: Stapler hepatectomy

The transectional line is marked and the liver capsule is cauterized. For subsequent transection of the hepatic parenchyma, the liver tissue is fractured with a vascular clamp in a stepwise fashion and subsequently divided using the Autosuture Endo Gia™ Universal Stapler and Endo Gia™ Universal Straight 60 mm loading units with 2.5 mm staples (Covidien). The hepatic veins and the portal triad are divided using the Autosuture Endo Gia™ Universal Stapler and Endo Gia™ Universal Angulating 45 mm loading units with 2.5 mm staples (Covidien).

Trial implementation

Patients scheduled for elective hepatic resection are screened consecutively for inclusion into the trial. All patients screened for the CRUNSH Trial are documented in the screening log. Patients meeting the inclusion criteria are enrolled in the trial. Informed consent has to be obtained at least on the day prior to surgery. Study visits within the CRUNSH Trial are displayed in Table 3.

Methods against Bias

Randomization

Patients are screened consecutively and all eligible patients are included into the trial. In order to achieve comparable groups and ensure allocation concealment patients are randomly allocated to the study groups. A block randomisation list is generated by the Institute for Medical Biometrics and Informatics (IMBI) applying SAS (SAS™ Version 9.1., SAS Institute Inc., Cary, USA). Randomization is carried out intraoperatively in case resectability is given. Randomization is carried out using opaque and sealed envelopes that are consecutively numbered. Block randomization will be performed for each center to achieve equal group sizes per center. The details of randomization will be kept in safe and confidential. Subjects withdrawn from the trial retain their identification codes (e.g. randomization number). New subjects receive a new identification code.

Blinding

Patients are blinded for the study intervention. Blinding of the surgeon and people in the operating room is not feasible. Therefore a third party blinded to patients' allocated treatment group assesses postoperative outcomes.

Standardization of care

To assure comparable treatment of patients, all surgeons who participate in this trial, will be instructed on both study interventions. Intra-and perioperative care is standardized. In particular, central venous pressure (CVP) will be lowered to < 5 mmHg for the period of parenchymal transection and resections in both study arms will be performed without routine use of the vascular control. Furthermore, the area of resection will be included in the multivariate analysis as a continuous covariate.

Sample size

The sample size is based on the primary outcome parameter and the primary analysis. Internal observations (Department of Surgery, University of Heidelberg) showed a mean intraoperative blood loss of 700 ml for patients undergoing stapler hepatectomy with a sample standard deviation of about 550 ml [19]. To detect a clinically relevant absolute difference reduction in intraabdominal blood loss of 280 ml with significance $\alpha = 5\%$ and a power of $(1-\beta) = 80\%$ $n = 122$ patients have to be randomized in the study ($n = 61$ patients per group) using two-sided t-test. Considering an estimated intraoperative drop-out rate of about 10% (e.g. unexpected death prior to beginning of transection, protocol violations) eight additional patients will be randomized and the total sample size accounts for $n = 130$ patients ($n = 65$ patients per group).

Table 3 Flow chart of the CRUNSH Trial

	Screening	Intervention		Follow Up	
	Visit 1 (up to 5 days before surgery)	Visit 2 (day of surgery)	Visit 3 (POD 1)	Visit 4 (POD 3)	Visit 5 (POD 7 or day of discharge)
Eligibility criteria Informed consent	•				
Medical history	•				
Demographics	•				
Physical examination	•				
Laboratory tests	•		•	•	•
Randomization		•			
Trial intervention		•			
Intraoperative parameters		•			
Postoperative parameters			•	•	•

POD, Postoperative day

Statistical analysis

Statistical methods are used to assess the quality of data, homogeneity of treatment groups, endpoints and safety of the two intervention groups. The confirmatory analysis is performed on the basis of an intention-to-treat (ITT) population and with respect to ITT principles.

Categorical data are summarized by means of absolute and relative frequencies (count and percent). Continuous data are presented by means of the following summary statistics: the number of observations, median, minimum, median and maximum. Wherever appropriate, data are visualized by box-whisker plots or histograms. The primary efficacy endpoint is amount of total intraoperative blood loss. The underlying two-sided null-hypothesis is that both study interventions lead to similar intraoperative blood loss:

$$H_0 : \mu 1 - \mu 2 = 0$$

The alternative is that one intervention performs better than the other:

$$H_1 : \mu 1 - \mu 2 \neq 0$$

A confirmatory intention-to-treat analysis (2-sided test), including all patients as randomized, is performed on the amount of intraoperative blood loss between the two groups. Analysis of covariance (ANCOVA) is used to detect possible treatment differences with intraoperative blood loss as dependent variable, area of resection and CVP during transection as continuous covariates and type of intervention as factor. The sample size calculation is based on a two-sided t-test, and it can be assumed that evaluation with analysis of covariance has the same or even higher power.

Secondary endpoints will be analyzed in an exploratory way, using appropriate statistical methods based on the underlying distribution of the data. All analysis will employ SASα Version 9.1.

Data management and quality assurance

The investigator or a designated representative enters all protocol-required information in the case report form (CRF). The CRF should be completed as soon as possible after the information is collected, preferably on the same day when a trial subject is seen for an examination, treatment, or any other trial procedure. The reason for missing data should be provided. The investigator is responsible for ensuring that all sections of the CRF are completed correctly and that entries can be verified in accordance with the source data.

The completed CRF must be reviewed and signed by the investigator named in the trial protocol or by a designated sub-investigator. The principle investigator will retain originals of all CRF at the end of the trial

Monitoring within the CRUNSH Trial is carried out by an independent investigator at the Department of Surgery, University of Heidelberg, who is not involved in the trial and in completing the CRFs. The basic data of all participating patients are completely checked, i.e. existing patient, patient number, initials, the availability of signed informed consent. For a proportion of 10% of the study participants (randomly selected) a complete check of all data in the CRF (i.e. a 100% clinical source data verification; SDV) is carried out. The extent of further SDV is dependent on the quality of the data and occurrence of protocol violations.

Ethical and legal considerations

The study is conducted in agreement with either the Declaration of Helsinki (Tokyo, Venice, Hong Kong, Somerset West and Edinburgh amendments) or the laws and regulations of the country, whichever provides the greatest protection of the patient. The protocol has been written, and the study will be conducted according to the ICH Harmonized Tripartite Guideline for Good Clinical Practice (ref: http://www.ich.org/fileadmin/

Public_Web_Site/ICH_Products/Guidelines/Efficacy/E6_R1/Step4/E6_R1__Guideline.pdf).

The trial protocol is approved by the local independent ethics committee of the University of Heidelberg approved the trial protocol, the patient information and informed consent sheet.

The CRUNSH Trial is registered at the ClinicalTrials.gov protocol registration system (NCT01049607).

All patients will be informed of the aims of the study, the possible adverse events, the procedures and possible hazards to which he/she will be exposed to, and the mechanism of treatment allocation. They will be informed as to the strict confidentiality of their patient data, but that their medical records may be reviewed for trial purposes by authorized individuals other than their treating physician. The signed consent document is kept by the investigator. A copy of the signed consent document is handed out to the subject or the subject's legally authorized representative.

It will be emphasized that the participation is voluntary and that the patient is allowed to refuse further participation in the study whenever he/she wants. This will not influence the patient's subsequent care. Documented informed consent must be obtained for all patients included in the study before they are registered or randomized in the study. This must be done in accordance with the national and local regulatory requirements.

It is the responsibility of the investigator to maintain patient's confidentiality. During the trial, patients will be identified solely by means of their initials, age and individual identification code (screening number, randomization number). Trial findings will be stored in accordance with local data protection law/ICH GCP Guidelines and will be handled in strictest confidence. For protection of these data, organizational procedures are implemented to prevent distribution of data to unauthorized people.

The investigator will maintain a personal subject identification list (screening numbers with the corresponding subject names) to enable records to be identified.

Abbreviations

ALT: Alanine aminotransferase; **AST**: Aspartate aminotransferase; **ANCOVA**: Analysis of covariance; **CRF**: Case Report Form; **CV**: Curriculum vitae; **CVP**: Central venous pressure; **GCP**: Good Clinical Practice; **GGT**: Gamma glutamyl transpeptidase; **ICH**: International Conference on Harmonization of Technical Requirements for Registration of Pharmaceuticals for Human Use; **INR**: International normalized ratio; **IVC**: Inferior vena cava; **POD**: Postoperative day; **PRBC**: Packed red blood cells; **RCT**: Randomized controlled trial; **SDV**: Source Data Verification

Acknowledgements

We are grateful to our patients who support scientific progress without private benefit.

Author details

[1]Department of General, Visceral and Transplant Surgery, University of Heidelberg, Germany. [2]Institute of Medical Biometry and Informatics, University of Heidelberg, Germany.

Authors' contributions

This study was designed by NNR, HE and JW who also wrote the article. TB performed the sample size calculation and planned the statistical analyses. MK, PV, FS, PS, AM and MWB are involved in trial implementation and critically revised the manuscript. All authors have read and approved the manuscript.

Competing interests

The authors declare that they have no competing interests.

References

1. Poon RT, Fan ST, Lo CM, Liu CL, Lam CM, Yuen WK, Yeung C, Wong J: **Improving perioperative outcome expands the role of hepatectomy in management of benign and malignant hepatobiliary diseases: analysis of 1222 consecutive patients from a prospective database.** *AnnSurg* 2004, **240(4)**:698-708.
2. Jarnagin WR, Gonen M, Fong Y, DeMatteo RP, Ben-Porat L, Little S, Corvera C, Weber S, Blumgart LH: **Improvement in perioperative outcome after hepatic resection: analysis of 1,803 consecutive cases over the past decade.** *AnnSurg* 2002, **236(4)**:397-406.
3. Reissfelder C, Rahbari NN, Koch M, Kofler B, Sutedja N, Elbers H, Buchler MW, Weitz J: **Postoperative course and clinical significance of biochemical blood tests following hepatic resection.** *Br J Surg* 2011, **98(6)**:836-844.
4. Pianka F, Baumhauer M, Stein D, Radeleff B, Schmied BM, Meinzer HP, Muller SA: **Liver tissue sparing resection using a novel planning tool.** *Langenbecks Arch Surg* 2011, **396(2)**:201-208.
5. Takahashi K, Sasaki R, Kondo T, Oda T, Murata S, Ohkohchi N: **Preoperative 3D volumetric analysis for liver congestion applied in a patient with hilar cholangiocarcinoma.** *Langenbecks Arch Surg* 2010, **395(6)**:761-765.
6. Rahbari NN, Wente MN, Schemmer P, Diener MK, Hoffmann K, Motschall E, Schmidt J, Weitz J, Buchler MW: **Systematic review and meta-analysis of the effect of portal triad clamping on outcome after hepatic resection.** *BrJSurg* 2008, **95(4)**:424-432.
7. Rahbari NN, Reissfelder C, Koch M, Elbers H, Striebel F, Buchler MW, Weitz J: **The Predictive Value of Postoperative Clinical Risk Scores for Outcome After Hepatic Resection: A Validation Analysis in 807 Patients.** *Ann Surg Oncol* 2011.
8. Wei AC, Tung-Ping PR, Fan ST, Wong J: **Risk factors for perioperative morbidity and mortality after extended hepatectomy for hepatocellular carcinoma.** *BrJSurg* 2003, **90(1)**:33-41.
9. Poon RT: **Current techniques of liver transection.** *HPB (Oxford)* 2007, **9(3)**:166-173.
10. Rahbari NN, Koch M, Schmidt T, Motschall E, Bruckner T, Weidmann K, Mehrabi A, Buchler MW, Weitz J: **Meta-analysis of the clamp-crushing technique for transection of the parenchyma in elective hepatic resection: back to where we started?** *AnnSurgOncol* 2009, **16(3)**:630-639.
11. McEntee GP, Nagorney DM: **Use of vascular staplers in major hepatic resections.** *Br J Surg* 1991, **78(1)**:40-41.
12. Voyles CR, Vogel SB: **Hepatic resection using stapling devices to control the hepatic veins.** *Am J Surg* 1989, **158(5)**:459-460.
13. Fong Y, Blumgart LH: **Useful stapling techniques in liver surgery.** *J Am Coll Surg* 1997, **185(1)**:93-100.
14. Schemmer P, Bruns H, Weitz J, Schmidt J, Buchler MW: **Liver transection using vascular stapler: a review.** *HPB (Oxford)* 2008, **10(4)**:249-252.
15. Gurusamy KS, Pamecha V, Sharma D, Davidson BR: **Techniques for liver parenchymal transection in liver resection.** *CochraneDatabaseSystRev* 2009, , **1**: CD006880.
16. Jurim O, Colonna JO, Colquhoun SD, Shaked A, Busuttil RW: **A stapling technique for hepatic resection.** *J Am Coll Surg* 1994, **178(5)**:510-511.
17. Delis SG, Bakoyiannis A, Karakaxas D, Athanassiou K, Tassopoulos N, Manesis E, Ketikoglou I, Papakostas P, Dervenis C: **Hepatic parenchyma**

resection using stapling devices: peri-operative and long-term outcome. *HPB (Oxford)* 2009, **11(1)**:38-44.

18. Balaa FK, Gamblin TC, Tsung A, Marsh JW, Geller DA: **Right hepatic lobectomy using the staple technique in 101 patients.** *J Gastrointest Surg* 2008, **12(2)**:338-343.
19. Schemmer P, Friess H, Hinz U, Mehrabi A, Kraus TW, Z'Graggen K, Schmidt J, Uhl W, Buchler MW: **Stapler hepatectomy is a safe dissection technique: analysis of 300 patients.** *World JSurg* 2006, **30(3)**:419-430.
20. Schemmer P, Friess H, Dervenis C, Schmidt J, Weitz J, Uhl W, Buchler MW: **The Use of Endo-GIA Vascular Staplers in Liver Surgery and Their Potential Benefit:A Review.** *DigSurg* 2007, **24(4)**:300-305.
21. Rahbari NN, Zimmermann JB, Koch M, Bruckner T, Schmidt T, Elbers H, Reissfelder C, Weigand MA, Buchler MW, Weitz J: **IVC CLAMP: infrahepatic inferior vena cava clamping during hepatectomy–a randomised controlled trial in an interdisciplinary setting.** *Trials* 2009, **10**:94.
22. Rahbari NN, Koch M, Zimmermann JB, Elbers H, Bruckner T, Contin P, Reissfelder C, Schmidt T, Weigand MA, Martin E, Büchler MW, Weitz J: **Infrahepatic Inferior Vena Cava Clamping for Reduction of Central Venous Pressure and Blood Loss During Hepatic Resection: A Randomized Controlled Trial.** *Ann Surg* 2011.
23. Rahbari NN, Garden OJ, Padbury R, Maddern G, Koch M, Hugh TJ, Fan ST, Nimura Y, Figueras J, Vauthey JN, Rees M, Adam R, Dematteo RP, Greig P, Usatoff V, Banting S, Nagino M, Capussotti L, Yokoyama Y, Brooke-Smith M, Crawford M, Christophi C, Makuuchi M, Büchler MW, Weitz J: **Post-hepatectomy haemorrhage: a definition and grading by the International Study Group of Liver Surgery (ISGLS).** *HPB (Oxford)* 2011, **13(8)**:528-535.
24. Koch M, Garden OJ, Padbury R, Rahbari NN, Adam R, Capussotti L, Fan ST, Yokoyama Y, Crawford M, Makuuchi M, Christophi C, Banting S, Brooke-Smith M, Usatoff V, Nagino M, Maddern G, Hugh TJ, Vauthey JN, Greig P, Rees M, Nimura Y, Figueras J, DeMatteo RP, Büchler MW, Weitz J: **Bile leakage after hepatobiliary and pancreatic surgery: a definition and grading of severity by the International Study Group of Liver Surgery.** *Surgery* 2011, **149(5)**:680-688.
25. Rahbari NN, Garden OJ, Padbury R, Brooke-Smith M, Crawford M, Adam R, Koch M, Makuuchi M, Dematteo RP, Christophi C, Banting S, Usatoff V, Nagino M, Maddern G, Hugh TJ, Vauthey JN, Greig P, Rees M, Yokoyama Y, Fan ST, Nimura Y, Figueras J, Capussotti L, Büchler MW, Weitz J: **Posthepatectomy liver failure: a definition and grading by the International Study Group of Liver Surgery (ISGLS).** *Surgery* 2011, **149(5)**:713-724.

A case report of primary neuroendocrine carcinoma of the perihilar bile duct

Yasuhiro Kihara[1*], Hiroshi Yokomizo[1], Takahiro Urata[2], Michiko Nagamine[3] and Toshihiko Hirata[1]

Abstract

Background: Although neuroendocrine tumors are most commonly found in the digestive system, neuroendocrine tumors originating from the bile duct are rare, and neuroendocrine carcinomas derived from the perihilar bile duct are extremely rare. This report presents the clinical course and clinicopathological features of neuroendocrine carcinomas arising from the extrahepatic bile duct.

Case presentation: A 70-year-old Japanese woman was preoperatively diagnosed with perihilar cholangiocarcinoma, and a radical resection with an extended left hepatic lobectomy and a choledochojejunostomy was performed. From the histopathological findings, we diagnosed the tumor as a neuroendocrine carcinoma of the bile duct (small cell type) with lymph node metastasis. The patient was treated with the same adjuvant chemotherapy as that used for small cell carcinoma of the lung. At 10 months after surgery, there was no recurrence of the disease.

Conclusion: Neuroendocrine carcinoma of the extrahepatic biliary tracts is a very rare and highly malignant disease with a poor prognosis. A multidisciplinary approach could improve the prognosis for this neoplasm.

Keywords: Neuroendocrine carcinoma, Bile duct, Small cell carcinoma

Background

The World Health Organization (WHO) classification system (2010) defines neoplasms with neuroendocrine differentiation as neuroendocrine tumors (NETs). These are stratified as NET Grade 1 (G1), NET Grade 2 (G2), and neuroendocrine carcinoma (NEC) [1]. Although NETs are most commonly found in the digestive system, NETs originating from the extrahepatic bile duct are rare, and NECs arising from the perihilar bile duct are extremely rare [2]. In this report, we present the clinical course and clinicopathological features of a case of NEC originating from the extrahepatic bile duct, as well as the results of a literature review on this subject.

Case presentation

A 70-year-old Japanese woman presented to our hospital for investigation of a chief complaint of jaundice. The patient had no family history of cancer. A physical examination revealed no remarkable findings. Laboratory data showed abnormally elevated levels of total bilirubin (3.6 mg/dL; normal, 0.2-1.0 mg/dL), AST, ALT, and γ-GTP. The serum level of CEA was normal; however, the CA19-9 was above the normal range (47 U/ml; normal, 0–37 U/ml). An abdominal computed tomography (CT) scan revealed a 3 cm enhancing mass located in the hilar bile duct extending to the left hepatic duct (Fig. 1a) and an enlarged regional lymph node along the common bile duct (Fig. 1b). In recent years, for the preoperative biliary drainage in patients with malignant biliary tract obstruction, we prefer endoscopic retrograde drainage rather than percutaneous transhepatic drainage in regard to adverse events, such as vascular injury and cancer dissemination. Therefore, an endoscopic retrograde cholangiopancreatography (ERCP) was performed, and cholangiography revealed the obstruction of the hilar to upper portion of bile duct (Fig. 2). And endoscopic retrograde biliary drainage (ERBD) tube was placed. A bile duct brush cytologic specimen obtained at the time of ERCP showed small clusters of relatively small atypical cells with hyperchromatic nuclei and scant cytoplasm. A salt-and-pepper chromatin pattern and cell molding, which are typical in

* Correspondence: flinge21@yahoo.co.jp
[1]Division of General Surgery, Japanese Red Cross Kumamoto Hospital, Nagamineminami 2-1-1, Higashiku, Kumamoto city, Kumamoto 861-8520, Japan
Full list of author information is available at the end of the article

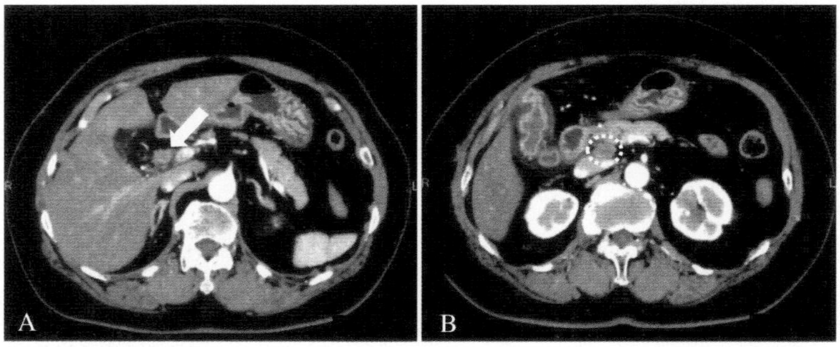

Fig. 1 CT findings. Abdominal enhanced computed tomography showed an enhanced tumor located in the hilar bile duct to the left hepatic duct (**a**: *arrow*). The encircled area indicated the regional lymph node metastasis located along the common bile duct (**b**)

neuroendocrine tumors, were not apparent. The cytologic diagnosis at this point was adenocarcinoma, possibly poorly differentiated. The patient was diagnosed with hilar cholangiocarcinoma with regional lymph node involvement. Abdominal and chest CT scans showed no other neoplastic lesions. A radical resection was performed, including an extended left hepatic lobectomy, excision of the caudate lobe and the extrahepatic bile duct, dissection of the regional lymph nodes, and a choledochojejunostomy.

In the resected specimen, the mucosa of the perihilar bile duct was diffusely rough, and the duct wall was thickened in a 3 cm portion of the proximal common hepatic duct. Microscopically, the thickened bile duct wall was infiltrated by irregular islands and nests of cells with hyperchromatic nuclei and a high nuclear-to- cytoplasmic ratio (Fig. 3a). The tumor cells were relatively small, approximately 2 to 3 times larger than the background lymphocytes (Fig. 3b). Rosette-like structures were not seen. Numerous mitotic figures and apoptotic bodies were present. Immunohistochemical stains showed the tumor cells to be positive for synaptophysin (Fig. 3c) and CD56 (Fig. 3d), and focally positive for chromogranin A. The Ki-67/MIB-1 Labeling Index was 70 % (Fig. 3e). Based on these findings, a pathological diagnosis of small cell neuroendocrine carcinoma was established. Two out of 8 regional lymph nodes were positive for metastatic carcinoma.

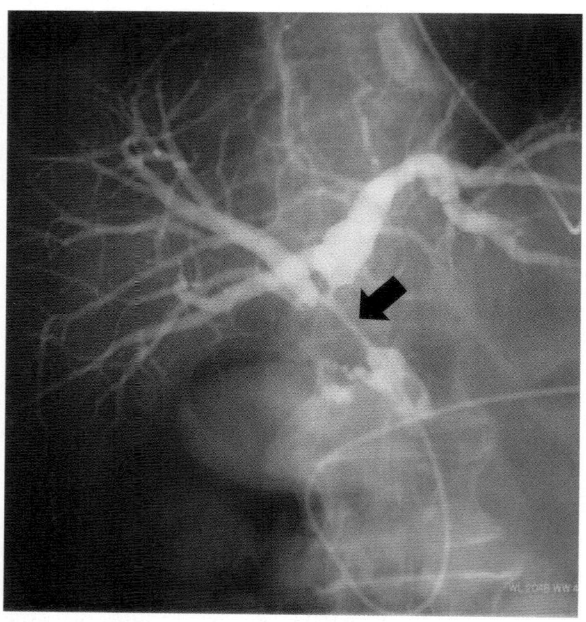

Fig. 2 Cholangiography. Cholangiography revealed the obstruction of the hilar to upper portion of bile duct (*arrow*)

There were no postoperative complications, and the patient received 4 courses of adjuvant chemotherapy with a regimen of irinotecan (50 mg/m^2) and carboplatin (5 AUC/body). Ten months after surgery, there was no recurrence of the disease.

Discussion

NECs were previously classified as small cell carcinomas (SCCs), large cell neuroendocrine carcinomas, or poorly differentiated neuroendocrine carcinomas [3]. NEC is a poorly differentiated, high-grade, malignant neoplasm composed of small cells or intermediate to large cells. In the digestive system, NECs have been reported in the esophagus, the ampulla of Vater [4], the pancreas [5], and the gallbladder [6]. However, NECs in the bile duct are extremely rare.

We conducted a PubMed systematic literature search (1985–2014) using keywords such as "neuroendocrine carcinoma," "small cell," and "biliary tract," and found only 23 reported cases of NEC of the extrahepatic biliary tracts, excluding the intrahepatic bile duct, the gallbladder, and the ampulla of Vater (Table 1, [7–29]). SCC was the most common histologic subtype of NEC of the extrahepatic bile ducts (19 of 23 cases; Table 1). There were only 3 cases of

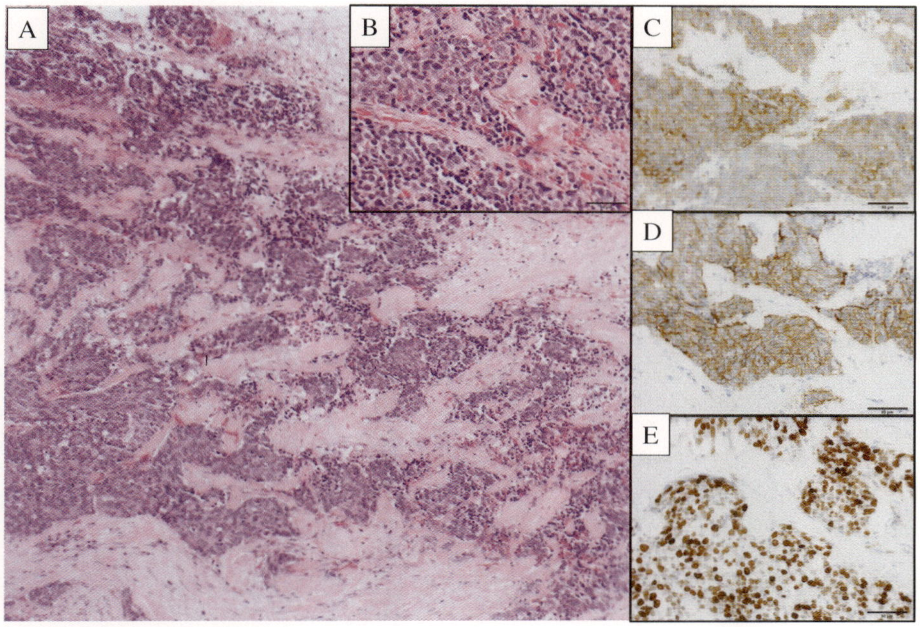

Fig. 3 Pathological findings. Hematoxylin-eosin stained histologic sections of the resected perihilar bile duct. The tumor cells were arranged in the cellular nests and cords infiltrating the bile duct wall. The mucosa epithelium was mostly eroded (*upper right*) (**a**: ×100). The tumor cells were round or oval with scant cytoplasm. Numerous mitotic figures and apoptotic bodies are noted (**b**: ×400). In the immunohistochemical studies, the tumor cells were diffusely positive for synaptophysin (**c**: ×400), and CD56 (**d**: ×400). Approximately 70 % of the tumor cells were positive for Ki-67 (**e**: ×400)

large cell carcinomas of the common bile duct (cases 21 to 23, Table 1). NEC can occur anywhere in the extrahepatic bile duct, but the middle portion of the common bile duct appears to be the most common site of involvement. The prognosis for NEC of the bile duct appears to be poor. Of the 23 cases with follow-up data, 57 % (12/23) of the patients died 3 to 20 months after surgery, and only 2 patients were reported to have survived more than 2 years. NEC of the biliary system has a high incidence of distant metastasis [15, 16, 19, 20, 22, 24–29]. Consequently, it has a poor prognosis, and surgical resection alone is not an effective treatment. A report by Levenson revealed that there is no survival benefit from using surgery to treat either small cell lung cancer or extrapulmonary SCC [30]. This may be because the most important prognostic factor is the extent of disease at diagnosis, and most patients with extrapulmonary SCC already have occult metastasis [30]. Of the 12 patients died within 20 months after surgery, 9 cases were identified their recurrence pattern and all of them were distant metastases [15, 16, 19, 20, 22, 24, 26, 28, 29]. Meanwhile, the long survival 2 cases had locoregional lymph node metastases without distant metastasis [13, 27]. Since NEC of the biliary system had a high incidence of distant metastasis, locolegional lymph node metastasis could not be a prognostic factor. In the report of 37 cases of neuroendocrine tumor of ampulla of Vater, the authors did not find any prognostic value of the locoregional lymph node metastases and lymphadenectomy [31].

If there is a biopsy-proven preoperative diagnosis of NEC, then preoperative chemotherapy can improve the prognosis in comparison to surgery alone or surgery with adjuvant chemotherapy. Hazama et al. revealed that neoadjuvant chemotherapy followed by surgery resulted in an excellent response for SCC of the common bile duct [15]. Okamura et al. reported that multidisciplinary management, consisting of preoperative chemotherapy, a curative resection, adjuvant chemotherapy, and radiation therapy, may scontribute to a prolonged survival for SCC of the common bile duct [26]. In most cases of NEC of the biliary system diagnosed from pathological findings of resected specimens, surgical resection followed by adjuvant chemotherapy is the generally accepted optimal treatment.

Although there is no established standard treatment for extrapulmonary SCC, chemotherapy should be attempted, if possible, because SCC is often chemosensitive [32]. The recommended chemotherapy regimen for extrapulmonary SCC is the same as that for small cell lung cancer. For patients with a diagnosis of the small cell type of NEC who are able to undergo surgical resection, adjuvant chemotherapy consisting of cisplatin and

Table 1 Neuroendocrine carcinoma of the extrahepatic bile duct. Review of the literature

No.	Author	Age	Sex	Histology	Location	Size	Treatment	Prognosis
1	Sabanathan (1988)	67	M	Small cell	Bm	5 cm	Palliative bypass and chemo.	6 months, alive
2	Van der Wal (1990)	55	M	Small cell + Adenoca.	Bm	4 cm	Resection	N.A.
3	Nishihara (1993)	64	M	Small cell + Adenoca.	Bh-Bs	1.9 cm	Resection	8 months, alive
4	Yamamoto (1998)	71	F	Small cell + Adenoca.	Bh	6 cm	Resection	8 months, dead
5	Kim (2000)	64	M	Small cell + Adenoca.	Bm	3 cm	Resection	1 month, alive
6	Miyashita (2001)	85	F	Small cell	Bi	3 cm	Palliative bypass	5 months, dead
7	Edakuni (2001)	82	F	Small cell + Adenoca.	Bm	6 cm	Resection	45 months, alive
8	Kuraoka (2003)	75	M	Small cell	Bi	4.5 cm	Resection	5 months, alive
9	Hazama (2003)	60	M	Small cell	CBD	0.3 cm	NAC and resection	12 months, dead
10	Arakura (2003)	70	F	Small cell	Bm	3 cm	Resection and chemo.	14 months, dead
11	Park (2004)	60	F	Small cell	Bs-Bm	3 cm	Resection	5 months, dead
12	Thomas (2005)	54	M	Small cell	Bh-CBD	N.A.	Resection	6 months, alive
13	Kaiho (2005)	66	F	Small cell + Adenoca.	Bm	3.5 cm	Resection and chemo.	8 months, dead
14	Sato (2006	68	M	Large cell + Adenoca.	Bi	2 cm	Resection and chemo.	3 months, dead
15	Viana Miguel (2006)	76	M	Small cell	Bm	N.A.	Resection, chemo. and irraiation	5 months, alive
16	Jeon (2006)	65	M	Small cell	Bs-Bm	2 cm	Resection and chemo.	12 months, dead
17	Nakai (2008)	32	M	Small cell	CBD	N.A.	N.A.	N.A.(autopsy)
18	Arakura (2008)	75	M	Small cell	Bh-Bs	6.5 cm	Chemo. and irradiation	10 months, dead
19	Hosonuma (2008)	69	F	Small cell	Bs-Bm	3 cm	Biliary drainage	2 months, alive
20	Okamura (2009)	62	M	Small cell	Bm	3 cm	NAC, resection and irradiation	20 months, dead
21	Yamaguch (2009)	77	F	NEC	Bi	N.A.	Resection and chemo.	27 months, alive
22	Demoreuil (2009)	73	M	Large cell + Adenoca.	Bh-Bs	3 cm	Resection and chemo.	12 months, dead
23	Sasatomi (2013)	76	M	Large cell	Bh-Bs	5 cm	Resection	21 days, dead
24	Current report (2014)	70	F	Small cell	Bh	5 cm	Resection and chemo.	10 months, alive

NEC neuroendocrine carcinoma, *NAC* neo adjuvant chemotherapy, *Adenoca.* adenocarcinoma, *CBD* common bile duct, *Bh* hilar bile duct, *Bs* superior portion of common bile duct, *Bm* mid portion of bile duct, *Bi* inferior portion of bile duct, *chemo.* chemotherapy, *N.A.* not available, *M* male, *F* female

etoposide is also recommended for prevention of systemic recurrence [33, 34].

Conclusion

In summary, neuroendocrine carcinoma of the extrahepatic biliary tracts is a very rare and highly malignantdisease with a poor prognosis. Although treatment strategies have not yet been established, a multidisciplinary approach at diagnosis of NEC of the biliary system, as well as further studies on therapeutic management could improve the prognosis of this highly malignant neoplasm.

Abbreviations

CA19-9: carbohydrate antigen 19–9; CEA: carcinoembryonic antigen; ERCP: endoscopic retrograde cholangiopancreatography; NEC: neuroendocrine carcinoma; NET: neuroendocrine tumour; SCC: small cell carcinoma.

Competing interests

The authors declare that they have no competing interests.

Authors' contributions

YK performed the surgery, wrote the case report, made literature review and drafted the manuscript. HY is the senior surgeon who performed all operations assisted by the authors, and revised the manuscript. TU is the gastroenterologist and performed preoperative examination. MN is the pathologist, performed conventional and immunohistochemical staining of NEC of extrahepatic biliary tract, and revised the manuscript. TH is the chief of our division of general surgery, and revised the manuscript. All authors read and approved the final manuscript.

Acknowledgement

The authors acknowledge all the medical and surgical staff that took care of the patient. All authors report no source of funding for conducting this manuscript.

Author details

[1]Division of General Surgery, Japanese Red Cross Kumamoto Hospital, Nagamineminami 2-1-1, Higashiku, Kumamoto city, Kumamoto 861-8520, Japan. [2]Division of Gastroenterology, Japanese Red Cross Kumamoto Hospital, Kumamoto, Japan. [3]Division of Diagnostic Pathology, Japanese Red Cross Kumamoto Hospital, Kumamoto, Japan.

References

1. Komminoth P, Arnold R, Capella C, Klimstra DS, Kloppel G, Rindi G, et al. Neuroendocrine neoplasms of the gallbladder and extrahepatic bile ducts. In: Bosman FT, Carneiro F, Hruban RH, Theise ND, editors. WHO Classification of Tumours of the Digestive System. Lyon, France: IARC Press; 2010. p. p274–6.
2. Chamberlain RS, Blumgart LH. Carcinoid tumors of the extrahepatic bile duct. A rare cause of malignant biliary obstruction. Cancer. 1999;86: 1959–65.
3. Rindi G, Arnold R, Bosman FT, Capella C, Klimstra DS, Kloppel G, et al. Nomenclature and classification of neuroendocrine neoplasms of the digestive system. In: Bosman FT, Carneiro F, Hruban RH, Theise ND, editors. WHO Classification of Tumours of the Digestive System. Lyon, France: IARC Press; 2010. p. 13–4.
4. Suzuki S, Tanaka S, Hayashi T, Harada N, Suzuki M, Hanyu F, et al. Small-cell neuroendocrine carcinoma of the ampulla of Vater. J Hepatobiliary Pancreat Surg. 2006;13:450–3.
5. Nakamura Y, Tajiri T, Uchida E, Arima Y, Aimoto T, Katsuno A, et al. Changes to levels of serum neuron-specific enolase in a patient with small-cell carcinoma of the pancreas. J Hepatobiliary Pancreat Surg. 2005;12:93–8.
6. Eriguchi N, Aoyagi S, Noritomi T, Imamura M, Sato S, Fujiki K, et al. Adeno-endocrine cell carcinoma of the gallbladder. J Hepatobiliary Pancreat Surg. 2000;7:97–101.
7. Sabanathan S, Hashimi H, Nicholson G, Edwards AS. Primary oat cell carcinoma of the common bile duct. J R Coll Surg Edinb. 1988;33:285–6.
8. Van der Wal AC, Van Leeuwen DJ, Walford N. Small cell neuroendocrine (oat cell) tumour of the common bile duct. Histopathology. 1990;16:398–400.
9. Nishihara K, Tsuneyoshi M, Niiyama H, Ichimiya H. Composite glandular-endocrine cell carcinoma of the extrahepatic bile duct: immunohistochemical study. Pathology. 1993;25:90–4.
10. Yamamoto J, Abe Y, Nishihara K, Katsumoto F, Takeda S, Abe R, et al. Composite glandular-neuroendocrine carcinoma of the hilar bile duct: report of a case. Surg Today. 1998;28:758–62.
11. Kim SH, Park YN, Yoon DS, Lee SJ, Yu JS, Noh TW. Composite neuroendocrine and adenocarcinoma of the common bile duct associated with Clonorchis sinensis: a case report. Hepatogastroenterology. 2000;47: 942–4.
12. Miyashita T, Konishi K, Noto M, Taniguchi K, Kaji M, Kimura H, et al. A case of small cell carcinoma of the common bile duct. Nihon Shokakibyo Gakkai Zasshi. 2001;98:1195–8.
13. Edakuni G, Sasatomi E, Satoh T, Tokunaga O, Miyazaki K. Composite glandular-endocrine cell carcinoma of the common bile duct. Pathol Int. 2001;51:487–90.
14. Kuraoka K, Taniyama K, Fujitaka T, Nakatsuka H, Nakayama H, Yasui W. Small cell carcinoma of the extrahepatic bile duct: case report and immunohistochemical analysis. Pathol Int. 2003;53:887–91.
15. Hazama K, Suzuki Y, Takahashi M, Takahashi Y, Yoshioka T, Takano S, et al. Primary small cell carcinoma of the common bile duct, in which surgical treatment was performed after neoadjuvant chemotherapy: report of a case. Surg Today. 2003;33:870–2.
16. Arakura N, Hasebe O, Yokosawa S, Imai Y, Furuta S, Hosaka N. A case of small cell carcinoma of the extrahepatic bile duct which could be diagnosed before operation. Nihon Shokakibyo Gakkai Zasshi. 2003;100: 190–4.
17. Park HW, Seo SH, Jang BK, Hwang JY, Park KS, Cho KB, et al. A case of primary small cell carcinoma in the common bile duct. Korean J Gastroenterol. 2004;43:260–3.
18. Thomas NE, Burroughs FH, Ali SZ. Small-cell carcinoma of the extrahepatic bile duct and concurrent clonorchiasis. Diagn Cytopathol. 2005;32:92–3.
19. Kaiho T, Tanaka T, Tsuchiya S, Yanagisawa S, Takeuchi O, Miura M, et al. A case of small cell carcinoma of the common bile duct. Hepatogastroenterology. 2005;52:363–7.
20. Sato K, Waseda R, Tatsuzawa Y, Fujinaga H, Wakabayashi T, Ueda Y, et al. Composite large cell neuroendocrine carcinoma and adenocarcinoma of the common bile duct. J Clin Pathol. 2006;59:105–7.
21. Viana Miguel MM, García-Plata Polo E, Vidal Doce O, Aldea Martínez J, de la Plaza GM, Santamaría García JL. Oat cell carcinoma of the common bile duct. Cir Esp. 2006;80:43–5.
22. Jeon WJ, Chae HB, Park SM, Youn SJ, Choi JW, Kim SH. A case of primary small cell carcinoma arising from the common bile duct. Korean J Gastroenterol. 2006;48:438–42.
23. Nakai N, Takenaka H, Hamada S, Kishimoto S. Identical p53 gene mutation in malignant proliferating trichilemmal tumour of the scalp and small cell carcinoma of the common bile duct: the necessity for therapeutic caution? Br J Dermatol. 2008;159:482–5.
24. Arakura N, Muraki T, Komatsu K, Ozaki Y, Hamano H, Tanaka E, et al. Small cell carcinoma of the extrahepatic bile duct diagnosed with EUS-FNA and effectively treated with chemoradiation. Intern Med. 2008;47:621–5.
25. Hosonuma K, Sato K, Honma M, Kashiwabara K, Takahashi H, Takagi H, et al. Small-cell carcinoma of the extrahepatic bile duct: a case report and review of the literature. Hepatol Int. 2008;2:129–32.
26. Okamura Y, Maeda A, Matsunaga K, Kanemoto H, Boku N, Furukawa H, et al. Small-cell carcinoma in the common bile duct treated with multidisciplinary management. J Hepatobiliary Pancreat Surg. 2009;16:575–8.
27. Yamaguchi Y, Shimizu H, Yoneda E. A case of recurrent endocrine cell carcinoma of the common bile duct successfully treated by hepatic artery infusion with CPT-11 and CDDP. Gan To Kagaku Ryoho. 2009;36:823–5.
28. Demoreuil C, Thirot-Bidault A, Dagher C, Bou-Farah R, Benbrahem C, Lazure T, et al. Poorly differentiated large cell endocrine carcinoma of the extrahepatic bile ducts. Gastroenterol Clin Biol. 2009;33:194–8.
29. Sasatomi E, Nalesnik MA, Marsh JW. Neuroendocrine carcinoma of the extrahepatic bile duct: Case report and literature review. World J Gastroenterol. 2013;19(28):4616–23.
30. Levenson RM, Ihde DC, Matthews MJ, Cohen MH, Gazdar AF, Bunn PA, et al. Small cell carcinoma presenting as an extrapulmonary neoplasm: sites of origin and response to chemotherapy. J Natl Cancer Inst. 1981;67:607–12.
31. Dumitrascu T, Dima S, Herlea V, Tomulescu V, Ionescu M, Popescu I. Neuroendocrine tumours of the ampulla of Vater: clinico-pathological features, surgical approach and assessment of prognosis. Langenbecks Arch Surg. 2012;397(6):933–43.
32. Kim JH, Lee SH, Park J, Kim HY, Lee SI, Nam EM, et al. Extrapulmonary small-cell carcinoma: a single-institution experience. Jpn J Clin Oncol. 2004;34:250–4.
33. Hogan BA, Thornton FJ, Brannigan M, Browne TJ, Pender S, O'Kelly P, et al. Hepatic metastases from an unknown primary neoplasm (UPN): survival, prognostic indicators and value of extensive investigations. Clin Radiol. 2002;57:1073–7.
34. Quoix E, Breton JL, Daniel C, Jacoulet P, Debieuvre D, Paillot N, et al. Etoposide phosphate with carboplatin in the treatment of elderly patients with small-cell lung cancer: a phase II study. Ann Oncol. 2001;12:957–62.

8

An atypical presentation of intrahepatic perforated cholecystitis: a modern indication to open cholecystectomy

Marcello Donati*, Antonio Biondi, Francesco Basile and Salvatore Gruttadauria

Abstract

Background: Intrahepatic gallbladder perforation with chronic liver abscess formation was anecdotically reported in the literature. The aim of this work is to report a case of intrahepatic gallbladder perforation and its atypical clinical presentation.

Case presentation: A 62-year-old male patient came to our observation; his medical history showed intermittent fever up to 39-40°C of about 2 weeks and anorexia, with an overall weight loss of about 12 Kg. Physical examination of the abdomen was negative. An ultrasound of the liver and an abdominal CT angiogram detected a disomogeneous hypoechoic-hypodense area in the 5th segment of the liver. Differential diagnosis between hepatic abscess or gallbladder cancer remained open. A surgical exploration was planned. After laparoscopic exploration, a conversion to open procedure with an atypical resection of the 5th hepatic segment was performed. Histologic examination of the specimen showed an intrahepatic chronic perforation of the gallbladder with intrahepatic abscess.

Conclusion: To the best of our knowledge, 18 cases have been reported in the literature as a Niemeier type I perforation. Clinical presentation, even in its extreme rarity, is more often acute. Differential diagnosis between gallbladder cancer versus liver abscess remains controversial. Open approach is mandatory in such cases.

Keywords: Intrahepatic perforation, Hepatic abscess, Chronic perforation, Chronic cholecystitis

Background

Perforation of the gallbladder has become a relatively uncommon complication of the natural history of cholelithiasis during acute cholecystitis (0.8-3.2% in recent reviews) [1]. It usually bursts with an acute abdomen and must be operated as a surgical emergency before causing septic peritonitis. Gallbladder perforations were classified following Niemeir's proposal of 1934 [2]. Gallbladder can perforate freely in the abdominal cavity or in a neighboring organ causing many different clinical situations [3]. The intrahepatic perforation causing a liver abscess is an extremely rare condition, anedoctically reported in the world literature, even in the rare type II or III perforation (subacute or acute perforation) [4]. Liver abscess caused by gallbladder perforation can be a a life-threatening complication (5.6% mortality) [5]. Current management of intrahepatic or hepatic abscess is to submit the patient to a percutaneous drainage supported by intravenous antibiotic therapy, when abscess size does not exceed 5 cm, otherwise surgical exploration and drainage remains the first line treatment option for pyogenic liver abscess [6,7]. In cases of gallbladder perforation cholecystectomy is, of course, the treatment of choice, even if in these cases the laparoscopic approach can be problematic [8]. The aim of this work is to report on an intrahepatic type I perforation of the gallbladder leading to a chronic hepatic abscess, causing a very rare and atypical clinical picture.

Case presentation

A 62-year-old male patient came to our observation with an initial diagnosis of clinically silent long-term inguinal hernia. His medical history showed intermittent fever and anorexia had been present for one year. In detail, the patient reported that over the previous year he had had alternating intermittent fever up to 39-40°C of about 2 weeks with quiescence periods of about 20–30 days,

* Correspondence: mdonati@unict.it
Department of Surgery. General and Oncologic Surgery Unit, Vittorio-Emanuele University Hospital of Catania, via Plebiscito 628, 95122 Catania, Italy

every few months together with an overall weight loss of about 12 Kg. These symptoms were not associated with any other abdominal or thoracic signs. Physical examination of the abdomen was negative. The fever disappeared after an empiric antibiotic therapy with third generation cephalosporins (1 gr. for 12 days) was started. Laboratory blood samples obtained when the patient was febrile, showed 12,000 WBC count; liver function tests were in the normal range and serologic screening for Salmonella and Brucella antibodies were negative. Blood cultures, antibiograms and tumor markers were also negative (CEA, CA 19.9).

An ultrasound scan of the liver and an abdominal CT scan (Figure 1A) detected a disomogeneous hypoechoic-hypodense mass with many internal hyperechoic/hyperdense stones in the 5th segment of the liver. In addition, a cholelithiasis with two small stones in the common bile duct was present. Differential diagnosis between hepatic abscess or gallbladder cancer remained open. An abdominal MRI scan confirmed the above mentioned findings with the evidence of a few bubbles of free air suggesting spontaneous perforation of the gallbladder (B). An ERCP was then performed and the choledocolithiasis was resolved through a papillotomy. Afterwards a surgical exploration was planned. The operation started with a laparoscopic approach to confirm the suspected diagnosis and exclude tumor diagnosis and even more important peritoneal tumor spread that would be a contraindication to radical R0-surgical resection. Laparoscopy showed a bulging lesion involving the gallbladder, liver, great omentum and duodenum, (Figure 2A) while no signs of peritoneal carcinomatosis were detected. We then decided to convert to open procedure due to uncertain anatomical limits of the lesion in front of the duodenum and the liver hilar structures. After resection of the omental adhesions and the spearing of the duodenum, the bulging was resected en-bloc with the gallbladder (Figures 2B-3) and gallbladder bed performing an atypical resection of the 5th hepatic segment. Opening the large abscess we found more than

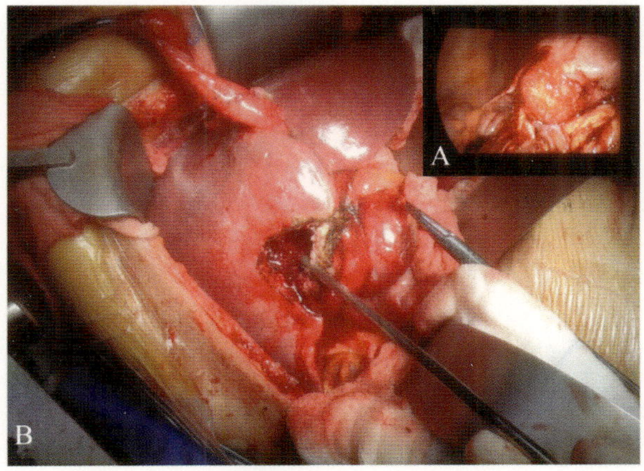

Figure 2 Intraoperative finding: Intrahepatic perforation of the gallbladder. Due to strong hilar adhesions and structure visualization difficulties in laparoscopic view **(A)**, a conversion to "open" approach was decided **(B)**.

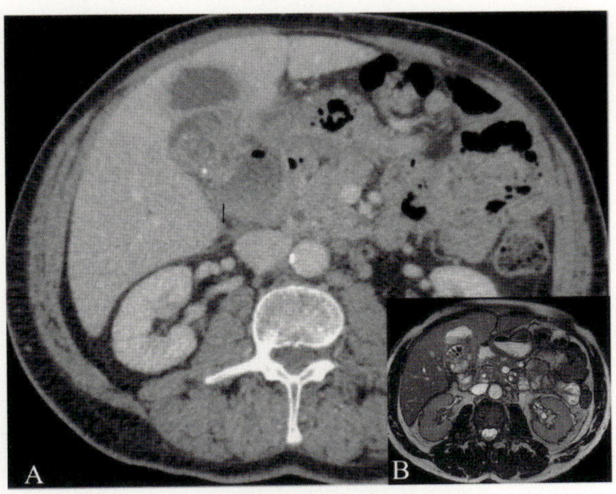

Figure 1 Preoperative Diagnostic. (A) Preop.-CT scan. A hypodense pseudocystic mass on the 5th liver segment, mimicking abscessed gallbladder cancer (bile stones are recognizable on the hilar part of the tumor). **(B)** MRI scan. Bubbles of free air inside the "tumour".

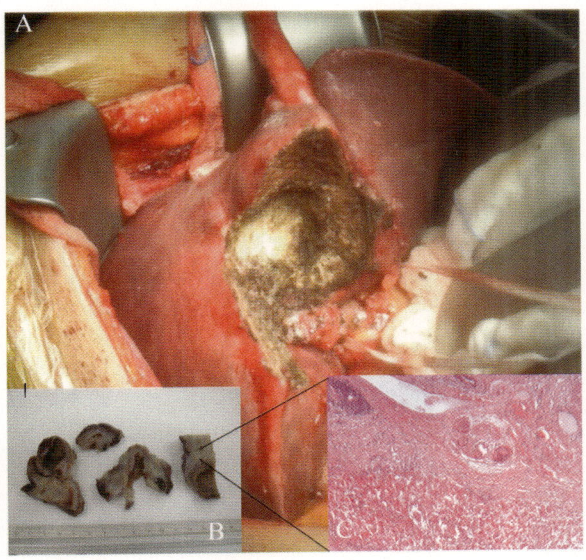

Figure 3 Specimen examination. A) A typical partial resection of the 5th Segment *en-bloc* with the gallbladder. Intrahepatic position of the gallbladder. **B)** Macroscopic details of the pathologic specimen: intrahepatic position of the gallbladder. **C)** Microscopic detail of the specimen (Zoom 10 X): chronic inflammatory cells (giant plurinucleated cells) mixed with hepatic regeneration nodes in the context of a granuloma under the gallbladder bed, effect of intrahepatic perforation. (Courtesy of Dr. Loredana Villari. Pathology Institute. Vittorio-Emanuele Hospital. Catania.).

20 biliary stones that had migrated intra-hepatically. The phlogistic nature of the tumor was histologically confirmed by three intra-operative sections (later frozen) and on the definitive histologic examination (Figure 3B, C). The post–operative course was uneventful and the patient was discharged on the 4th post-operative day completely afebrile and in good general condition.

Intra-hepatic gallbladder perforation is generally considered to be a very rare evolution of cholelithiasis, in fact, to date, performing a Pubmed search using as key words: "Intrahepatic abscess, intrahepatic gallbladder perforations, Neimeir's type I perforation, chronic gallbladder perforation" and then using "related articles" and "see reviews" functions of the database, 20 articles were selected but after reading them and avoiding the well-known confusion [9] and mistakes of reporting Neimeir's classification [4,10], only 18 cases of chronic gallbladder perforation with formation of intrahepatic abscess were found to be reported in the literature [4,11]; therefore following the original classification they should be considered as Niemeier type I perforations (chronic perforation with fistula) [2]. Despite chronic processes with fistula formation, its clinical presentation, even in its rarity, is more often acute (nausea, vomiting, upper quadrant pain, fever, altered mental status, and septic shock) [12,13], or the consequence of an acute perforation [10]. The diagnosis is usually made by US or CT scan. In our case CT scan was not able to exclude a tumor in the 5th hepatic segment. The lack of acute abdomen symptoms characterized our case and this clinical presentation is to be considered exceptional, while usually such a perforation leads to an emergency operation [4]. This subtle clinical picture can be misleading for the physician causing a delay in obtaining prompt imaging tests. Some reports have highlighted the difficult differential diagnosis between gallbladder cancer versus liver abscess [12,14,15]. Because of the very few reports to date, there is no consensus on the standard treatment of such a rare condition [15,16]. Simple puncture and drainage in these cases seems to not be an effective option [15]. An endoscopic examination could be an option, even if in this case laparoscopic cholecystectomy could not be performed due to technical reasons (many adhesions, not clear anatomy, high risk of damage to hilar structures). Some Authors question whether this rare condition is more common in patients with an intrahepatic gallbladder [17]. Therefore chronic liver abscess due to gallbladder perforation is a rare evolution of cholelithiasis.

Conclusions

Intrahepatic gallbladder perforation with abscess formation should be considered an exceptional clinical entity. Despite new diagnostic tools, differential diagnosis with cancer sometimes remains challenging.

It is our opinion that an open approach or early conversion should, in these cases, as in other Niemeier's perforation type I [3], still be the preferred surgical treatment.

Abbreviations

Kg: Kilograms; Gr: Grams; CEA: Carcioembriogenic Antigen; WBC: White blood cells; CT: Computed tomography; US: Ultrasound scan; MRI: Magnetic resonance imaging; ERCP: Endoscopy retrograde colangiopancreatography.

Competing interests

Marcello Donati, Antonio Biondi, Francesco Basile and Salvatore Gruttadauria have no conflict of interests.

Authors' contributions

DM wrote the paper and made the final revision. BA collected data and reviewed the text. FB designed the study, chose figures and reviewed the paper. GS coordinated the study, performed the operation, made style and language revision. All authors read and approved the final manuscript.

Acknowledgments

We would like to thank Dr. Loredana Villari (Pathology Institute. Vittorio-Emanuele Hospital. Catania.) for the images of this work.

References

1. Göbel T, Kubitz R, Blondin D, Häussinger D: **Intrahepatic type II gallbladder perforation by a gallstone: in a CAPD patient.** *Eur J Med Res* 2011, **16**:213–216.
2. Niemeier OW: **Acute free perforation of the gallbladder.** *Ann Surg* 1934, **99**(6):922–924.
3. Donati M, Cardì F, Brancato G, Calò P, Donati A: **The surgical treatment of a rare complication: gallstone ileus.** *Ann Ital Chir* 2010, **81**(1):57–62.
4. Kochar K, Vallance K, Mathew G, Jadhav V: **Intrahepatic perforation of the gall bladder presenting as liver abscess: case report, review of literature and Niemeier's classification.** *Eur J Gastroenterol Hepatol* 2008, **20**(3):240–244.
5. Meddings L, Myers RP, Hubbard J, Shaheen AA, Laupland KB, Dixon E, Coffin C, Kaplan GG: **A population-based study of pyogenic liver abscesses in the United States: incidence, mortality, and temporal trends.** *Am J Gastroenterol* 2010, **105**(1):117–124.
6. Lok KH, Li KF, Li KK, Szeto ML: **Pyogenic liver abscess: clinical profile, microbiological characteristics, and management in a Hong Kong hospital.** *J Microbial Immunol Inf* 2008, **41**:483–490.
7. Ch Yu S, Hg Lo R, Kan PS, Metreweli C: **Pyogenic liver abscess treatment with needle aspiration.** *Clin Radiol* 1997, **52**:912–916.
8. Lo HC, Wang YC, Su LT, Hsieh CH: **Can early laparoscopic cholecystectomy be the optimal management of cholecystitis with gallbladder perforation? A single institute experience of 74 cases.** *Surg Endosc* 2012, **26**(11):3301–3306.
9. Singal R, Mittal A, Gupta S, Singh B, Jain P: **Management of gall bladder perforation evaluation on ultrasonography: report of six rare cases with review of literature.** *J Med Life* 2011, **4**(4):364–371.
10. Date RS, Thrumurthy SG, Whiteside S, Umer MA, Pursnani KG, Ward JB, Mughal MM: **Gallbladder perforation: case series and systematic review.** *Int J Surg* 2012, **10**(2):63–68.
11. Derıcı H, Kamer E, Kara C, Ünalp HR, Tansuğ T, Bozdağ AD, Nazli O: **Gallbladder perforation: clinical presentation, predisposing factors, and surgical outcomes of 46 patients.** *Turk J Gastroenterol* 2011, **22**(5):505–512.
12. Teebken OE, Bartels M, Fangmann J, Nagel E, Klempnauer J: **Chronische Cholezystitis imponierend als Gallenblasen-tumor mit Leberabszess.** *Swiss Surg* 2001, **7**(1):28–31.
13. Alkofer B, Dufay C, Parienti JJ, Lepennec V, Dargere S, Chiche L: **Are pyogenic liver abscesses still a surgical concern? A Western experience.** *HPB Surg* 2012, **2012**:316013.
14. Singla SL, Garg P, Tahlan RN: **Gallbladder carcinoma presenting as liver abscess.** *Indian J Gastroenterol* 1998, **17**(2):68.
15. Bakalakos EA, Melvin WS, Kirkpatrick R: **Liver abscess secondary to intrahepatic perforation of the gallbladder, presenting as a liver mass.** *Am J Gastroenterol* 1996, **91**(8):1644–1646.

Combined measurements of tumor number and size helps estimate the outcome of resection of Barcelona clinic liver cancer stage B hepatocellular carcinoma

Xin Wang[1], Zusen Wang[1] and Liqun Wu[1,2*]

Abstract

Background: Although the Barcelona Clinic Liver Cancer (BCLC) staging system suggests that patients with stage B hepatocellular carcinoma (HCC) should be treated with transcatheter arterial chemoembolization instead of surgical treatment, recent studies indicated that the prognosis of surgical resection for patients with BCLC stage B HCC was better than that of TACE. However, the portion of patients with stage B that will achieve better outcomes from surgical treatment remains unclear. In this study, we identified risk factors that influence the prognosis of BCLC stage B HCC after R0 surgical resection to determine whether some patients with stage B HCC may benefit more from R0 resection than other patients and to provide a guideline to estimate the tendency.

Methods: The clinical data of 78 patients with BCLC stage B HCC after R0 surgical treatment within 11 years were analyzed retrospectively, using relapse or death as the endpoint. Kaplan-Meier survival and Cox regression analyses were used to study prognosis (disease-free survival, DFS and overall survival, OS) and independent risk factors.

Results: For all stage B patients, 1-, 2-, and 5-year DFS rates were 62.5, 36.4, and 16.6 %, respectively. Cumulative tumor size >5.0 cm and tumor number ≥4 were independent prognostic risk factors for DFS. The 1-, 2-, and 5- year DFS rates and OS rates of patients with at least one of these two factors were 49.0, 17.2, and 7.4 % (for DFS), and 78.6, 54.8, and 13.4 % (for OS), respectively, which were significantly lower than patients without these two factors (77.8, 58.3, and 27.2 % for DFS, and 94.4, 83.3,and 51.8 % for OS, respectively, $P < 0.01$).

Conclusions: The analyses indicated that the outcomes of R0 resection were much better for patients with BCLC stage B HCC with two or three tumors and cumulative tumor sizes of ≤5.0 but >3.0 cm than other patients with stage B.

Keywords: BCLC staging, Hepatocellular carcinoma, Prognosis, R0 surgical treatment, Risk factors

Background

Hepatocellular carcinoma (HCC) is one of the five most common malignancies worldwide. Each year, more than 690,000 people die from liver cancer, and the number is increasing every year [1]. HCC is also the third most frequent cause of tumor-related death [2]. The clinical staging system of HCC has an important function for selecting treatment modes and evaluating prognosis, and in recent years, the Barcelona Clinic Liver Cancer (BCLC) staging system has received more attention. According to the BCLC staging system, only patients with very early stage and stage A (early stage) HCC should undergo surgical resection, ablation, or liver transplantation. Patients with stage B HCC should be treated with transcatheter arterial chemoembolization (TACE) [3]. However, many studies have indicated that for patients with BCLC stage B HCC, the prognosis of surgical resection is better than that of TACE [4–7], indicating that it is feasible and applicable for some patients with BCLC stage B HCC to undergo R0 section. However, the portion of patients with stage B that will achieve better outcomes from surgical treatment remains unclear. Moreover, the standard

* Correspondence: wulq5810@126.com
[1]Department of Hepatobiliary and Pancreatic Surgery, Affiliated Hospital of Qingdao University, Qingdao 266000, China
[2]Jiangsu Road 16, Qingdao 266000, China

indicators or influencing risk factors for selection of HCC patients with stage B toward surgical resection have not yet been established. Therefore, study of the risk factors for prognosis of BCLC stage B after surgical treatment has profound significance in forming a guideline for clinical treatment of this sort of patients. Clarification of major factors influencing curative efficiency will enable clinicians to estimate whether a patient with BCLC stage B HCC may achieve a better prognosis from R0 resection and identification of those patients with non-improved outcomes should be more carefully monitored after resection. This study aims to provide surgeons with a guideline to estimate clinical treatment and predict prognosis to guide postoperative treatment.

Methods

Case data

From 2001 to 2012, 827 patients with HCC underwent R0 hepatic resection in the Affiliated Hospital of Qingdao University, China and 78 patients suffered BCLC stage B HCC disease. We declare that informed consents for the use of their clinical data in this study were obtained from all participants or their next of kin before follow up and before the study began. We thank them a lot for their consent of this study. BCLC staging was determined using liver ultrasonography or computed tomography (CT) and thorough clinical assessment. All the patients had 2–5 cancerous nodules with a cumulative tumor size of >3.0 cm, a Child-Pugh score of A-B, and performance status of 0, and thus, were classified as BCLC stage B. Pathological diagnoses were made for all patients. There were 66 men and 12 women (ratio 5.5:1) and their age ranged 33–80 years old, with an average of 55.9 years. The clinicopathological features of the 78 patients are shown in Table 1. The collection of clinical data was approved by the Ethic Committee of Affiliated Hospital of Qingdao University.

Surgical methods

All 78 cases underwent liver resection in accordance with the Couinaud segmentation method to implement hepatic segmentectomy or combined resection for adjacent liver segments (anatomical resection) or partial hepatectomy containing tumor (nonanatomical resection). R0 hepatic resection means there were no residual cancer cells present in the surgical margin when checked

Table 1 Clinicopathological features of 78 patients with Barcelona Clinic Liver Cancer stage B hepatocellular carcinoma

Factors	Median (range or proportion)
Sex (male/female)	66:12 (84.6 %:15.4 %)
Age (years)	56.0 (33–80)
Alcohol consumption (no/yes)[a]	56:20 (73.7:26.3)
Preoperative TACE (no/yes)	67:11 (85.9 %:14.1 %)
HBsAg (negative/positive)	7:71 (9.0 %:91.0 %)
Anti-HCV (negative/positive)	76:2 (97.4 %:2.6 %)
ALT (U/L)	45.5 (12–191)
GGT (U/L)	49.5 (15–395)
Child–Pugh Classification (A/B)	76:2 (97.4 %:2.6 %)
Cirrhosis (no/yes)	5:73 (6.4 %:93.6 %)
Portal hypertension (no/yes)	65:13 (83.3 %:16.7 %)
Liver resection range (hepatic segment)	2 (1–4)
Resection margin (mm)[a]	5 (0–30)
Anatomical resection (yes/no)	18:60 (23.1 %:76.9 %)
Hepatic inflow occlusion (no/yes)	33:45 (42.3:57.7)
Intraoperative blood loss (mL)	300 (100–3500)
Blood transfusion (mL)	0.0 (0–1100)
Preoperative alpha-fetoprotein (μg/L)	17.8 (1.1–1211.0)
Cumulative tumor size (cm)	5.0 (2.5–20.0)
Tumor number	3 N
Differentiation (high/middle and low/necrosis)	3:73:2 (3.8 %:93.6 %:2.6 %)
Liver capsule invasion (no/yes)	12:66 (15.4 %:84.6 %)

ALT alanine aminotransferase, *GGT* gamma glutamyltransferase, *HBsAg* hepatitis B surface antigen
[a]Some patients lack data

microscopically and no tumor visible with the naked eyes.

Follow-up study

Serum alpha-fetoprotein, liver function tests, liver ultrasonography or CT and lung CT scan were performed monthly for 3 months after surgical resection. The time of recurrence after resection was adjudged by the presence of clear masses on imaging examination. The follow-up ended on 31 December 2015 or when patients died. The median follow-up time was 31.4 months (ranging 3.3–113.2 months).

Statistical analysis

All the data were statistically analyzed with SPSS Statistics software for Windows, Version 13.0 (SPSS Inc., Chicago, IL, USA). The Kaplan-Meier survival analysis (log-rank test) was used to analyze disease-free survival (DFS) and overall survival (OS). The factors with $P < 0.05$ were enrolled in the Cox regression hazard model. $P < 0.05$ was considered significant.

Results

Risk factors for DFS and OS

Seventy-eight patients with BCLC stage B HCC underwent R0 hepatic resection. The OS rates for1, 2 and 5 years were 85.9, 67.9 and 29.8 %, respectively; the median OS was 35.0 months [95 % confidence interval (CI) = 29.4–40.6 months]. The DFS rates for 1, 2 and 5 years were 62.5, 36.4 and 16.6 %, respectively; and the median DFS was 15.0 months (95 % CI = 10.7–19.3 months).

In Table 2, we analyzed the relation of selected factors with the DFS with Kaplan-Meier analysis. The result showed that cumulative tumor size >5.0 cm and tumor number ≥4 were important risk factors that significantly influenced DFS ($P < 0.01$). Then the two factors were enrolled into Cox regression hazard model analysis which showed that the cumulative tumor size and tumor number were two significant independent risk factors for DFS ($P < 0.05$).

Relationship between recurrence and tumor number

Patients with BCLC stage B HCC were divided into three groups according to tumor numbers which included 2, 3

Table 2 Factors influencing disease-free survival (DFS) for patients with Barcelona Clinic Liver Cancer stage B hepatocellular carcinoma after R0 resection

Factors	Kaplan–Meier analysis		Cox regression hazard model	
	Median DFS (mo)	*P* value	HR(95 % CI)	*P* value
Sex (male/female)	15.0/13.0	0.771		
Age (≤60/>60 years)	15.0/13.0	0.530		
Alcohol consumption (no/yes)[a]	15.0/18.0	0.463		
Preoperative TACE (no/yes)	13.0/33.0	0.058		
HBsAg (negative/positive)	8.0/18.0	0.267		
Anti-HCV (negative/positive)	15.0/11.4	0.529		
ALT (≤50/>50 U/L)	23.0/11.4	0.076		
GGT (≤64/>64 U/L)	19.0/13.0	0.096		
Child–Pugh classification (A/B)	15.0/5.7	0.288		
Cirrhosis (no/yes)	25.0/15.0	0.317		
Portal hypertension (no/yes)	15.0/23.0	0.769		
Liver resection range (≤2/>2 segments)	17.0/8.0	0.084		
Resection margin (<5/≥5 mm)[a]	13.0/19.0	0.573		
Anatomical resection (yes/no)	14.6/15.0	0.783		
Hepatic inflow occlusion (no/yes)	13.0/19.0	0.223		
Intraoperative blood loss (≤1000/>100 mL)	18.0/13.0	0.282		
Blood transfusion (yes/no)	17.0/15.0	0.732		
Preoperative alpha-fetoprotein (≤20/>20 μg/L)	14.6/18.0	0.273		
Cumulative tumor size (≤5/>5 cm)	25.0/13.0	0.009	1.685 (1.011–2.808)	0.045
Tumor number (≤3/≥4)	23.0/10.1	0.000	2.681 (1.506–4.770)	0.001
Differentiation (high/middle and low/necrosis)	24.0/15.0/19.2	0.671		
Liver capsule invasion (no/yes)	13.0/17.0	0.882		

[a]Some patients lacked data

Table 3 Disease-free survival of patients with different tumor number

No of tumors.	*n*	Median (months)	1 year (%)	2 years (%)	5 years (%)	*P*
2	39	28.8	76.9	53.8	23.1	0.001
3	17	19.0	58.8	25.3	22.1	
≥4	22	10.1	38.5	4.8	0.0	

and more than 4 tumors, respectively. Kaplan-Meier survival analysis was used to analyze the DFS for the three groups. The median DFS time and the DFS rate for1, 2 and 5 years decreased as tumor number increased ($P < 0.01$; Table 3).

Then, the receiver operating characteristic (ROC) curve was applied for further analysis. The tumor number was regarded as a test variable while the recurrence a state variable. The area under the curve was 69.4 % ($P = 0.024$) and the Youden index was 2.5 (specificity = 78.6 %, sensitivity = 56.3 %) (Fig. 1). We took the tumor number of 3 as the critical value according to the Youden index. The 1-, 2-, and 5-year DFS rates for the patients with tumor number ≤ 3 (56 cases) and ≥4 (22 cases) were 71.4, 48.2, and 23 % (for number ≤3), and 38.5, 4.8 and 0 % (for number ≥4), respectively ($P = 0.000$) (Fig. 2). These analytic data clearly indicate that the patients with 2 to 3 tumor number survived better with much lower recurrence rates than those with tumor number ≥4.

Relationship between recurrence and tumor size

On the basis of the cumulative tumor size, patients were divided into two groups, ≤5 cm (45 cases) and > 5 cm (33 cases). Kaplan-Meier analysis was performed to analyze the DFS for the patients in the two groups. The 1-, 2- and 5-year DFS rates were 70.6 , 50.1 and 22 % for the ≤5 cm group, and 51.5, 18.2 and 9.1 % for the > 5 cm group, respectively ($P = 0.009$, Fig. 3), indicating that the patients with cumulative tumor size ≤5 but >3 cm showed significant lower recurrence rates than those with cumulative tumor size > 5 cm.

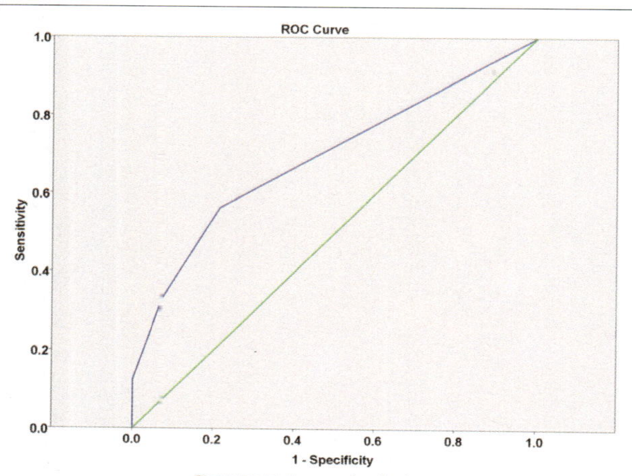

Fig. 1 ROC curves of tumor number and recurrence

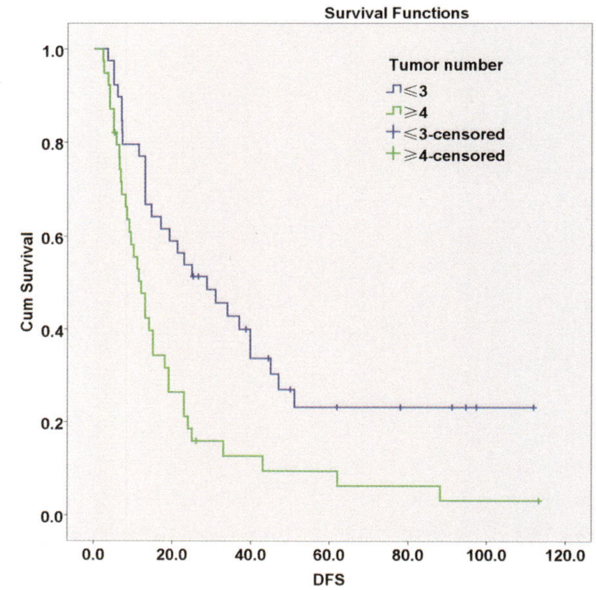

Fig. 2 Disease-free survival (DFS) curves of tumor number ≤3 and ≥4. The upper curve represents DFS of patients with ≤3 tumors, while the lower curve represents DFS of patients with ≥4 tumors

Comparison of DFS and OS between high-risk and non-high-risk groups

Patients with tumor number ≥4 and cumulative tumor size >5 cm were classified as the high-risk group (42 cases) while the other 36 patients as the non-high-risk group. Kaplan-Meier survival analysis was performed to

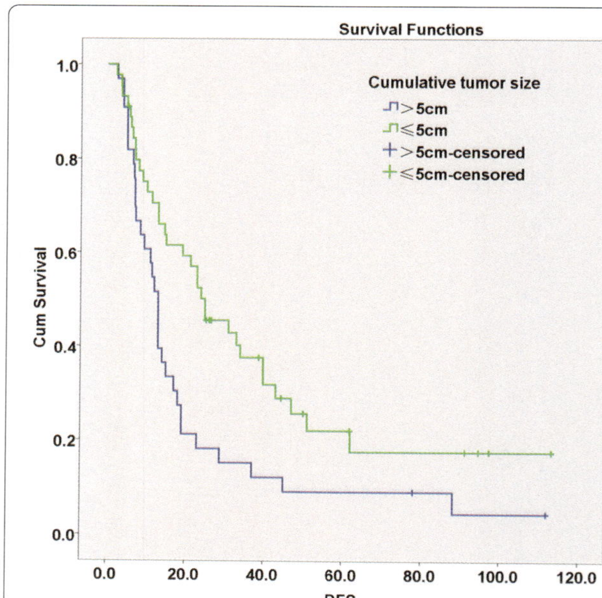

Fig. 3 Disease-free survival (DFS) curves of cumulative tumor size ≤5 cm and >5 cm. The upper curve represents DFS of patients with a cumulative tumor size of ≤5.0 cm, while the lower curve represents DFS of patients with a cumulative tumor size >5.0 cm

analyze the DFS. For patients in the high-risk and non-high-risk groups, the 1-, 2-, and 5-year DFS rates were 49, 17.2 and 7.4 (for high-risk), and 77.8, 58.3 and 27.2 % (for non-high-risk), respectively ($P = 0.001$); the OS rates at 1, 2. and 5 years were 78.6, 54.8 and 13.4 % (for high-risk), and 94.4, 83.3 and 51.8 % (for non-high-risk), respectively ($P = 0.000$) (Fig. 4). The significance of the analytic results was in line with those in 3.2 and 3.3 sections, i.e., the recurrence rates of the non-high-risk group were significantly lower than those of the high-risk group.

Discussion

Tumor recurrence after resection is an important factor affecting the prognosis of patients with HCC. The BCLC staging system was proposed in 1999 by Llovet et al. [8] and modified by the American Association for the Study of Liver Diseases in 2005 [9]. This staging system

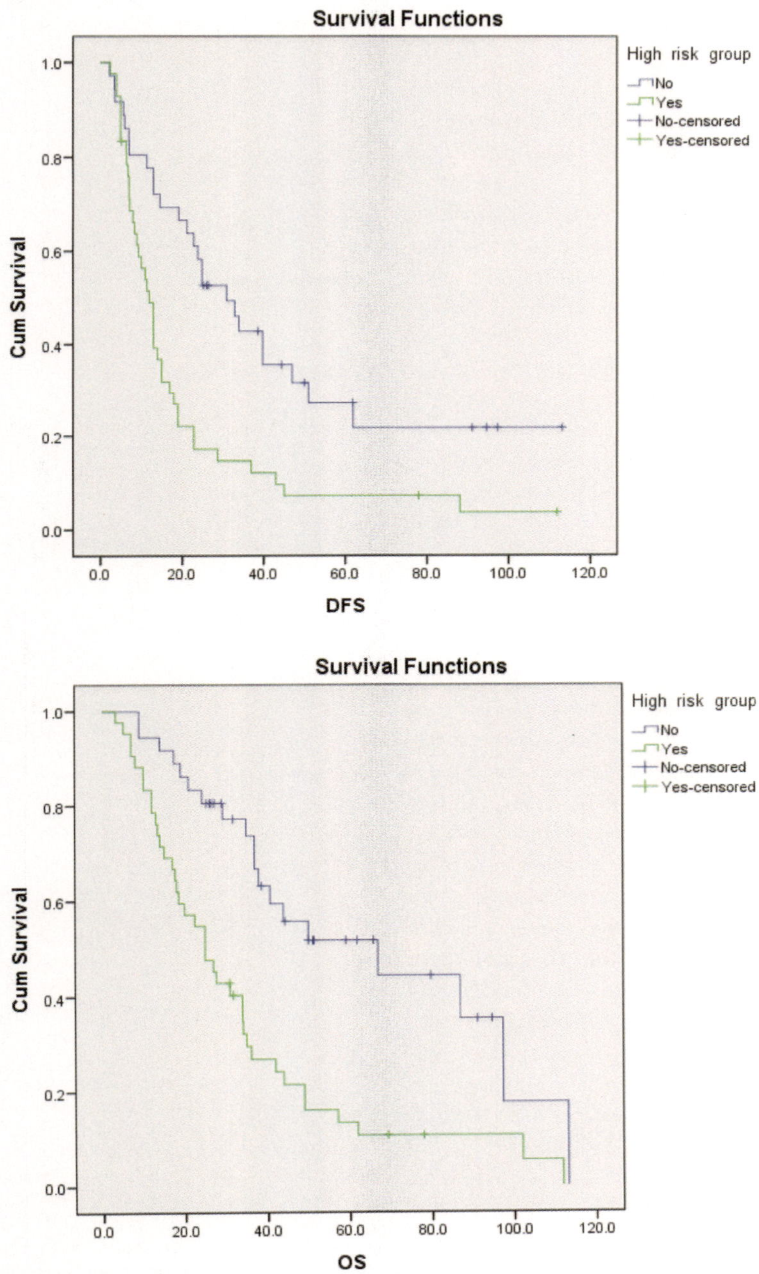

Fig. 4 Disease-free survival (DFS) and overall survival (OS) curves of high-risk and non-high-risk group. The upper curves represent the DFS and OS of the non-high-risk group, while the lower curves are DFS and OS of the high-risk group

comprehensively considers tumor size and number, vascular invasion, liver function, and general condition. It has been accepted worldwide at present. The system recommends that patients with stage B HCC should be treated with TACE. However, many studies have indicated that for patients with BCLC stage B HCC, the prognosis for surgical resection treatment is superior to that for TACE. For example, from 171 patients with BCLC stage B HCC, Lin [5] found that the 1-, 2- and 3-year OS rates after surgical resection or TACE was 83, 62 and 49 % or 39, 5 and 2 %, respectively. The prognosis of surgical resection was obviously better than that of TACE.

Considering that patients with BCLC stage B HCC frequently have multiple tumors with or without vascular invasion and intrahepatic metastasis, we think that it is necessary to explore further the indicators of surgical resection for this stage HCC to obtain a better prognosis. In this study, we identified that tumor number ≥4 and cumulative tumor size >5 cm were independent risk factors influencing the prognosis of BCLC stage B HCC after R0 liver resection. Median DFS and OS in patients with these two factors were 12.0 and 25.0 months, respectively, which were significantly lower than those of patients with tumor number 2 or 3 and cumulative tumor size ≤5 cm (31.0 and 67.0 months, $P < 0.01$). In keeping with our current study, many studies have proved that tumor number [10–14] and tumor size [10, 11, 15–17] can affect prognosis after resection of HCC. For example, Shah et al. [10] discovered that multiple tumors and large tumor size are independent risk factors of postoperative recurrence of HCC.

It is clinically significant that tumor number and size have been identified as two independent risk factors. The blood supply of HCC is mainly from the hepatic artery and portal vein. Therefore, large tumors always have a more abundant blood supply, grow faster, break through the capsule more easily and transfer to and infiltrate the surrounding liver tissue readily. Large tumors also more easily cause invasion of the portal vein, increasing the probability of postoperative intrahepatic recurrence. Multiple tumors in the liver are mostly due to intrahepatic metastasis, and an increase in tumor number usually indicates more rapid metastasis. For these patients, even if the visible tumors are totally removed, small metastases may also be present in the liver, resulting in recurrence of HCC, which is consistent with the finding of this study that patients with HCC stage B with ≥4 tumors or a cumulative tumor size of >5.0 cm had higher postoperative recurrence rates.

Our study was limited by the small sample size and regional area, which may not be representative of patients with BCLC stage B HCC in other areas. Moreover, the follow-up period for some patients was relatively short. Nonetheless, these patients were included in the analysis because they meet the BCLC stage B-staging standard, although they had many significant risk factors reported already, e.g., age of >60 years; 4–5 nodules; tumor size of >5.0 cm; significant amount of perioperative blood loss; and much higher AFP, ALT, and GGT levels than normal. In spite of these limitations, the results of this study revealed that both tumor number and tumor size were the main staging indicators of BCLC stage B HCC. Therefore, our study has important significance in estimating clinical treatment and predicting the prognosis to guide postoperative treatment.

Competing interests

The authors declare that they have no competing interests.

Authors' contributions

WX collected and analyzed the data. WZ collected and analyzed the data. WL collected the data and wrote the manuscript. All authors read and approved the final manuscript.

Acknowledgments

We thank Dr. Zhiqiang Qu (Center for Medical Research, Affiliated Hospital of Qingdao University) for critical revision and comments on the manuscript. This project was supported by the Funding for Excellent Departments (Qingdao University) to WL.

References

1. Marrero JA. Multidisciplinary management of hepatocellular carcinoma: where are we today? Semin Liver Dis. 2013;33(S1):S3–10.
2. Ferlay J, Shin HR, Bray F, et al. Estimates of worldwide burden of cancer in 2008: GLOBOCAN 2008. Int J Cancer. 2010;127(12):2893–917.
3. Bruix J, Llovet JM. Prognostic prediction and treatment strategy in hepatocellular carcinoma. Hepatology. 2002;35(3):519–24.
4. Torzilli G, Belghiti J, et al. A snapshot of the effective indications and results of surgery for hepatocellular carcinoma in tertiary referral centers: is it adherent to the EASL/AASLD recommendations?: an observational study of the HCC East-west study group. Ann Surg. 2013;257(5):929–37.
5. Lin CT, Hsu KF, et al. Comparing hepatic resection andtranscatheterarterial chemoembolization for Barcelona Clinic Liver Cancer (BCLC) stage B hepatocellular carcinoma: change for treatment of choice? World J Surg. 2010;34(9):2155–61.
6. Wang JH, Chang CS, Hu TH, et al. The efficacy of treatment schedules according to Barcelona clinic liver cancer staging for hepatocellular carcinoma: survival analysis of 389 patients. Eur J Cancer. 2008;44(7):1000–6.
7. Jianyong L, Lunan Y, et al. Barcelona clinic liver cancer stage B hepatocellular carcinoma: transcatheterarterial chemoembolization or hepatic resection? Medicine. 2014;93(26):180.
8. Llovet JM, Bru C, Bruix J. Prognosis of hepatocellular carcinoma: the BCLC staging classification. Semin Liver Dis. 1999;19(3):329–38.
9. Bruix J, Sherman M. Management of hepatocellular carcinoma. Hepatology. 2005;42(5):1208–36.
10. Shah SA, Cleary SP, et al. Recurrence after liver resection for hepatocellular carcinoma: risk factors, treatment, and outcomes. Surgery. 2007;141(3):330–9.
11. Cha C, Fong Y, et al. Predictors and patterns of recurrence after resection of hepatocellular carcinoma. J Am Coll Surg. 2003;197(5):753–8.
12. Ruzzenente A, Capra F, Pachera S, et al. Is liver resection justified in advanced hepatocellular carcinoma? Results of an observational study in 464 patients. J Gastrointest Surg. 2009;13(7):1313–20.
13. Nojiri K, Tanaka K, et al. The efficacy of liver resection for multinodular hepatocellular carcinoma. Anticancer Res. 2014;34(5):2421–6.
14. Jun CH, da Sim W, et al. Risk factors for patients with stage IVB hepatocellular carcinoma and extension into the heart: prognostic and therapeutic implications. Yonsei Med J. 2014;55(2):379–86.
15. Yip VS, Gomez D. Tumour size and differentiation predict survival after liver resection for hepatocellular carcinoma arising from non-cirrhotic and nonfibrotic liver: a case-controlled study. Int J Surg. 2013;11(10):1078–82.

Laparoscopic liver resection as a safe and efficacious alternative to open resection for colorectal liver metastasis

Yanming Zhou[1*†], Yaqing Xiao[2†], Lupeng Wu[1], Bin Li[1] and Hua Li[2*]

Abstract

Background: The safety and efficacy of laparoscopic liver resection (LLR) for colorectal liver metastasis (CLM) remain to be established. A meta-analysis was undertaken to compare LLR and open liver resection (OLR) for CLM with respect to surgical and oncologic outcomes.

Methods: An electronic search was performed to retrieve all relevant articles published in the English language by the end of March 2013. Data were analyzed using Review Manager version 5.0.

Results: A total of 8 nonrandomized controlled studies with 695 subjects were analyzsed. Intra-operative blood loss, the proportion of patients requiring blood transfusion, morbidity and the length of hospital stay were all significantly reduced after LLR. Postoperative recurrence, 5-year overall and disease-free survivals were comparable between two groups.

Conclusions: LLR for CLM is safe and efficacious. It improves surgical outcomes and uncompromises oncologic outcomes as compared with OLR.

Keywords: Laparoscopic liver resection, Colorectal liver metastasis, Meta-analysis

Background

Colorectal cancer (CRC) is among the most frequently encountered malignant neoplasms in the world. Approximately 50% CRC patients developed liver metastasis during disease evolution, which is a major cause of cancer death [1]. Conventional open liver resection (OLR) is an effective treatment for colorectal liver metastasis (CLM), offering a 5-year survival of 16-74% and a 10-year survival of 9-69% [2].

Lparoscopic liver resection (LLR) was first reported as a minimally invasive procedure two decades ago [3], but many surgeons are reluctant to accept it as an alternative to an open approach due to the potential risks of intraoperative complications and oncologic adequacy. With tremendous instrumental and technological advances in the laparoscopic field in recent years, increased numbers of reports on LLR have been published [4]. A number of case-series reports and comparative trials have demonstrated the potential benefits, safety and feasibility of LLR for CLM [5-16]. However, no related evidence has been reviewed systematically. In accordance with recommendations of the Preferred Reporting Items for Systematic Reviews and Meta-Analyses (PRISMA) Statement [17], we made a meta-analysis to provide a better quality of evidence in the literature to support the recommendation of LLR as an alternative option for CLM treatment.

Methods

Study selection and data extraction

A MEDLINE, EMBASE, OVID, and Cochrane database were searched to identify all clinical trials published as full papers in the English language that compared LLR and OLR for CLM between July 1992 and March 2013. The following Mesh search headings were used: "laparoscopic liver resection", "colorectal cancer", and "colorectal liver metastases". The bibliographies of relevant

* Correspondence: zhouymsxy@sina.cn; endohlihua@126.com
†Equal contributors
1Department of Hepatobiliary & Pancreatovascular Surgery, Oncologic Center of Xiamen, First affiliated Hospital of Xiamen University, Xiamen, China
2Department of Digestive Diseases, First affiliated Hospital of Xiamen University, Xiamen, China
Full list of author information is available at the end of the article

articles were reviewed manually to identify additional trials.

The following parameters were extracted from each study and tabulated by two investigators (BL and LPW) independently: name of first authors, year of publication, study design, number of patients in each arm, patient baseline characteristics, and outcomes of interest. All relevant texts, tables and figures were reviewed for data extraction. If the study provided medians and interquartile ranges instead of means and SDs, the means and SDs were imputed as described by Hozo *et al.* [18]. Discrepancies between the reviewers were resolved by discussion and consensus.

Outcomes of interests

Surgical outcomes: operative parameters (duration of operation, intra-operative blood loss, and need for blood transfusion), postperative adverse events (morbidity and mortality rates), and postoperative recovery (hospital stay, time to bowel movement, time to oral intake, and requirement for analgesia).

Oncologic outcomes: resection margin, recurrence, 5-year overall survival (OS) and disease-free survival (DFS).

Criteria for inclusion and exclusion

To be included in the analysis, a study had to compare LLR and OLR for CLM. If dual (or multiple) studies were reported by the same institution, only the most recent was used. Unpublished studies, abstracts, letters, proceedings from scientific meetings, editorials and expert opinions, reviews without original data, case reports and studies lacking control groups were excluded. Trials that involved heterogeneous groups of patients with a variety of hepatic disesase were also excluded.

Qualitative analysis

The methodological quality of the included trials was assessed according to the Newcastle-Ottawa Scale (NOS), which scores patient selection, comparability of the two study groups, and assessment of outcomes [19]. Studies achieving more than 6 points (maximum 11) were defined as higher quality.

Statistical methods

All data were analyzed using the Review Manager version 5.0 (The Cochrane Collaboration, Software Update, Oxford) and $P < 0.05$ was considered statistically significant. Analyses were performed using odds ratios (OR) with a 95% confidence interval (95% CI) for dichotomous variables and weighted mean differences (WMD) with a 95% CI for continuous variables. Heterogeneity was evaluated by χ^2 and I^2. Data that were not significantly heterogeneous ($P > 0.1$) were calculated using a fixed effects model, and heterogeneous data ($P < 0.1$) were calculated using a random-effects model. Publication bias was assessed visually using a funnel plot for standard error by effect size (log OR).

Results

Eligible studies

Figure 1 demonstrates a flow chart of the selection process that yielded a total of 8 non-randomized comparative studies published between 2002 and 2013 that matched the criteria of inclusion and exclusion and were included in the current meta-analysis [9-16]. The characteristics of these 8 studies are summarized in Table 1. The 8 studies included a total of 695 patients: 268 in LLR group and 427 in OLR group. Two studies were conducted in the United States [13,15], one in Norway [9],

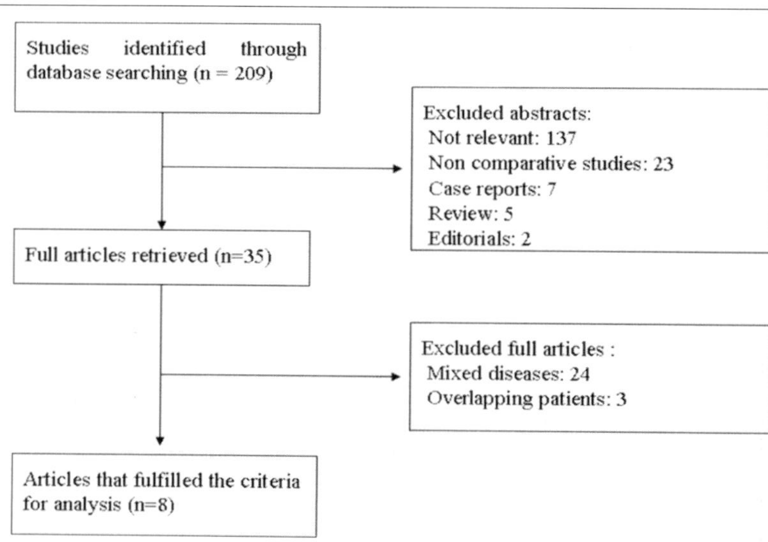

Figure 1 Selection flow diagram.

Table 1 Baseline characteristics of the studies included in the meta-analysis

Author	Year	Country	Group	No. of patients	M/F	Age, year (range and/or SD)	MH	Tumor size, cm (range and/or SD)	No. of tumor (range and/or SD)	Conversions (n [%])	Study quality
Mala *et al.* [9]	2002	Norway	LLR	13	4/9	68 (55–73)	2	2.6 (1–6)	2 (1–7)	0	*****
			OLR	14	4/10	59 (24–74)	2	3 (1.5-9)	1 (1–4)		
Castaing *et al.* [10]	2009	France	LLR	60	37/23	62 ± 11	26	3.3 ± 1.1	2.2 ± 2.3	6 (10)	*******
			OLR	60	37/23	62 ± 11	24	4.4 ± 3.8	2.2 ± 1.98		
Abu *et al.* [11]	2010	United Kingdom	LLR	50	28/22	66 (42–85)	19	3.15 (0.3–9)	1 (1–3)	6 (12)	******
			OLR	85	55/30	67 (47–86)	46	–	–		
Cheung *et al.* [12]	2012	Hong Kong	LLR	20	13/7	57.5 (42–74)	1	1.5 (0.5–4.5)	1 (1–2)	0	*******
			OLR	40	29/11	64 (29–83)	2	2.2 (0.5–7)	1 (1–2)		
Cannon *et al.* [13]	2012	United States	LLR	35	–	62 ±10	19	4 ±3	1 ± 1	–	*******
			OLR	138	–	62 ±11	71	5 ± 3	1 ± 1		
Topal *et al.* [14]	2012	Belgium	LLR	20	10/10	57.6	20	4 (0.4–7)	2 (1–6)	–	******
			OLR	20	8/12	66.0	20	3.2 (1–12.5)	2 (1–14)		
Guerron *et al.* [15]	2013	United States	LLR	40	21/19	66.2 ± 1.9	5	3.3 ± 0.3	1.3 ± 0.1	2 (5)	*******
			OLR	40	15/25	62.2 ± 1.8	9	3.2 ± 0.3	1.7 ± 0.1		
Qiu *et al.* [16]	2013	China	LLR	30	14/16	52.5 ± 11.5	2	2.5 ± 2.0	≥2 (n=10)	2 (6.6)	********
			OLR	30	15/15	–	5	2.8 ± 1.5	≥2 (n=9)		

LLR laparoscopic liver resection, *OLR* open liver resection, *M/F* Male/Female, *MH* major hepatectomy (≥ 3 segments of the liver). *Newcastle-Ottawa Scale.

Table 2 Results of a meta-analysis comparing laparoscopic versus open liver resection for colorectal liver metastasis

Outcome of interest	No. of studies	No. of participants	OR/WMD	95% CI	*P*-value	I^2 (%)
Operative outcomes						
Operative time	7 [9-12,14-16]	LLR = 235, OLR= 289	1.91	−15.92, 19.75	0.83	49
Blood loss	7 [9,11-16]	LLR = 210, OLR= 367	−173.08	−297.52, -48.64	0.006	83
Blood transfusions requirement	4 [10,12,13,15]	LLR = 155, OLR= 278	0.35	0.20, 0.64	< 0.001	0
Overall morbidity	8 [9-16]	LLR = 270, OLR= 427	0.56	0.39, 0.82	0.003	0
Mortality	8 [9-16]	LLR = 268, OLR= 427	0.69	0.13, 3.75	0.67	0
Hospital stay	6 [9,10,12,14-16]	LLR = 185, OLR= 204	−3.54	−5.12, -1.96	< 0.001	75
Oncologic outcomes						
Negative surgical margin	6 [9-11,13,14,16]	LLR = 208, OLR= 347	2.97	1.53, 5.78	0.001	0
Recurrence	3 [10,11,15]	LLR = 150, OLR = 185	0.68	0.41, 1.14	0.14	0
5-year overall survival	4 [10,12-14]	LLR = 135, OLR= 258	1.33	0.86, 2.07	0.20	41
5-year disease-free survival	4 [10,12-14]	LLR = 135, OLR= 258	1.48	0.89, 2.44	0.13	45

OR odds ratio, *WMD* weighted mean difference, *CI* confidence interval.

one in France [10], one in the United Kingdom [11], one in Hong Kong [12], one in Belgium [14], and one in Mainland China [16]. The sample size of the included studies ranged from 27 to 173 patients. The patient baseline characteristics including sex, age, and the number and size of metastases were well matched between the two groups in all the 8 studies. Only one study conducted by Cannon *et al.* [13] had differences in type of resections. In their series, left lateral segmentectomy was significantly more common in the laparoscopic group, while wedge resection/bisegmentectomy was significantly more common in the open group.

The methods of patient selections and indications for LLR were reported in four studies [10,11,13,16]. In general, patients with centrally located lesions such as those near the hilum or in proximity to the hepatic veins were considered unsuitable for the laparoscopic approach.

Six of the 8 studies reported on the conversion rate in LLR group, which ranged from 0 to 12% [9-12,15,16]. The overall conversion rate was 8.2% (16/193). The reasons for conversion were bleeding (n=5), massive adhesions (n=4), inadequate hemostasis (n=2), peritoneal tumor implants (n=1), control of the right or middle hepatic vein (n=2), multiple hepatic metastases (n=1), and diagnostic uncertainty (n =1).

Meta-analysis of surgical outcomes

Table 2 presents a summary of outcomes. Regarding the operative parameters, differences in the duration of operation were not statistically significant (7 trials reported this datum, WMD: 1.91, 95% CI: -15.92 to 19.75; P =0.83), while intra-operative blood loss was significantly lower in LLR group (7 trials reported this datum, WMD: -173.08, 95% CI: -297.52 to −48.64; P = 0.006). Consequently, the proportion of patients requiring blood transfusion was lower in LLR group (4 trials reported this datum, OR: 0.35, 95% CI: 0.20 to 0.64; P <0.001). Significant heterogeneity of difference in operation duration and blood loss was observed between the studies (P < 0.1).

Regarding the postoperative adverse events, patients in the laparoscopic group had lower morbidity than those in the open resection group (all 8 trials reported this datum, 21.1% vs. 33.7%; P = 0.003) (Figure 2). Overall, postoperative mortality occurred only in one patient in

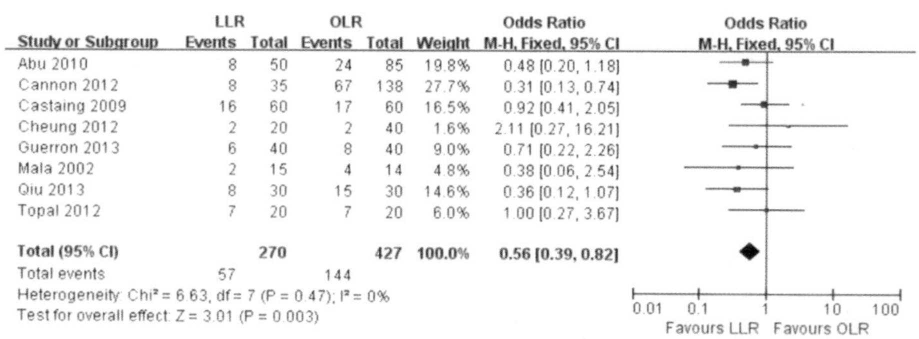

Figure 2 Forest plot displaying the results of the meta-analysis on postoperative morbidity.

Study or Subgroup	LLR Mean	LLR SD	LLR Total	OLR Mean	OLR SD	OLR Total	Weight	Mean Difference IV, Random, 95% CI
Castaing 2009	10	11.2	60	11	7.2	60	13.0%	-1.00 [-4.37, 2.37]
Cheung 2012	4.5	13.2	20	7	23.5	40	2.6%	-2.50 [-11.80, 6.80]
Guerron 2013	3.7	0.5	40	6.5	0.5	40	32.0%	-2.80 [-3.02, -2.58]
Mala 2002	3.7	1.3	15	11.2	4.5	14	18.1%	-7.50 [-9.95, -5.05]
Qiu 2013	7.5	1.5	30	11.5	3	30	27.1%	-4.00 [-5.20, -2.80]
Topal 2012	8	11.5	20	8	3.5	20	7.0%	0.00 [-5.27, 5.27]
Total (95% CI)			**185**			**204**	**100.0%**	**-3.54 [-5.12, -1.96]**

Heterogeneity: Tau² = 2.01; Chi² = 19.87, df = 5 (P = 0.001); I² = 75%
Test for overall effect: Z = 4.40 (P < 0.0001)

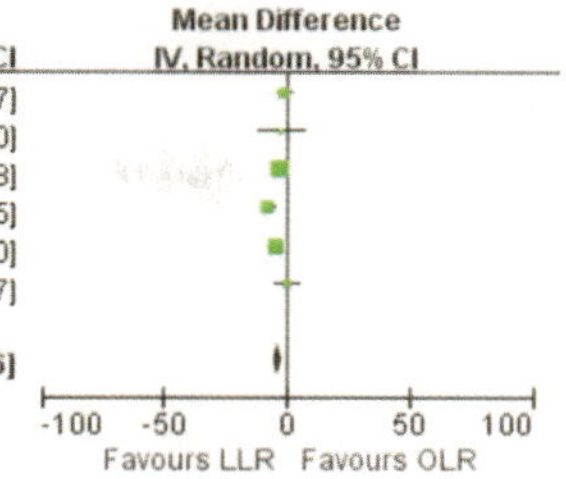

Figure 3 Forest plot displaying the results of the meta-analysis on hospital stay.

LLR group vs. four patients in OLR group (all 8 trials reported this datum, 0.3% vs. 0.9%; $P = 0.67$). There was no significant heterogeneity between studies in reporting these two outcomes.

Regarding postoperative recovery, Mala *et al.* [9] reported the median duration of postoperative usage of analgesia, which was 1 (0–7) days in laparoscopic resection group compared with 5 (2–11) days in the open group ($P < 0.001$). Qiu *et al.* [16] reported that the total dosage and frequency of analgesic administration in LLR group were significantly lower than those in OLR group (30.2 ± 20.8 vs. 70.3 ± 38.5mg, $P < 0.001$; 2.0 ± 0.5 vs. 4.0 ± 0.8, $P < 0.001$). They also found that the time to the return of bowel function, passage of feces and soft diet tolerance occurred significantly earlier in LLR group (1.0 ± 0.9 vs. 2.4 ± 1.8 days, $P < 0.001$; 2.2 ± 0.7 vs. 4.0 ± 1.5 days, $P < 0.001$; 1.8 ± 1.2 vs. 3.2 ± 1.0 days, $P < 0.001$). All studies reported on the length of hospital stay, and two studies were excluded due to present data as median without range [11,13]. The pooled analysis of the 6 studies showed that hospital stay was shorter in the laparoscopic group (WMD: -3.54, 95% CI: -5.12 to −1.96; $P < 0.001$) with significant heterogeneity ($I^2 = 75\%$, $P = 0.001$) (Figure 3).

Meta-analysis of oncologic outcomes

Six of the 8 studies reported the pathological resection margin status [9-11,13,14,16]. The pooled analysis showed that patients undergoing laparoscopic resection had a higher incidence of negative margin resection than patients in the open group (93.7 % vs. 84.4%; $P = 0.001$) (Figure 4). Regarding recurrence, pooled data on three studies showed no difference between two groups (33.3% vs. 37.3%; $P = 0.14$). No recurrence at laparoscopic port sites was reported in all 8 included studies.

Regarding survival, four studies reported 5-year OS and DFS [10,12-14], both of which were comparable between two groups (51.8% vs. 39.9%; $P = 0.20$; 28.8% vs. 20.5%; $P = 0.13$, respectively). In one study, 2-year OS was 89 % for LLR and 81% for open resection ($P = 0.283$). Median DFS was also similar in the two groups (23 vs. 23 months; $P = 0.904$) [15].

Publication bias

The funnel plot of standard of error by effect estimate of morbidity showed none of the studies lay outside the limits of the 95% CI, indicating no evidence of publication bias (Figure 5).

Discussion

Compared with open surgery, the laparoscopic approach confers patients with benefits such as diminished postoperative pain, less operative trauma, faster recovery, and shorter hospital stay. During the two decades, minimally invasive surgery has been applied to various abdominal surgical procedures. Initial evidence in support of LLR for CLM was mostly from case series and thus limited by small sample size and the lack of a comparator [5-8]. In 2007, Simillis *et al.* [20] performed the first meta-analysis by comparing LLR with OLR for benign and malignant tumors in 8 studies published between 1998 and 2005. Subsequently, two updated meta-

Study or Subgroup	LLR Events	LLR Total	OLR Events	OLR Total	Weight	Odds Ratio M-H, Fixed, 95% CI
Abu 2010	48	50	80	85	20.3%	1.50 [0.28, 8.04]
Cannon 2012	34	35	112	138	11.1%	7.89 [1.03, 60.33]
Castaing 2009	52	60	43	60	49.1%	2.57 [1.01, 6.53]
Mala 2002	12	13	12	14	7.6%	2.00 [0.16, 25.11]
Qiu 2013	30	30	27	30	3.8%	7.76 [0.38, 157.14]
Topal 2012	19	20	19	20	8.1%	1.00 [0.06, 17.18]
Total (95% CI)		**208**		**347**	**100.0%**	**2.97 [1.53, 5.78]**
Total events	195		293			

Heterogeneity: Chi² = 2.66, df = 5 (P = 0.75); I² = 0%
Test for overall effect: Z = 3.20 (P = 0.001)

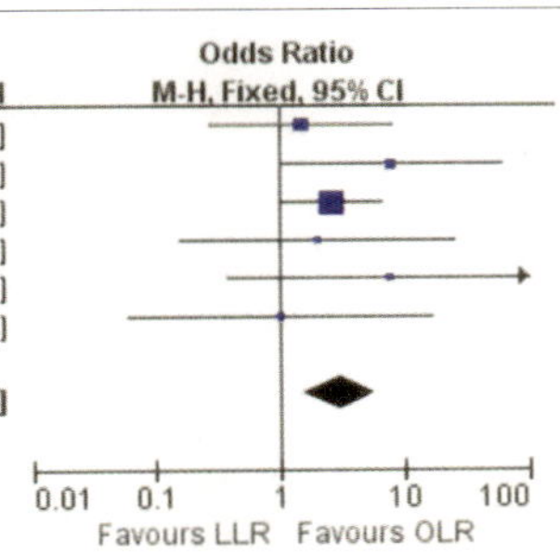

Figure 4 Forest plot displaying the results of the meta-analysis on negative margin resection.

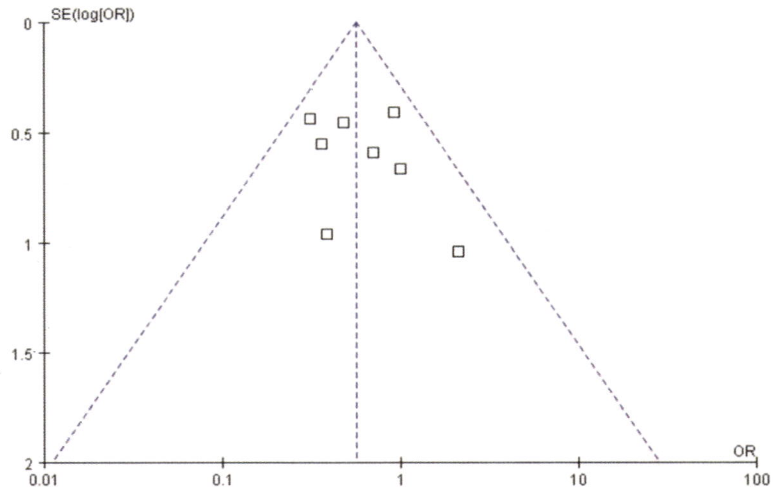

Figure 5 Funnel plot analysis of publication bias.

analyses on this topic have been published [21,22]. However, only one study with CLM only was included in the three meta-analyses [9]. In the present meta-analysis, we included 8 studies covering 695 patients, which may represent the largest body of information so far available for the comparison of LLR and OLR for CLM in the literature.

With respect to operative parameters, blood loss and transfusion requirements for LLR were significantly lower than those of OLR. This difference can be attributed to the magnification of images and more meticulous dissection, pneumoperitoneum, and less blood loss from the abdominal wall provided by the laparoscopic approach [23]. As both the amount of blood loss and the need for transfusion have been associated with increased postperative morbidity [24], it is reasonable to note that patients in the laparoscopic group had lower morbidity.

Concerning postoperative recovery, patients undergoing laparoscopic resection required smaller doses and less frequency of analgesic administration, and experienced more rapid recovery of bowel function [9,16]. As expected, LLR significantly reduced the length of hospital stay by 3.5 days.

LLR is associated with reduced postoperative morbidity and a shorter length of hospital stay. Hence, LLR may very likely outweigh the higher costs of the laparoscopic technique. Although we did not compare the costs between the two procedures due to inadequate data, a recent deviation-based cost modeling study compared the economic impact of laparoscopic versus open left lateral sectionectomy and found that the cost of each patient undergoing LLR was US $ 2,939 less than that of a patient undergoing a similar open operation on average [25].

The most important question regarding the use of LLR for the treatment of CLM is its oncologic efficiency. Port-site tumor metastasis in early repots of other types of gastrointestinal malignancy has increased the doubt about the oncologic safety of the laparoscopic approach [26]. However, port-site tumor metastasis or peritoneal carcinomatosis was not identified in any of the 8 included studies. Meticulous intraoperative manipulation, adoption of no-touch technique, and use of plastic bags to retrieve the specimen would prevent the port-site tumor metastasis. Currently, complete macroscopic removal of all lesions with negative resection margins is established as the gold standard of care of CLM. In our analysis, negative margins were achieved in 93.6% of the patients, and such an excellent result may be attributed to the routine use of intraoperative ultrasonography. Finally, our study showed that the 5-year OS, DFS and postoperative recurrence did not differ significantly between the two groups. Therefore, the laparoscopic approach has no negative effect on oncologic outcomes of surgery for CLM.

After hepatic resection, approximately 60% of the patients with CLM would develop recurrent disease, often isolated to the liver. Repeat hepatectomy is an effective treatment that offers long-term survival for these patients. However, peri-hepatic adhesions caused by the initial operation may prolong the operative duration and increase blood loss [27]. Given its advantage of minimal adhesion formation, laparoscopic techniques facilitate repeat hepatectomy, and the procedure is better tolerated by patients [23].

Approximately 25% of CRC patients have synchronous CLM at the time of diagnosis. Laparoscopy could facilitate the operative approach of a simultaneous procedure. Several case reports and small series have demonstrated the safety and benefit as well as good oncologic outcome of this strategy [28-31].

The results of this meta-anaysis should be interpreted with caution for several reasons. First, it should be noted that patients who underwent LLR were a highly selected population. In general, lesions located in the antero-lateral segments of the liver are good candidates for LLR. In contrast, lesions located adjacent to major vessels or requiring vascular or biliary reconstruction are inappropriate for LLR. Second, all the trials available are observational in nature, which inevitably introduces selection bias and may produce confounding results. However, it would be difficult to recruit patients for conducting a prospective randomized controlled trial to compare a less invasive procedure versus an invasive procedure. Third, the included number of patients was relatively small, which could reduce the reliability and validity of results. However, encouraging data of LLR for CLM also have been reported in recently published two large cohort studies involving more than 100 patients [23,32]. Kazaryan and colleagues, in a single center study of 122 LLRs for CLM, reported that the morbidity and mortality rates were 14.3% and 0%, respectively, and the 5-year actuarial overall and disease-free survivals were 51% and 42%, respectively [23]. Nguyen and colleagues, in a retrospective study of 109 LLRs for CLM in 5 medical centers, reported that the morbidity and mortality rates were 12% and 0%, respectively, and the 5-year overall and disease-free survivals were 50% and 43%, respectively [32]. Finally, LLR is suggested as a more technically demanding procedure and is associated with a learning curve, especially in cases that need more major resections. A study involving 74 patients who underwent LLR indicates that increased experience confers better results in terms of the conversion rate, operative time, blood loss and morbidity. The studies included in our analysis did have surgeons of varying experience with LLR [33], but unfortunately none of these studies reported on their initial experience of this technique. Therefore, we were unable to perform a subgroup analysis regarding the effect of learning curve on surgical outcomes.

Conclusions

Our meta-analysis has shown that LLR for CLM is associated with improved surgical outcomes and uncompromising oncologic outcomes compared to OLR. These findings provide evidence to support its use as a safe and efficacious alternative to open resection for CLM.

Competing interests

The authors declare that they have no competing interests.

Authors' contributions

YZ participated in the design and coordination of the study, carried out the critical appraisal of studies and wrote the manuscript. LW and YX developed the literature search, carried out the extraction of data, assisted in the critical appraisal of included studies and assisted in writing up. HL and BL carried out the statistical analysis of studies. All authors read and approved the final manuscript.

Acknowledgements

We thank Doctor Yanfang Zhao (Department of Health Statistics, Second Military Medical University, Shanghai, China) for her critical revision of the meta-analysis section.

Author details

[1]Department of Hepatobiliary & Pancreatovascular Surgery, Oncologic Center of Xiamen, First affiliated Hospital of Xiamen University, Xiamen, China. [2]Department of Digestive Diseases, First affiliated Hospital of Xiamen University, Xiamen, China.

References

1. Mohammad WM, Balaa FK: **Surgical management of colorectal liver metastases.** *Clin Colon Rectal Surg* 2009, **22:**225–232.
2. Kanas GP, Taylor A, Primrose JN, *et al*: **Survival after liver resection in metastatic colorectal cancer: review and meta-analysis of prognostic factors.** *Clin Epidemiol* 2012, **4:**283–301.
3. Reich H, McGlynn F, DeCaprio J, *et al*: **Laparoscopic excision of benign liver lesions.** *Obstet Gynecol* 1991, **78:**956–958.
4. Nguyen KT, Gamblin TC, Geller DA: **World review of laparoscopic liver resection-2,804 patients.** *Ann Surg* 2009, **250:**831–841.
5. Gigot JF, Glineur D, Santiago Azagra J, *et al*: **Laparoscopic liver resection for malignant liver tumors: preliminary results of a multicenter European study.** *Ann Surg* 2002, **236:**90–97.
6. O'Rourke N, Shaw I, Nathanson L, *et al*: **Laparoscopic resection of hepatic colorectal metastases.** *HPB (Oxford)* 2004, **6:**230–235.
7. Vibert E, Perniceni T, Levard H, *et al*: **Laparoscopic liver resection.** *Br J Surg* 2006, **93:**67–72.
8. Tang CN, Tsui KK, Ha JP, *et al*: **A single-centre experience of 40 laparoscopic liver resections.** *Hong Kong Med J* 2006, **12:**419–425.
9. Mala T, Edwin B, Gladhaug I, *et al*: **A comparative study of the short-term outcome following open and laparoscopic liver resection of colorectal metastases.** *Surg Endosc* 2002, **16:**1059–1063.
10. Castaing D, Vibert E, Ricca L, *et al*: **Oncologic results of laparoscopic versus open hepatectomy for colorectal liver metastases in two specialized centers.** *Ann Surg* 2009, **250:**849–855.
11. Abu Hilal M, Underwood T, Zuccaro M, *et al*: **Short- and medium-term results of totally laparoscopic resection for colorectal liver metastases.** *Br J Surg* 2010, **97:**927–933.
12. Cannon RM, Scoggins CR, Callender GG, *et al*: **Laparoscopic versus open resection of hepatic colorectal metastases.** *Surgery* 2012, **152:**567–573.
13. Cheung TT, Poon RT, Yuen WK, *et al*: **Outcome of laparoscopic versus open hepatectomy for colorectal liver metastases.** *ANZ J Surg* 2012. Epub ahead of print.
14. Topal H, Tiek J, Aerts R, *et al*: **Outcome of laparoscopic major liver resection for colorectal metastases.** *Surg Endosc* 2012, **26:**2451–2455.
15. Guerron AD, Aliyev S, Agcaoglu O, *et al*: **Laparoscopic versus open resection of colorectal liver metastasis.** *Surg Endosc* 2013, **27:**1138–1143.
16. Qiu J, Chen S, Pankaj P, *et al*: **Laparoscopic hepatectomy for hepatic colorectal metastases - a retrospective comparative cohort analysis and literature review.** *PLoS One* 2013, **8:**e60153.
17. Moher D, Liberati A, Tetzlaff J, Altman DG, PRISMA Group: **Preferred reporting items for systematic reviews and meta-analyses: the PRISMA statement.** *PLoS Med* 2009, **6:**e1000097.
18. Hozo SP, Djulbegovic B, Hozo I: **Estimating the mean and variance from the median, range, and the size of a sample.** *BMC Med Res Methodo* 2005, **5:**13.
19. Athanasiou T, Al-Ruzzeh S, Kumar P, *et al*: **Off-pump myocardial revascularization is associated with less incidence of stroke in elderly patients.** *Ann Thorac Surg* 2004, **77:**745–753.
20. Simillis C, Constantinides VA, Tekkis PP, *et al*: **Laparoscopic versus open hepatic resections for benign and malignant neoplasms–a meta-analysis.** *Surgery* 2007, **141:**203–211.
21. Croome KP, Yamashita MH: **Laparoscopic vs open hepatic resection for benign and malignant tumors: An updated meta-analysis.** *Arch Surg* 2010, **145:**1109–1118.
22. Mirnezami R, Mirnezami AH, Chandrakumaran K, *et al*: **Short- and long-term outcomes after laparoscopic and open hepatic resection: systematic review and meta-analysis.** *HPB (Oxford)* 2011, **13:**295–308.

23. Kazaryan AM, Marangos IP, Røsok BI, *et al*: **Laparoscopic resection of colorectal liver metastases: surgical and long-term oncologic outcome.** *Ann Surg* 2010, **252**:1005–1012.
24. Wu WC, Smith TS, Henderson WG, *et al*: **Operative blood loss, blood transfusion, and 30-day mortality in older patients after major noncardiac surgery.** *Ann Surg* 2010, **252**:11–17.
25. Vanounou T, Steel JL, Nguyen KT, *et al*: **Comparing the clinical and economic impact of laparoscopic versus open liver resection.** *Ann Surg Oncol* 2010, **17**:998–1009.
26. Reza MM, Blasco JA, Andradas E, *et al*: **Systematic review of laparoscopic versus open surgery for colorectal cancer.** *Br J Surg* 2006, **93**:921–928.
27. Antoniou A, Lovegrove RE, Tilney HS, *et al*: **Meta-analysis of clinical outcome after first and second liver resection for colorectal metastases.** *Surgery* 2007, **141**:9–18.
28. Leung KL, Lee JF, Yiu RY, *et al*: **Simultaneous laparoscopic resection of rectal cancer and liver metastasis.** *J Laparoendosc Adv Surg Tech A* 2006, **16**:486–488.
29. Geiger TM, Tebb ZD, Sato E, *et al*: **Laparoscopic resection of colon cancer and synchronous liver metastasis.** *J Laparoendosc Adv Surg Tech A* 2006, **16**:5153.
30. Lupinacci RM, Machado MA, Lupinacci RA, *et al*: **Simultaneous left colectomy and standard hepatectomy reformed by laparoscopy.** *Rev Col Bras Cir* 2011, **38**:139–141.
31. Polignano FM, Quyn AJ, Sanjay P, *et al*: **Totally laparoscopic strategies for the management of colorectal cancer with synchronous liver metastasis.** *Surg Endosc* 2012, **26**:2571–2578.
32. Nguyen KT, Laurent A, Dagher I, *et al*: **Minimally invasive liver resection for metastatic colorectal cancer: a multi-institutional, international report of safety, feasibility, and early outcomes.** *Ann Surg* 2009, **250**:842–848.
33. Vigano L, Laurent A, Tayar C, *et al*: **The learning curve in laparoscopic liver resection: improved feasibility and reproducibility.** *Ann Surg* 2009, **250**:772–782.

Early complications after biliary enteric anastomosis for benign diseases

Syed Nabeel Zafar[1], Muhammad Rizwan Khan[1*], Rushna Raza[1], Muhammad N Khan[1], Mahwash Kasi[2], Ammar Rafiq[2] and Omer H Jamy[2]

Abstract

Background: Biliary-enteric anastomosis (BEA) is a common surgical procedure performed for the management of biliary obstruction or leakage that results from a variety of benign and malignant diseases. Complications following BEA are not rare. We aimed to determine the incidence and the factors associated with early complications occurring after BEA for benign diseases.

Methods: We reviewed the medical records of all patients who underwent BEA for benign diseases at our institution between January 1988 and December 2009. The primary outcome was early post operative complication. Logistic regression analysis was done to identify factors predicting the occurrence of complications.

Results: Records of 79 patients were reviewed. There were 34 (43%) males and 45 (57% females). Majority (53%) had choledocholithiasis with impacted stone or distal stricture, followed by traumatic injury to the biliary system (33%). Thirty-four patients (43%) underwent a hepaticojejunostomy, 19 patients (24%) underwent a choledochojejunostomy, and choledochoduodenostomy was performed in 26 patients (33%). Early complications occurred in 39 (49%) patients - 41% had local complications and 25% had systemic complications. Most frequent complications were wound infection (23%) and bile leak (10%). Four (5%) patients died. On multivariate analysis, low serum albumin level (odds ratio = 16, 95% CI = 1.14-234.6) and higher ASA levels (odds ratio = 7, 95% CI: 1.22-33.34) were the independent factors predicting the early complications following BEA.

Conclusions: Half of the patients who underwent BEA for benign diseases had complications in our population. This high incidence may be explained by the high incidence of hypoalbuminemia and the high-risk group who underwent operation.

Background

Biliary-enteric anastomosis (BEA) is a common surgical procedure performed for a variety of indications. This includes bypass or reconstruction following resection of malignant or benign biliary obstruction, primary biliary stones, iatrogenic bile duct injury, liver transplantation; and a number of biliary tract problems that are benign but have malignant potential such as primary sclerosing cholangitis, choledochal cyst, and hepatolithiasis. Surgical options for these diverse conditions include hepaticojejunostomy, choledochoenterostomies and cholecystoenterostomies. Biliary-enteric surgery is an essential surgical procedure even for a benign disease etiology [1,2].

Post-operative complications following BEA including anastomotic leak, hemorrhage, wound infection, cholangitis, intra-abdominal abscess/biloma and stricture formation have been reported [3-5]. These complications are sometimes serious enough to warrant a repeat surgery and at times result in serious long-term morbidity. A few studies have looked at factors associated with the development of these complications [6,7]. Patient's age, co-morbid conditions, nutritional status, pre-operative serum bilirubin, associated chronic liver disease, nature

* Correspondence: doctormrkhan@yahoo.com
[1]Dertment of Surgery, Aga Khan University, Stadium Road, Karachi - 74800, Pakistan
Full list of author information is available at the end of the article

and extent of the primary disease and type of anastomosis performed have been proposed to influence the outcome of BEA [7,8]. We aimed to determine the incidence and factors associated with complications following BEA for a group of benign diseases.

Methods

We retrieved and reviewed the medical records of all patients who underwent BEA for benign diseases at the Aga Khan University Hospital (AKUH), Karachi, Pakistan between January 1988 and December 2009. Since the study spanned over a long period of time, the records with incomplete information were excluded from the study. AKUH is one of the largest private tertiary care hospitals in Pakistan.

Data pertaining to patient demographics, medical history, primary diagnosis, operative procedure, intra-operative details and post-operative outcome were retrieved. The diagnosis of benign disease was identified by pathology records and the hospital coding system. Early complications were defined as any untoward event occurring within 30 days of surgery. Selection of the type of bypass was based on surgeon's preference. All surgeries were performed by consultant general surgeons. There was no established hepatobiliary service at AKUH during the study period.

The primary outcome of early complications was divided into local (wound infection, biliary leak, cholangitis or persistent jaundice, delayed gastric emptying, pancreatic fistula, hemorrhage and pancreatitis) and systemic complications (chest infection, urinary tract infection, venous thromboembolism, pulmonary edema, acute myocardial infarction, renal failure and systemic sepsis). All complications were clumped into a single dichotomous variable called early complication (yes/no), which was used for further analysis as a categorical variable.

Descriptive analysis was performed by calculating proportions for categorical variables and means (with standard deviations) for continuous variables. Univariate and multivariate logistic regression analysis were performed to determine the predictors of early complications. The multivariate model analyzed variables that had a p value of ≤ 0.1 on univariate analysis; in addition to age, gender, American Association of Anesthesiologists (ASA) class, and Charlson Index, which were determined a priori to be clinically significant variables [9].

This research project was a retrospective review of medical records and in accordance with the ethical principles laid forth by the Declaration of Helsinki, retrospective reviews of medical records are exempt from formal ethical review by the ethical review committee of the AKUH. Consent from individual patients was not sought. No identifying information was recorded by the research team.

Results

A total of 79 adult patients underwent a BEA for a benign pathology. Out of these 79 patients, 45 (57%) were women and 34 (43%) were men. Twenty three (29%) patients had a BMI above 25 Kg/m^2. Most patients scored 0 (22%) or 1-2 (54%) on the Charlson co-morbidity index, indicating no or mild co-morbidities. The primary diagnosis in most cases (53%) was choledocholithiasis with impacted stone or distal stricture, followed by traumatic injury to the CBD (33%). Seven patients (5.5%) had a benign inflammatory mass resulting in obstruction, while 2 patients each (2.5%) had a choledochal cyst and Mirrizi's syndrome.

The surgical procedures included a hepaticojejunostomy in 34 (43%) patients, choledochojejunostomy in 19 (24%) patients, and choledochoduodenostomy in 26 (33%) patients. Majority of the patients (81%) who underwent a choledochoduodenostomy had a primary diagnosis of choledocholithiasis with or without a distal stricture, while most of the patients (60%) who underwent a hepaticojejunostomy had a diagnosis of traumatic injury to the CBD. Whipple pancreaticoduodenectomy was performed in 4 patients when there was a strong suspicion of malignancy on preoperative assessment. Final histopathology revealed a benign inflammatory mass in 2 cases and benign CBD stricture in 2 cases.

The jejunum was used as a Roux-en-Y loop with end to side anastomosis in 41 (77%) patients and as a loop in 12 (23%). The duodenal anastomoses were fashioned in the usual side to side manner. Majority (65%) of the anastomoses were single layered with interrupted sutures. Eighteen (23%) patients underwent a pre-operative drainage procedure. A stent was used in 28 (35%) patients. Intra-operative bile culture was sent in 77 cases and a positive bacterial growth was documented in 24 (31%) cases.

Early complications occurred in 39 (49%) patients; out of which 18 had more than one complication. Local complication occurred in 32 (41%) patients. The most common local complication was wound infection, followed by biliary leak, as shown in table 1. Systemic complications occurred in 20 (25%) patients. Of the eight patients with biliary leak, one underwent a re-exploration and later on expired of sepsis. The other seven patients were managed either by image guided percutaneous approaches (2 patients) or conservatively (5 patients), and one of them died. Post-operative hemorrhage occurred in two patients - one had an intraperitoneal bleed requiring re-operation, while the other patient developed intra-luminal bleeding and improved on conservative management.

The total average duration of hospital stay was 17 (± 12) days with a mean stay of 6 (± 7) days pre-operatively. Postoperatively the mean stay was 12 (± 9) days

Table 1 Frequency of complications after biliary enteric anastomosis for a benign disease

Complications	N (%)
Local	
Wound infection	18 (22.8)
Biliary leak	8 (10)
Cholangitis/persistent jaundice	7 (8.9)
Delayed gastric emptying	7 (8.9)
Pancreatic fistula	2 (2.5)
Hemorrhage	2 (2.5)
Pancreatitis	1 (1.3)
Systemic	
Chest infection	5 (6.3)
Pulmonary edema	3 (3.8)
Acute myocardial infarction	3 (3.8)
Systemic sepsis	3 (3.8)
Renal Failure	2 (2.5)
Mortality	4 (5.1)

with a mean stay of 2.2 (± 6) days in the intensive care unit and 3.6 (± 3) days in the special care unit. Four patients (5%) died during hospital stay. Two of these patients underwent Whipple's procedure. Both of these patients had multiple local and systemic complications including bile leak and chest infection, and subsequently died of systemic sepsis with organ failure. The other two patients who died developed wound infection and systemic sepsis; one had concomitant renal failure while the other developed chest infection. A total of 5 patients developed chest infection and 3 of them died, making it the most dreaded systemic complication.

The occurrence of complications was not affected by patient demographic factors, year of surgery, diagnosis or operative technique. The incidence of complications remained similar over the 22-year period. Upon univariate analysis (table 2), patients with albumin levels lower than 3.5 g/dl were 10 times more likely to have a complication (95% CI = 1.10, 98.20). Multivariate analysis (table 3) demonstrated that after adjusting for age, gender, Charlson score and ASA class, patients with an albumin lower than 3.5 g/dl were 16 times more likely to suffer a complication than those with higher albumin levels. Similarly after adjusting for age, gender, Charlson score and albumin level, patients with an ASA class of > 2 were 7 times more likely to suffer a complication than those with a higher ASA class (95% CI: 1.22, 33.34).

Discussion

A high number (49%) of our patients suffered at least one complication after the anastomotic procedure and majority of these were managed conservatively. Complications after biliary-enteric anastomotic procedures have ranged from 3% to 43% in the previous reports [5,10].

Table 2 Uni-variate logistic regression analysis of factors associated with early complications in patients undergoing biliary enteric anastomotic surgery for a benign disease

Variable	Category	OR	95% CI
Age (ref: < 50 years)	> 50 years	0.96	0.39, 2.31
Gender (ref: male)	Female	0.78	0.32, 1.90
BMI (ref: ≤25)	> 25 Kg/m^2	0.86	0.29, 2.53
Albumin (ref: > 3.5)	≤3.5	10.4	1.10, 98.20
Charlson score (re: = 0)	1-2	1.24	0.40, 3.87
	3 and above	2.45	0.64, 9.37
ASA class (ref: 1-2)	> 2	1.30	0.52, 3.33
Primary diagnosis	CBD stones ± stricture	1	-
	Traumatic CBD injury	1.09	0.29, 4.13
	Others	1.4	0.34, 5.77
Surgery	Hepaticojejunostomy	1	-
	Choledochoduoenostomy	0.87	0.31, 2.46
	Choledochojejunostomy	2.26	0.66, 7.76
	Whipple	3.69	0.34, 39.8
Year of Surgery	2003-2009	1	-
	1998-2002	1.17	0.33, 4.12
	1993-1997	1.2	0.31, 4.61
	1988-1992	0.75	0.22, 2.58
Layers of anastomosis (ref: 1 layer)	2 layer	0.95	0.36, 2.55
Stent Placement (ref: yes)	No	1	0.38, 2.62
Sutures (ref: continuous)	Interrupted	1.12	0.44, 2.99
Level of duct (ref: hepatic)	CBD	1.45	0.59, 3.54
Loop (Ref: jejunum)	Duodenum	1.53	0.59, 3.94
Pre -operative drainage (ref: yes)	No	0.46	0.15, 1.43
T Tube placement (ref: yes)	No	0.84	0.28, 2.49
Bile Culture positive (ref: positive)	Negative	1.04	0.40, 2.72

However, most of these studies are specific to BEA due to iatrogenic biliary tract injuries. The differing disease etiology, surgery performed and definition of 'complications' make it difficult to make logical comparisons. The largest and most recent of these studies by Sicklick *et al*

Table 3 Multivariate logistic regression analysis of factors associated with early complications in patients undergoing biliary enteric anastomotic surgery for a benign disease

Variable	Category	OR	95% CI
Age (ref: < 50 years)	> 50 years	0.49	0.09, 2.61
Gender (ref: male)	Female	0.52	0.11, 2.61
Albumin (ref: > 3.5)	≤3.5	16.3	1.14, 234.6
ASA class (ref: 1-2)	> 2	6.67	1.22, 33.34
Charlson score (re: = 0)	1-2	0.59	0.07, 5.08
	3 and above	3.5	0.26, 46.3

consisted of 175 patients who underwent biliary reconstruction for the iatrogenic bile duct injury following laparoscopic cholecystectomy found a complication rate of 43% [5]. In another study by Tocchi *et al* consisting of 84 patients undergoing hepaticojejunostomy for benign biliary stricture found a rate of complication of 21% [3]. Even though, there were patients with biliary stricture due to a number of reasons including choledocholithiasis, trauma and choledochal cyst, a hepaticojejunostomy was performed in less than half (43%) of our patients. Also we have included a wider range of conditions in our definition of 'complications', which may have led to higher rates.

Our study included four patients who underwent Whipple pancreaticoduodenectomy due to a strong preoperative suspicion for a malignant disease. All four of these patients had complications during hospital stay. Our patient population consisted of all patients who underwent BEA with a final diagnosis of a benign disease condition and therefore those four that underwent the Whipple's procedure were included in the analysis. The authors believe that this is a more 'real life' representation as pancreaticoduodenectomies for benign conditions is not a rarity in the literature, and a recent study reviewing 459 pancreaticoduodenectomies for a suspected malignant disease found 11% of them to have a final benign histology [11]. Type of surgery which included a category for 'Whipple's procedure' was not found to be significantly associated with incidence of early complications, however this may be due to lack of power. Furthermore we did perform sensitivity analysis after excluding patients that underwent Whipple's procedure and the results were similar with the incidence of early and local complications being 48% and 39% respectively.

Our study demonstrated a higher incidence of wound infection (23%) as compared to other studies [5]. In both studies by Sicklick et al and Tochi et al, wound infection was the most frequent complication, 8% and 12% respectively [3,5]. Biliary leak occurred in 10% of our patients while it has been reported to occur in 3-8% of patients in previous studies [3,8]. Patients in Pakistan generally present late, are malnourished and thus sicker when compared to patients in the Western world. This is a possible reason for the higher rates of surgical complications in our study. In fact, 87% of our patients had low pre-operative albumin levels (< 3.5 g/dl) and multivariate analysis demonstrated low albumin levels to be an independent predictor of post-operative complications. Previous studies have also shown hypoalbuminemia to influence on in-hospital complications, mortality and long term survival [6,7].

The association between higher ASA classes and the occurrence of complications to the best of our knowledge has not been studied for BEA. ASA class is a measure of functional status of the patient and higher ASA class has been known to lead to a higher rate of complication in other gastrointestinal surgeries [12,13]. ASA class, but not the Charlson score, was shown to be significantly associated to the outcome in our study; we believe this may be reflective of inadequate optimization of patients prior to surgery. To note, none of the other demographic, clinical or operative variables were significantly associated with the outcome. This is similar to other reports [3].

The mortality in our study was 5%. Mortality after BEA for benign biliary stricture has fallen over the years from 10% to 1% in the recent years [3,5,6,8,10]. Half of the deaths in our study occurred in patients who underwent Whipple's pancreaticoduodenectomy; this has not been included in the previous studies. The remaining deaths occurred in patients with multiple complications including renal failure and chest infection. Both of these patients had low pre-operative albumin levels. Due to the small number of deaths (n = 4) we were unable to determine independent factors associated with mortality.

There is no dedicated hepatobiliary service at present at AKUH and all surgeries were performed by the general surgery service. The surgeries were performed by 16 different surgeons over the course of 22 years. Limitations in both financial and human resources make it difficult for institutions in underdeveloped countries to maintain dedicated sub-specialty surgical services. However this may be an important factor contributing to the higher rate of complications as most other reports are from dedicated hepatobiliary centers. Higher volumes of surgery has been associated with better outcomes [14]. A dedicated service offers higher volume to the surgeon and the team. We are currently in the process of developing a number of subspecialty services including pancreatobiliary surgery. It will be interesting to see how outcomes change in the following decades.

The inherent limitation of the retrospective study design made it difficult to account for all potential confounders or study every possible variable that may be related to rate of complications. For example we were unable to retrieve data on time since biliary injury, local ischemia, evolution of surgical technique or other similar factors. However, as we have discussed above, previous studies have also not found an association between other operative, clinical and demographic factors. It would have been interesting to look at factors responsible for specific complications for example wound infection and biliary leak. However in our analysis we did not have enough power to test for these associations. A related limitation is that of the small sample size, we were only able to report on 79 cases; however this is still the largest report of this kind from an underdeveloped country. A larger study looking for associations with specific complications should be conducted.

Conclusion

BEA for benign conditions has a high rate of post operative complications. Operative technique and type of surgery was not associated with occurrence of complications. Independent factors associated with a high rate of complications are low albumin levels and a higher ASA class. Populations from developing countries may benefit from pre-operative nutritional screening and enhancement.

Acknowledgements
None
Funding
No funding was received from any resource for this research project.

Author details
[1]Dertment of Surgery, Aga Khan University, Stadium Road, Karachi - 74800, Pakistan. [2]Medical College, Aga Khan University, Stadium Road, Karachi - 74800, Pakistan.

Authors' contributions
MRK and RR were involved in the concept and design of the study. SNZ and MRK were involved data analysis, interpretation and manuscript writing. RR, MNK, AR, AHJ, MK retrieved data from medical records. All authors have reviewed and approved of the final manuscripts.

Competing interests
The authors declare that they have no competing interests.

References

1. Pitt HA, Kaufman SL, Coleman J, White RI, Cameron JL: **Benign postoperative biliary strictures. Operate or dilate?** *Ann Surg* 1989, **210(4)**:417-425, discussion 426-417.
2. Nealon WH, Urrutia F: **Long-term follow-up after bilioenteric anastomosis for benign bile duct stricture.** *Ann Surg* 1996, **223(6)**:639-645, discussion 645-638.
3. Tocchi A, Mazzoni G, Liotta G, Lepre L, Cassini D, Miccini M: **Late development of bile duct cancer in patients who had biliary-enteric drainage for benign disease: a follow-up study of more than 1,000 patients.** *Ann Surg* 2001, **234(2)**:210-214.
4. Parrilla P, Ramirez P, Sanchez Bueno F, Perez JM, Candel MF, Muelas MS, Robles R: **Long-term results of choledochoduodenostomy in the treatment of choledocholithiasis: assessment of 225 cases.** *Br J Surg* 1991, **78(4)**:470-472.
5. Sicklick JK, Camp MS, Lillemoe KD, Melton GB, Yeo CJ, Campbell KA, Talamini MA, Pitt HA, Coleman J, Sauter PA, *et al*: **Surgical management of bile duct injuries sustained during laparoscopic cholecystectomy: perioperative results in 200 patients.** *Ann Surg* 2005, **241(5)**:786-792, discussion 793-785.
6. Chapman WC, Halevy A, Blumgart LH, Benjamin IS: **Postcholecystectomy bile duct strictures. Management and outcome in 130 patients.** *Arch Surg* 1995, **130(6)**:597-602, discussion 602-594.
7. Pottakkat B, Vijayahari R, Prakash A, Singh RK, Behari A, Kumar A, Kapoor VK, Saxena R: **Factors predicting failure following high bilio-enteric anastomosis for post-cholecystectomy benign biliary strictures.** *J Gastrointest Surg* **14(9)**:1389-1394.
8. Blankensteijn JD, Terpstra OT: **Early and late results following choledochoduodenostomy and choledochojejunostomy.** *HPB Surg* 1990, **2(3)**:151-158.
9. Hosmer DW, Lemeshow S: **Applied logistic Regression.** John Wiley & Sons, Inc; 2 2000.
10. Laasch HU, Martin DF: **Management of benign biliary strictures.** *Cardiovasc Intervent Radiol* 2002, **25(6)**:457-466.
11. Manzia TM, Toti L, Lenci I, Attia M, Tariciotti L, Bramhall SR, Buckels JA, Mirza DF: **Benign disease and unexpected histological findings after pancreaticoduodenectomy: the role of endoscopic ultrasound fine needle aspiration.** *Ann R Coll Surg Engl* **92(4)**:295-301.
12. Garcea G, Ganga R, Neal CP, Ong SL, Dennison AR, Berry DP: **Preoperative early warning scores can predict in-hospital mortality and critical care admission following emergency surgery.** *J Surg Res* **159(2)**:729-734.
13. Story DA, Leslie K, Myles PS, Fink M, Poustie SJ, Forbes A, Yap S, Beavis V, Kerridge R: **Complications and mortality in older surgical patients in Australia and New Zealand (the REASON study): a multicentre, prospective, observational study*.** *Anaesthesia* 2010, **65(10)**:1022-30.
14. Birkmeyer JD, Stukel TA, Siewers AE, Goodney PP, Wennberg DE, Lucas FL: **Surgeon volume and operative mortality in the United States.** *N Engl J Med* 2003, **349(22)**:2117-2127.

Clinical score to predict the risk of bile leakage after liver resection

Takahiro Kajiwara[1], Yutaka Midorikawa[1*], Shintaro Yamazaki[1], Tokio Higaki[1], Hisashi Nakayama[1], Masamichi Moriguchi[1], Shingo Tsuji[2] and Tadatoshi Takayama[1]

Abstract

Background: In liver resection, bile leakage remains the most common cause of operative morbidity. In order to predict the risk of this complication on the basis of various factors, we developed a clinical score system to predict the potential risk of bile leakage after liver resection.

Methods: We analyzed the postoperative course in 518 patients who underwent liver resection for malignancy to identify independent predictors of bile leakage, which was defined as "a drain fluid bilirubin concentration at least three times the serum bilirubin concentration on or after postoperative day 3," as proposed by the International Study Group of Liver Surgery. To confirm the robustness of the risk score system for bile leakage, we analyzed the independent series of 289 patients undergoing liver resection for malignancy.

Results: Among 81 (15.6 %) patients with bile leakage, 76 had grade A bile leakage, and five had grade C leakage and underwent reoperation. The median postoperative hospital stay was significantly longer in patients with bile leakage (median, 14 days; range, 8 to 34) than in those without bile leakage (11 days; 5 to 62; $P = 0.001$). There was no hepatic insufficiency or in-hospital death. The risk score model was based on the four independent predictors of postoperative bile leakage: non-anatomical resection (odds ratio, 3.16; 95 % confidence interval [CI], 1.72 to 6.07; $P < 0.001$), indocyanine green clearance rate (2.43; 1.32 to 7.76; $P = 0.004$), albumin level (2.29; 1.23 to 4.22; $P = 0.01$), and weight of resected specimen (1.97; 1.11 to 3.51; $P = 0.02$). When this risk score system was used to assign patients to low-, middle-, and high-risk groups, the frequency of bile leakage in the high-risk group was 2.64 (95 % CI, 1.12 to 6.41; $P = 0.04$) than that in the low-risk group. Among the independent series for validation, 4 (5.7 %), 16 (10.0 %), and 10 (16.6 %) patients in low-, middle, and high-risk groups were given a diagnosis of bile leakage after operation, respectively ($P = 0.144$).

Conclusions: Our risk score model can be used to predict the risk of bile leakage after liver resection.

Keywords: Postoperative complication, Bile leakage, Risk score

Background

Liver resection is widely accepted as the only potentially curative treatment for primary or metastatic liver malignancy. In high-volume centers, the mortality rate associated with liver resection has decreased [1–3]. However, the incidence of bile leakage, one of the most common complications after liver resection, remains high, ranging from 3.6 to 12.9 % [3–12].

Many different definitions of bile leakage have been proposed [3–12], most of which were based on both the bilirubin concentration and the amount of drain fluid. We previously defined bile leakage as continuous drainage with a bilirubin level of 5 mg/dl or higher beyond 1 week [13]. A bilirubin concentration of 20 mg/dl in drain fluid persisting for 2 weeks has also been proposed [5]. On the basis of drain fluid volume, bile leakage has been defined as the drainage of ≥50 ml of bile for longer than 1 to 3 days [8, 14]. On the other hand, some authors have defined bile leakage as the intra-abdominal accumulation of bile confirmed at reoperation or on percutaneous drainage or as the presence of cholangiographic

* Correspondence: mido-tky@umin.ac.jp
[1]Department of Digestive Surgery, Nihon University School of Medicine, 30-1 Oyaguchikami-cho, Itabashi-ku, Tokyo 173-8610, Japan
Full list of author information is available at the end of the article

evidence of biliary leakage. Finally, a uniform definition ("a drain discharge with a bilirubin concentration 3 times the serum level on after postoperative day 3") and grading of bile leakage were established by the International Study Group of Liver Surgery (ISGLS) [15].

Despite the use of various procedures to decrease the risk of bile leakage, such as bile leakage tests [13], intraoperative cholangiography [16], and application of fibrin glue to the cut surface of the liver [17], this complication is not completely avoidable. Most cases of minor bile leakage are controllable and can be cured by conservative treatments [11]. On the other hand, the management of bile leakage is often difficult in patients with refractory ascites followed by the development of intra-abdominal sepsis after liver resection, resulting in a prolonged hospital stay or operative death [18]. Major bile leakage can lead to intractable ascites and liver failure unless it is treated appropriately. It is therefore clinically important to identify patients at high risk for bile leakage.

Despite the high incidence of bile leakage after liver resection, how to accurately assess the risk of this complication remains unclear. We therefore developed a risk score system for bile leakage on the basis of risk factors after liver resection.

Methods

Patients

Between 2008 and 2010, we performed curative liver resection without biliary reconstruction in 518 consecutive patients; this study received an approval (protocol number: RK-101208-6) by the institutional review boards of Nihon University, and each participant provided written informed consent. Clinical investigations were conducted according to the principles expressed in the Declaration of Helsinki. All the surgical procedures were performed via laparotomy. The diagnosis was hepatocellular carcinoma (HCC) in 364 patients, metastatic liver cancer in 130, intrahepatic cholangiocarcinoma in 14, liver invasion by an extrahepatic tumor in 2, malignant lymphoma in 1, and benign liver tumor in 7. There were 364 men and 154 women, with a median age of 68 years (range, 20 to 84).

To confirm the robustness of the risk score system for bile leakage (described below in detail), we analyzed the independent series of 289 patients undergoing liver resection for malignancy between 2011 and 2012.

Surgical procedures

The indications for surgical resection and the operative procedures were determined in accordance with Makuuchi's criteria [19]. Anatomic resection of Couinaud's segment was the first-line operative procedure for HCC. Non-anatomic resection was performed in patients with colorectal metastases. Minor liver resection was defined as limited resection or resection of up to two Couinaud's segments, and major liver resection was defined as resection of more than two segments. Hepatic parenchymal transection was guided ultrasonographically and performed by the clamp-crushing method with the inflow-blood-occlusion technique. Glisson's pedicles were tied with silk thread and divided [13, 20].

At the end of the resection procedure, bile leakage was checked by placing a piece of gauze on the transected surface of the liver to confirm the presence or absence of bile staining. In patients who underwent resection of multiple segments of the liver or hemi-hepatectomy, bile leakage tests were routinely performed through the cystic duct of the gallbladder [13]. A fibrin glue preparation (Beriplast®; CSL Bering, Ltd., Tokyo, Japan) was applied to the raw surface of the liver.

A silicone rubber, closed irrigation drain (inner diameter, 10 mm) with one hole at the tip and two side holes (Pleats drain®; Sumitomo Co., Ltd., Tokyo, Japan) was placed in each cut surface of the liver via the shortest route from the abdominal wall. Standard systemic antibiotic therapy with cefazolin was routinely administered immediately before surgery and then twice daily on postoperative day (POD) 1 to 3. The drainage tube was managed as described previously [21]. Briefly, the drains were removed on POD 3 if the drainage fluid bilirubin level was less than 5 mg/dl and bacteriological cultures were negative.

Two consultant surgeons (T.T. and T.H.) performed three quarters of the operations. The first had done 3,000 liver resections, and the second had performed 1,000. Five resident specialists did a quarter of the operations while being assisted by the consultant. Neither the surgical nor anesthetic technique was modified during the study period.

Definition of bile leakage

Bile leakage after liver resection was defined according to the criteria proposed by ISGLS [22]. Briefly, bile leakage was defined as a discharge of fluid with an increased bilirubin concentration via the intra-abdominal drains on or after POD 3 or as the need for radiologic intervention and relaparotomy for bile collection and bile peritonitis, respectively. An increased bilirubin concentration in the drain fluid was defined as a bilirubin concentration at least 3 times higher than the serum bilirubin concentration at the same time. Bile leakage was graded according to the system proposed by the ISGLS [15]. Grade A bile leakage has little or no impact on patients' clinical management, and additional diagnostic or therapeutic interventions are unnecessary. A bile leakage that requires a change in patients' clinical management, but can be treated without relaparotomy is defined as Grade B. A Grade A bile leakage requiring drainage for more than 1 week is also classified as

Grade B. Patients with Grade C bile leakage require relaparotomy to control this complication.

Reoperation was performed when the amount of a discharge of fluid with a bilirubin concentration more than 50 mg/dl via drains was more than 50 ml/day.

Risk score

Risk factors for bile leakage were defined as follows: clinicopathological factors that were associated with bile leakage on univariate analyses were included in logistic regression analysis (Table 1). Independent risk factors for bile leakage identified by the logistic regression model were weighted according to the odds ratios for postoperative bile leakage, and the point scores for variables related to bile leakage were calculated. Each patient was then assigned a total score.

Statistical analysis

Comparisons between variables collected from the patients who underwent liver resection were evaluated with Fisher's exact test for categorical variables and the Welch two sample *t*-test for ratios.

The durations of abdominal drainage and the hospital stay were calculated with the Kaplan-Meier method and were compared using the log-rank test. *P* values of less than 0.05 were considered to indicate statistical significance. All analyses were performed using a statistical software package (JMP version 8.0, SAS, NC).

Results

Bile leakage

Among the 518 patients who underwent liver resection for malignancy, bile leakage was diagnosed in 81 (15.6 %). Seventy-six of these patients did not require radiologic intervention or relaparotomy (94 %), and all of their drainage tubes were removed within 1 week (Grade A). The other five patients underwent relaparotomy to treat bile leakage (Grade C, 6 %) (Table 1).

The median time to removal of the drain after operation was significantly longer in patients with bile leakage (9 days; range, 8 to 34) than in those without bile leakage (5 days; 5 to 62, $P < 0.001$). The median day of discharge was POD 24 (range, 13 to 34) in the 5 patients who underwent reoperation, as compared with POD 14 (range, 8 to 28) in the 76 patients who did not undergo relaparotomy ($P < 0.001$).

Table 1 Bile leakage

	Healed spontaneously (*N* = 76)	Reoperation (*N* = 5)[a]	*P* value
Bilirubin concentration, mg/dl (range)	3.0 (1.4–42.1)	26.9 (5.3–55.2)	<0.001
Culture, n (%)	2 (2.6 %)	2 (40 %)	0.092
Discharge, day (range)	14 (8–28)	24 (13–34)	0.007
Drain removal	8 (4–191)	40 (14–107)	0.029

[a]one patient underwent both percutaneous drainage and reoperation

Postoperative course

The median day of drain removal was POD 5 (range, 2 to 65) in the patients without bile leakage and POD 10 (range, 4 to 191) in the patients with bile leakage ($P < 0.001$) (Fig. 1a). The median postoperative hospital stay was 11 days (range, 5 to 62) in the patients without bile leakage and 14 days (range, 8 to 34) in those with bile leakage ($P = 0.003$) (Fig. 1b). No patient had hepatic failure, and there was no operative or in-hospital death.

Risk factors

Among the 18 clinicopathological factors studied, indocyanine green clearance rate at 15 min (ICGR15) ($P = 0.02$), albumin level ($P = 0.04$), operation time ($P < 0.001$), ischemia time ($P = 0.008$), blood loss ($P = 0.004$), anatomical resection ($P = 0.01$), vascular invasion ($P = 0.04$), and weight of resected specimen ($P = 0.006$) were significantly related to bile leakage (Table 2).

On multivariate analysis (Table 3), the independent factors for bile leakage were non-anatomical resection (odds

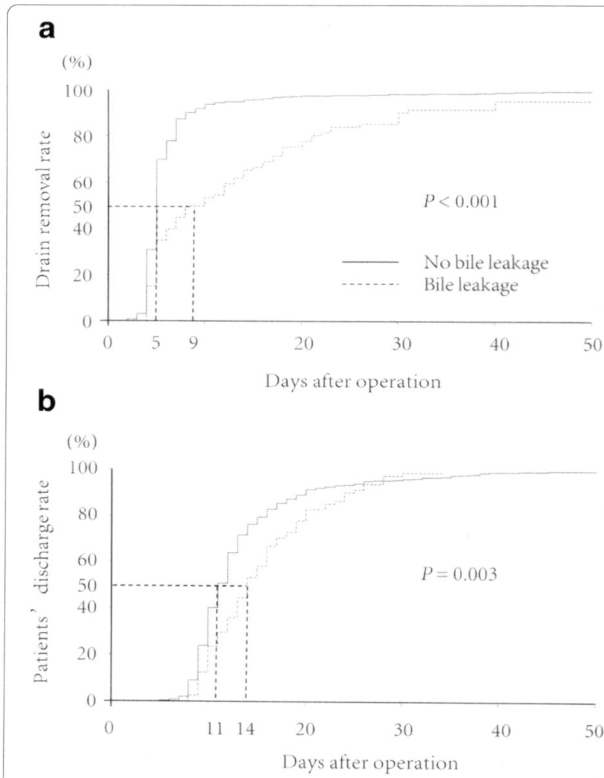

Fig. 1 Cumulative rates of the postoperative drain removal (**a**) and patients' discharge (**b**). There were significant differences between the two groups in both the duration of abdominal drainage ($P < 0.001$) and the discharge rate ($P = 0.003$)

Table 2 Univariate analyses

	Bile leakage ($n = 81$)	Control ($n = 437$)	P value
Age, years (range)	68 (44–84)	68 (20–84)	0.91
Background liver, NL/CH + LC	26/55	143/294	0.91
ICGR15, % (range)	9.95 (2.05–34.83)	11.38 (1.14–43.1)	0.03*
Child-Pugh, A/B	80/1	431/6	0.92
Diabetes mellitus (+/–)	22/59	118/319	0.92
Steatosis, +/–	31/50	137/300	0.29
Aspartate transamonase, IU/L (range)	28 (9–213)	32 (11–265)	0.06
Total bilirubin, μmol/L (range)	0.58 (0.19–1.62)	0.59 (0.19–3.51)	0.37
Platelet count, $\times 10^{5}$ (range)	17.9 (5–41.4)	16.4 (4.2–54.9)	0.26
Albumin, g/L (range)	3.8 (2.7–4.7)	4.1 (2.4–5.3)	0.04*
Operation time, min (range)	425 (141–752)	356 (115–803)	0.004*
Ischemia time, min (range)	91 (10–240)	72 (0–243)	0.008*
Intraoperative blood loss, ml (range)	407 (17–3777)	266 (10–850)	0.004*
Anatomic resection, +/–	16/65	144/293	0.01*
Primary/repeated	63/18	108/329	0.64
Resected number, single/multiple	59/22	321/116	0.9
Vascular invasion, +/–	20/61	62/375	0.04*
Weight of resected specimen, g	90 (10–730)	64.5 (2–1635)	0.006*

*significant difference between 2 groups
NL normal liver, *CH* chronic hepatitis, *LC* liver cirrhosis, *ICGR15* indocyanine green clearance rate at 15 min, *AST* aspartate aminotransferase, *HCC* hepatocellular carcinoma

ratio [OR], 3.16; 95 % confidence interval [CI], 1.72 to 6.07; $P < 0.001$), ICGR15 (2.43; 1.32 to 7.76; $P = 0.004$), albumin level (2.29; 1.23 to 4.22; $P = 0.01$), and weight of resected specimen (1.97; 1.11 to 3.51; $P = 0.02$).

Risk score system

In the risk score system, each of the following factors was assigned a score of 1 point: ICGR15 less than 15 %, serum albumin level less than 3.5 g/L, and weight of resected specimen less than 70 g. If non-anatomical resection was performed, two points were assigned because the odds ratio of this factor was much higher than that of the other risk factors (Table 3).

Patients with a risk score of 1 or less were assigned to the low-risk group, those with a risk score of 2 or 3 to the middle-risk group, and those with a risk score 4 or higher to the high-risk group (Table 4). Among the 122 (23.5 %) patients in the low-risk group, 316 (61.0 %) in the middle-risk group, and 80 (15.5 %) in the high-risk group, bile leakage was diagnosed after liver resection in 12 (9.8 %), 51 (16.1 %), and 18 (22.5 %) patients, respectively ($P = 0.04$).

The independent series for validation contained 69 (23.8 %) patients in the low-risk group, 160 (55.3 %) in the middle-risk group, and 60 (20.7 %) in the high-risk group, and 4 (5.7 %), 16 (10.0 %), and 10 (16.6 %) patients were given a diagnosis of bile leakage after operation, respectively ($P = 0.144$). Although there were no significant difference between each group, the patients in the high-risk group tended to suffer from bile leakage in the independent series of 289 patients.

Table 3 Multivariate analyses

	Odds ratio (95 % CI)	Score	P value
Non-anatomical resection	3.16 (1.72–6.07)	2	0.0001
ICGR15 (<15 %)	2.43 (1.32–7.76)	1	0.004
Albumin (g/L) (3.5≧)	2.29 (1.23–4.22)	1	0.01
Weight of resected specimen	1.97 (1.11–3.51)	1	0.02

95 % CI, 95 % confidence interval
ICGR15 indocyanine green clarance rate at 15 min

Table 4 Risk score for bile leakage

Risk score	No. of patients (%)	Bile leakage (%)	Odds ratio (95 % CI)[a]	P value
Low	122 (23.5)	12 (9.8)	1	0.04
Middle	316 (61.0)	51 (16.1)	1.76 (0.88–3.77)	
High	80 (15.5)	18 (22.5)	2.64 (1.12–6.45)	

Low risk, risk score 0 or 1; Middle risk, 2 or 3; High risk, 4 or 5, respectively
[a]Each odds ratio was calculated relative to the low-risk group

Discussion

In this study, we developed a risk score to identify patients at high risk for bile leakage after liver resection. Our system was based on four independent factors (non-anatomical resection, shorter ICGR15, low albumin level, and weight of resected specimen) in 518 patients undergoing liver resection that were found to be independently related to the risk of bile leakage, and was confirmed using the another series of 289 patients who underwent liver resection in the next 2 years.

Because a range of variables contribute to prediction models, empirical weights are necessary. Regression models generated by a mathematical approach are usually used to classify patients according to the risk of predefined events [23]. However, the complexity of regression models can make them unsuitable for clinical use [24]. In this study, we identified variables related to the risk of bile leakage and assigned these variables empirical weights in accordance with the odds ratios. This process simplified the regression model to facilitate routine clinical use. With the use of our scoring system, the patients were clearly divided into three risk groups for bile leakage.

We determined the extent of liver resection according to the Makuuchi criteria [19], which is based on only ICGR15, serum total bilirubin level, encephalopathy, and ascites. Therefore, a patient with a lower ICGR15 and serum albumin level could be a candidate for more extensive liver resection. In conjunction with weight of resected specimen more than 70 g [21], large resection of the liver for relatively poorer liver function could harbors high risk for bile leakage by the score system.

In this study, anatomical resection decreased the risk of bile leakage. This is because, in anatomical resection, Glisson's sheath is ligated at the central side, and the number of peripheral branches appearing in the cut surface is theoretically small [22]. Exposure of major Glisson's sheath is also rare, which was reported to be one of independent risk factors for bile leakage [7, 8, 25].

It has been reported that the use of a drainage tube is no longer necessary in patients who undergo liver resection [26, 27]. However, our results and those of previous studies have shown that bile leakage after liver resection is not a rare event, occurring in about 20 % of patients, and that high-risk patients can be identified by means of a clinical risk score. We therefore advocate that a drainage tube should be placed, especially in high-risk patients.

As for the management of bile leakage, Vigano et al. reported that conservative management was successful in 76 % of patients and that a drainage output of greater than 100 ml on POD 10 was a predictor of conservative management failure [11]. However, even patients in whom leakage spontaneously resolved had a median waiting time of 15 days, and the hospital stay in patients with no response to conservative treatment was prolonged. In our series, 5 of the 81 patients with bile leakage underwent reoperation. The median postoperative hospital stay in patients who underwent reoperation was 24 days, as compared with 14 days in patients who did not undergo reoperation. Given the results of a previous study of bile leakage treated conservatively [11], the postoperative hospital stay in patients who received reoperation was quite short. We therefore assume that patients who have major leakage that shows no improvement on POD 3 are good candidates for reoperation [11, 28].

Drainage after liver resection is controversial by recent randomized controlled trials [26, 27, 29]. However, our results show that there definitely exists a subgroup of patients at high risk for bile leakage and that this risk can be preoperatively predicted by the risk score system. Especially, bile leakage was observed within three postoperative days, and after drain removal, bile leakage in which treatments had been required did not occur. Therefore, we emphasize the need for drainage after liver resection, especially in high-risk patients, as well as early removal of prophylactic drains according to appropriate criteria and the risk score [21].

Conclusion

Our risk score system, simply based on four clinical factors, effectively predicted the risk of bile leakage after liver resection. Patients with a high-risk score thus require more meticulous management by an expert surgeon and the use of standardized techniques to avoid this complication.

Abbreviations

HCC: hepatocellular carcinoma; ICGR15: indocyanine green clearance rate at 15 min ; ISGLS: the International Study Group of Liver Surgery; POD: postoperative day.

Competing interests

The authors declare that they have no competing interests.

Authors' contributions

All authors were involved in the preparation of this manuscript. TT, TK, and YM participated in the design of the study and drafted the manuscript. SY, TH, HN, and MM helped with data collection. ST, TK, and YM analyzed the collected data. TK, TT, and YM participated in its design and coordination and helped to draft the manuscript. All authors have read and approved the final manuscript.

Acknowledgements

This work was mainly supported by a Grant-in-Aid for Scientific Research (A) 24249068 (T.T.) and (C) 15 K10152 (Y.M.) from the Ministry of Education, Culture, Sports, Science and Technology (MEXT), Japan.

Author details

[1]Department of Digestive Surgery, Nihon University School of Medicine, 30-1 Oyaguchikami-cho, Itabashi-ku, Tokyo 173-8610, Japan. [2]Genome Science Division, Research Center for Advanced Science and Technologies, University of Tokyo, 4-6-1 Komaba, Meguro-ku, Tokyo 153-8904, Japan.

References

1. Imamura H, Seyama Y, Kokudo N, Maema A, Sugawara Y, Sano K, et al. One thousand fifty-six hepatectomies without mortality in 8 years. Arch Surg. 2003;138:1198–206.
2. Makuuchi M, Sano K. The surgical approach to HCC: our progress and results in Japan. Liver Transpl. 2004;10:S46–52.
3. Takayama T. Surgical treatment for hepatocellular carcinoma. Jpn J Clin Oncol. 2011;41:447–54.
4. Benzoni E, Cojutti A, Lorenzin D, Adani GL, Baccarani U, Favero A, et al. Liver resective surgery: a multivariate analysis of postoperative outcome and complication. Langenbecks Arch Surg. 2007;392:45–54.
5. Capussotti L, Ferrero A, Viganò L, Sgotto E, Muratore A, Polastri R. Bile leakage and liver resection: Where is the risk? Arch Surg. 2006;141:690–4.
6. Kyoden Y, Imamura H, Sano K, Beck Y, Sugawara Y, Kokudo N, et al. Value of prophylactic abdominal drainage in 1269 consecutive cases of elective liver resection. J Hepatobiliary Pancreat Sci. 2010;17:186–92.
7. Lee CC, Chau GY, Lui WY, Tsay SH, King KL, Loong CC, et al. Risk factors associated with bile leakage after hepatic resection for hepatocellular carcinoma. Hepatogastroenterology. 2005;52:1168–71.
8. Lo CM, Fan ST, Liu CL, Lai EC, Wong J. Biliary complications after hepatic resection: risk factors, management, and outcome. Arch Surg. 1998;133:156–61.
9. Poon RT, Fan ST, Lo CM, Liu CL, Lam CM, Yuen WK, et al. Improving perioperative outcome expands the role of hepatectomy in management of benign and malignant hepatobiliary diseases: analysis of 1222 consecutive patients from a prospective database. Ann Surg. 2004;240:698–708.
10. Tanaka S, Hirohashi K, Tanaka H, Shuto T, Lee SH, Kubo S, et al. Incidence and management of bile leakage after hepatic resection for malignant hepatic tumors. J Am Coll Surg. 2002;195:484–9.
11. Viganò L, Ferrero A, Sgotto E, Tesoriere RL, Calgaro M, Capussotti L. Bile leak after hepatectomy: predictive factors of spontaneous healing. Am J Surg. 2008;196:195–200.
12. Virani S, Michaelson JS, Hutter MM, Lancaster RT, Warshaw AL, Henderson WG, et al. Morbidity and mortality after liver resection: results of the patient safety in surgery study. J Am Coll Surg. 2007;204:1284–92.
13. Ijichi M, Takayama T, Toyoda H, Sano K, Kubota K, Makuuchi M. Randomized trial of the usefulness of a bile leakage test during hepatic resection. Arch Surg. 2000;135:1395–400.
14. de Castro SM, Kuhlmann KF, Busch OR, van Delden OM, Laméris JS, van Gulik TM, et al. Incidence and management of biliary leakage after hepaticojejunostomy. J Gastrointest Surg. 2005;9:1163–71.
15. Koch M, Garden OJ, Padbury R, Rahbari NN, Adam R, Capussotti L, et al. Bile leakage after hepatobiliary and pancreatic surgery: a definition and grading of severity by the International Study Group of Liver Surgery. Surgery. 2011; 149:680–8.
16. Kubo S, Sakai K, Kinoshita H, Hirohashi K. Intraoperative cholangiography using a balloon catheter in liver surgery. World J Surg. 1986;10:844–50.
17. Kohno H, Nagasue N, Chang YC, Taniura H, Yamanoi A, Nakamura T. Comparison of topical hemostatic agents in elective hepatic resection: a clinical prospective randomized trial. World J Surg. 1992;16:966–9.
18. Yamashita Y, Hamatsu T, Rikimaru T, Tanaka S, Shirabe K, Shimada M, et al. Bile leakage after hepatic resection. Ann Surg. 2001;233:45–50.
19. Makuuchi M, Kosuge T, Takayama T, Yamazaki S, Kakazu T, Miyagawa S, et al. Surgery for small liver cancers. Semin Surg Oncol. 1993;9:298–304.
20. Imamura H, Takayama T, Sugawara Y, Kokudo N, Aoki T, Kaneko J, et al. Pringle's manoeuvre in living donors. Lancet. 2002;360:2049–50.
21. Yamazaki S, Takayama T, Moriguchi M, Mitsuka Y, Okada S, Midorikawa Y, et al. Criteria for drain removal following liver resection. Br J Surg. 2012;99:1584–90.
22. Takayama T, Makuuchi M, Kubota K, Harihara Y, Hui AM, Sano K, et al. Randomized comparison of ultrasonic vs clamp transection of the liver. Arch Surg. 2001;136:922–8.
23. Freedman DA. Statistical Models: Theory and Practice. New York: Cambridge University Press. 2009;41-60.
24. Infante-Rivard C, Esnaola S, Villeneuve JP. Clinical and statistical validity of conventional prognostic factors in predicting short-term survival among cirrhotics. Hepatology. 1987;7:660–4.
25. Yoshioka R, Saiura A, Koga R, Arita J, Takemura N, Ono Y, et al. Predictive factors for bile leakage after hepatectomy: analysis of 505 consecutive patients. World J Surg. 2011;35:1898–903.
26. Belghiti J, Kabbej M, Sauvanet A, Vilgrain V, Panis Y, Fekete F. Drainage after elective hepatic resection. A randomized trial. Ann Surg. 1993;218:748–53.
27. Liu CL, Fan ST, Lo CM, Wong Y, Ng IO, Lam CM, et al. Abdominal drainage after hepatic resection is contraindicated in patients with chronic liver diseases. Ann Surg. 2004;239:194–201.
28. Ishii H, Ochiai T, Murayama Y, Komatsu S, Shiozaki A, Kuriu Y, et al. Risk factors and management of postoperative bile leakage after hepatectomy without bilioenteric anastomosis. Dig Surg. 2011;28:198–204.
29. Fong Y, Brennan MF, Brown K, Heffernan N, Blumgart LH. Drainage is unnecessary after elective liver resection. Am J Surg. 1996;171:158–62.

Usefulness of CT-scan in the diagnosis and therapeutic approach of gallstone ileus: report of two surgically treated cases

Danzi Michele[1*], Grimaldi Luciano[1], Fabozzi Massimiliano[2], Reggio Stefano[1], Danzi Roberta[3], Soscia Ernesto[3], Amato Bruno[4]

From 26th National Congress of the Italian Society of Geriatric Surgery
Naples, Italy. 19-22 June 2013

Abstract

Background: Gallstone ileus is a rare cause of gastrointestinal obstruction, more frequent in elderly patients, whose treatment is essentially surgical, although some para-surgical and mini-invasive possibilities exist, allowing the solution of such obstructive condition in a completely non-invasive way.

Description In our study, after reporting two cases of biliary ileus managed by our surgical division, we will analyze the most suitable diagnostic procedures and the therapeutic approaches to this pathology.

Conclusions: Gallstone ileus is a quite rare pathology in population, but affects more frequently elderly people; The treatment of this disease is mainly surgical.

Background

Gallstone ileus, the intestinal obstruction due to the migration of gallstones into the intestine lumen, is a quite rare occurrence that must be taken into account in the differential diagnosis of mechanical intestinal obstructions, mainly those affecting small intestine and particularily in elderly patients. The diagnosis of this disease is often late, sometimes detected only during surgery, even if the current routine use of echography and, above all, of TC (more accurate) for abdominal emergencies, allows to detect such condition earlier.

The treatment is basically surgical and the kind of surgery must be chosen according to the risk: a radical surgery in one time should be reserved to selected patients (younger, satisfactory general conditions, absence of serious co-morbidities). The practice of only enterolithotomy is preferred in high risk patients, postponing to a second surgery the solution of the biliary-digestive fistula.

* Correspondence: michele.danzi@unina.it
[1]Department of Specialized Surgery - Division of Gastrointestinal Surgery Rehabilitation of Election and Emergency. "Federico II" University, Naples - Italy
Full list of author information is available at the end of the article

Clinical case 1

R.M., female, 74 years old, HCV+, with ischemic heart disease, came to our department in april 2009, complaining of 15 days of pain to right upper quadrant with nausea and vomit. After a time of apparent well-being by taking painkillers, the patient shows abundant biliary vomit with 38°C fever and pain. At a physical examination the abdomen is treatable but aching in the right upper quadrant and in the pancreatic duodenal area, peristalsis is present.

Blood test shows low sodium (128 mg/dl), low potassium (2,3 mg/dl), normal values for creatinine and urea, total bilirubin 1,3 mg/dl, 8000 leukocytes; the remaining values, including the most common tumor markers, are normal. TC with contrast to abdomen and pelvis, performed in emergency, shows a marked hydrogaseous distension of jejunum-ileal loops (Figure 1) extended distally up to the terminal ileum where a coarse endoluminal mass (max diam. 2,5 mm) can be detected (Figure 2), with calcium density, multilayered, that indicates a gallstone; it is also present hard gallbladder with thickened walls (Figure 3). The clinical - radiological situation of the patient indicates an intestine obstruction due to ileus

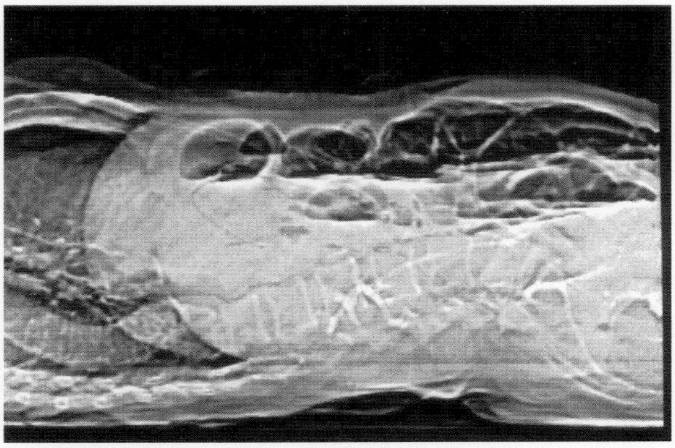

Figure 1 CT scan L-L: Marked hydro-gaseous distention of jejunum-ileal loops with multiples air-fluid levels.

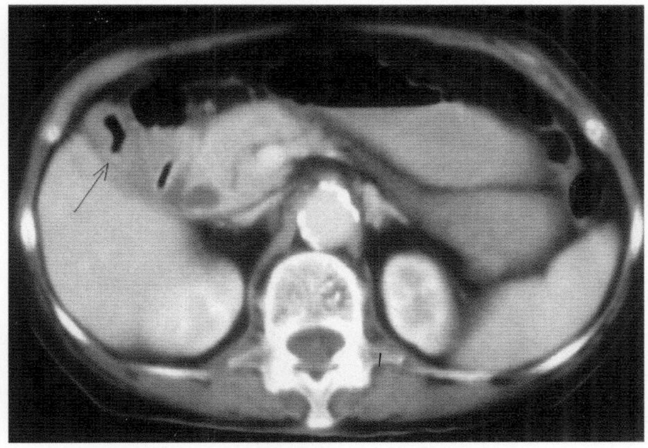

Figure 3 CT scan case 1: Gallbladder with thickened walls and with hydrogaseous levels.

gallstone; the patient is taken to the surgery theatre for the emergency laparotomy. A pararectal right-side incision is made; once the peritoneum is opened, many adhesions around gallbladder are visible and we proceed with the adhesiolysis and with the exploration of abdominal organs, that are free of neoplastic lesions. We identify a gallbladder-duodenal fistula, a diverticulum at about 70 cm from the ileocecal valve and a large gallstone formation at ileocecal valve level; we proceed with the enterotomy, with gallstone removal and diverticulum resection with TA. The post surgery course is normal, without complications, with regular discharge from hospital on day 13 after surgery. The patient enjoyed good health for one year and, after 20 months from the surgery, died because of heart disease.

Clinical case 2

On december 2003 A.T., 83 years old, came to our department complaining of biliary vomit, bloating and pain to the abdomen epi-mesogastric region. At physical examination, abdomen is aching when both deep and surface palpation to upper quadrants are carried out, and some pings (metallic noises) can be heard on auscultation. Blood test does not show significant alterations. An x-ray of the abdomen is performed in urgency and highlights the presence of multiple air-fluid levels; in order to achieve a better knowledge of the patient's situation, we decide to perform abdomen and pelvis TC with contrast which shows the classic triad of gallstone ileus: hard gallbladder, intestine loops distension and air-fluid levels, presence of gallstones in jejunum loops lumen (Figure 4). We decide for urgent surgery; through midline laparotomy we explore the peritoneal cavity and find the dilatation of jejunum-ileal loops that is due to an obstructing gallstone located approximately in the middle of ileum.We proceed cautiously to a mobilization in cranial direction and to ileotomy in healthy bowels, gallstone extraction and following ileotomy suture with

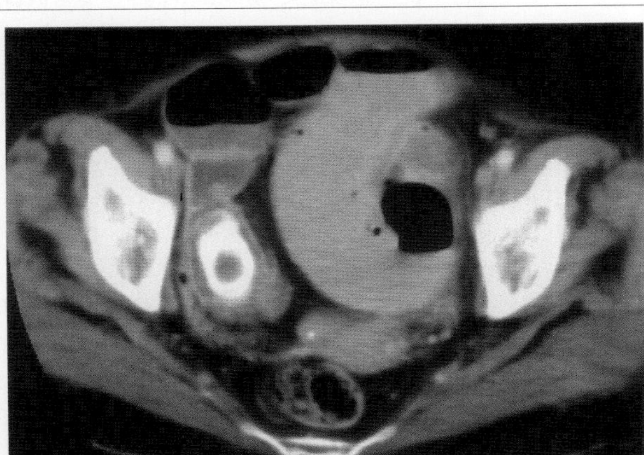

Figure 2 CT scan case 1: The gallstone is clearly detectable within the lumen of ileus.

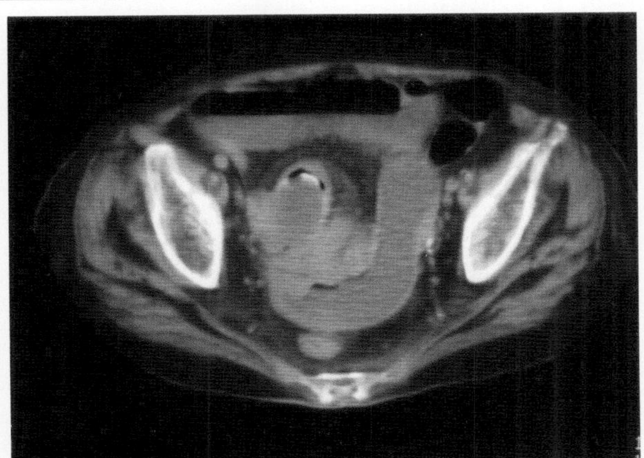

Figure 4 CT scan case 2: Intestin loops distention, with air-fluid levels and endoluminal gallstone.

an absorbable thread 2/0 single stitches suture. During liver area exploration are found strong gallbladder - duodenum adhesions, but further manipulations are avoided taking into account patient's age and general conditions, and a check of haemostasis and suture of abdomen layered wall is carried out. After 7 days of after-surgery hospitalization without complications, the patient is discharged in a good general condition.

Discussion

Gallstone ileus causes about 1-4% of intestine obstruction in population [1,2]; such percentage rises to almost 25% in patients older than 65 [3], being the third cause of obstruction after bridles and strangulated hernia. This data highlights the importance of age factor in this pathology: 70% of patients is over 65[4]. Another feature is the higher frequency in females: the average rate is 3,5:1 [5].The gallstone ileus symptoms have, at least at the beginning, their most peculiar expression in the "migrating pain", which is due to what is called "rolling phenomenon": the gallstone, driven by peristalsis, stops and then restarts its migration to a more distal section of intestine, stopping again and so causing the symptoms of an intermittent and discontinuous intestine obstruction [6]. The real disease beginning is at the occurrence of a very strong colic, localized in the right hypocondrium and epigastrium, which denounces the formation of a biliary-digestive fistula [7]; such symptoms tend to attenuate even up to their complete disappearing, but this is actually only momentary (from few hours to some days), after which arise repeated painful crises of the occlusive kind. On the contrary, if the gallstone is small, it can be expelled with no harm to the patient, leaving a biliary-digestive fistula that can remain unknown. Since it is quite difficult to recognize from clinical perspective this particular kind of intestine obstruction, which is often polymorphous, showing insidious onset, underestimated in patients already suffering from biliary colic, x-rays scan is very important (abdomen direct, ecography, TC), like endoscopic and laparoscopic tests which supply a way of diagnosis as well as therapy [8]. Gallstone ileus x-rays diagnostics is based essentially on the Rigler triad [9]: intestine loops dilatation and air-fluid levels (mainly if migrating, fluctuating and changing appearance) sign of intestine obstruction, aerobilia, visualization of a radiopaque image due to a gallstone mass in atypical position, position that can change during the following days. Such triad, actually, is present in less than a half of patients affected by gallstone ileus [10], and this makes infrequent a diagnosis after only x-rays to the abdomen [11]. Ecography is more sensitive than x-rays, since it can show the complete Rigler triad even when abdomen direct shows only the occlusion signs [12]; ultrasonography findings are made of: absent visualization of the gallbladder or presence of hyperechoic foci with posterior acoustic shadowing in the gallbladder bed, aerobilia, intralumen hyperechoic image with posterior acoustic shadowing (gallstone obstructing intestine lumen), image of intestine loops dilatation. TC has proved to be also for this pathology very sensitive and specific, showing the classical signs of Rigler triad even when neither x-rays, nor ultrasound scan could show them [13,14]. Besides the non-invasive techniques, endoscopy is very useful in diagnostics and treatment since it allows not only to detect biliary-digestive fistula, its position, the kind of tissue it is made of, but also to carry out a biopsy that can provide information about the neoplastic nature of the fistula [15]. In addition to this useful information for the diagnosis, endoscopy allows also the treatment of those gallstones that stopped at duodenum and colon level [16], either by extraction with the Dormia drum, or by breaking previously the gallstone with the lithotripter and then extracting the fragments [17]. Laparoscopy proved to be also very useful in the diagnostics of abdominal emergencies, allowing sometimes their treatment [18]. The prognosis of gallstone ileus, if it is not treated by surgery, is fatal; the recovery hope lays exclusively on surgery, which is not free of risk itself. Surgical treatment has some para-surgical and mini invasive alternatives, allowing the solution of such obstructive condition in a totally non invasive way [19]. Surgery performance is divided into two times: one is mandatory and is aimed to the intestine obstruction elimination, the other is not always possible, sometimes not advisable for opportunity reasons, and is aimed to the solution of the biliary-digestive fistula [1,20]. The first phase requires the search of the gallstone nested into the intestine and its extraction by enterotomy (to be carried out on healthy tissue, some centimeters from gallstone impact site, on the anti-mesenteric side, with longitudinal incision); in rare cases it is necessary a segmental resection of the intestinal tract due to the presence of necrosis and perforations. The second phase of surgery is aimed to the solution of biliary-digestive fistula, of the eventual residual gallstones, and final cholecistectomy; this is exactly the most discussed problem: whether to treat contemporarily both the obstruction and biliary fistula (one time treatment), or whether to treat the obstruction only and delay the fistula correction to a second time (two times treatment), or whether to treat the obstruction only, not correcting the fistula at all. Many studies [21,22] have analyzed the pros and cons of such different approaches and the conclusion was that:

- only carefully selected patients with low co-morbidity and good general conditions can stand a long lasting anesthesia and a wide dissection of surgery in one time;

- in case the patient treated with enterotomy only shows symptoms referable to the biliary tract and that cannot be treated differently, cholecistectomy is strongly advisable;
- considering the excellent tolerability of the biliary-digestive fistulas that are not spontaneously closed (event occurring 10% of cases) and the advantages of a treatment with only enterotomy, this seems to be the most suitable surgical treatment for gallstone ileus patients.

The most frequent complication is the wound infection [1,21,22] which occurs to about 30% of patients; the recurrence of gallstone ileus is an always pending risk, that's why abdomen exploration must always be accurate and complete (since recurrence is mainly due to the presence of multiple gallstones upstream or downstream the place where enterotomy is made). The appropriate use of endoscopy (alone or associated with mechanical lithotripsy or shock wave), of extracorporeal shock wave lithotripsy, and of laparoscopy are the new approaches to the treatment of gallstone ileus; such methods are sometimes alternative actions, sometimes first choice, with reference mainly to the patient's condition, to the gallstone ileus shape, to the possibility of using them in a short span of time and, if necessary, repeat them. Endoscopy treatment is possible when gallstones are positioned at gastro-duodenal level [16] or in colon; sometimes, when the gallstone is big, it is possible to use the mechanical lithotripsy (Endoscopic Mechanical Lithotripsy) [17], or, if the gallstone is too hard so that the mechanical lithotripsy is useless, it is possible to use the electrohydraulic kind (Endoscopic Electrohydraulic Lithotripsy). Sometimes it is possible to use the extracorporeal shock wave lithotripsy (Extracorporeal Shock Wave Lithotripsy) which allows to shatter gallstones so that they get to such dimensions as to be expelled with the feces [23]. This method requires some basic requirements: the gallstone must be visible on ultrasound scan (shock waves are reflected or attenuated by intestine gas, so that they are useless), absence of coagulopathy, absence of anenurysms, calcified vessels or bone tissue on the shock wave path. Collateral effects and complicances are really irrelevant. A further possibility of treatment is eventually given by laparoscopy, which has undoubted advantages due to the reduced occurrence of wound infection and a lower occurrence of respiratory problems; with respect to other treatments, laparoscopy approach allows, if carried out by expert hands, also a radical treatment of the disease, avoiding complications that could arise not correcting the biliary-digestive fistula [24-26].

Conclusions

Gallstone ileus is a quite rare pathology in population, but affects more frequently elderly people; symptoms have little typical elements so that the diagnosis is often late, even if the routine application of ultrasound scan and TC have reduced a lot such diagnosis delay. The treatment of this disease is mainly surgical even if recently some new therapeutic possibilities have been proposed (endoscopy with or without lithotripsy, laparoscopy, extracorporeal lithotripsy).

List of abbreviations used

CT: computed tomography; HCV: hepatitis C virus; TA: thoracic - abdominal stapler.

Competing interests

The authors declare that they have no competing interests.

Authors' contributions

D.M.: conception and design, interpretation of data, given final approval of the version to be published.
G.L.: critical revision, interpretation of data, given final approval of the version to be published.
F.M: acquisition of data, drafting the manuscript, given final approval of the version to be published.
R.S.: acquisition of data, drafting the manuscript, given final approval of the version to be published.
D.R.: acquisition of data, drafting the manuscript, given final approval of the version to be published.
S.E.: acquisition of data, drafting the manuscript, given final approval of the version to be published.
A.B.: conception and design, critical revision, given final approval of the version to be published.

Authors' information

DM: Assistant Professor of Surgery at University Federico II of Naples.
GL: MD, PhD, in Surgery at University Federico II of Naples.
FM: MD, PhD, in Surgery at U. Parini Hospital of Aosta
RS: Resident in Surgery at University Federico II of Naples.
DR: Resident in Radiology at University Federico II of Naples.
SE: MD, in Radiology at University Federico II of Naples.
AB: Associate Professor of Surgery at University "Federico II" of Naples.

Declarations

Funding for this article came from personal funds.
This article has been published as part of *BMC Surgery* Volume 13 Supplement 2, 2013: Proceedings from the 26th National Congress of the Italian Society of Geriatric Surgery. The full contents of the supplement are available online at http://www.biomedcentral.com/bmcsurg/supplements/13/S2

Authors' details

[1]Department of Specialized Surgery - Division of Gastrointestinal Surgery Rehabilitation of Election and Emergency. "Federico II" University, Naples - Italy. [2]Department of General Surgery. "U. Parini" Hospital, Aosta - Italy. [3]Department of Diagnostic Imaging and Radiotherapy. "Federico II" University, Naples - Italy. [4]Department of General, Geriatric, Oncologic Surgery and Advanced Technologies. "Federico II" University, Naples - Italy.

References

1. Doko M, Zovak M, Kopljar M, Glavan E, Ljubicic N, Hochstadter H: **Comparison of surgical treatments of gallstone ileus: preliminary report.** *WJS* 2003, **27**:400-404.

2. Tucker A, Garstin I: **A peculiar case of bowel obstruction.** *Int J Surg Case Report* 2013, **4(5)**:473-476.
3. Kirchmayr W, Mulhmann G, Zitt M, Bodner J, Weiss H, Klaus A: **Gallstone ileus: rare and still controversial.** *ANZ J Surg* 2005, **75**:234-238.
4. Ayantunde AA, Agrawal A: **Gallstone ileus: Diagnosis and Management.** *WJS* 2007, **31**:1292-1297.
5. Nakao A, Okamoto Y, Sunami M, Fujita T, Tsuji T: **The oldest patient with gallstone ileus: report of a case and review of 176 cases in Japan.** *Kurume Med J* 2008, **55(1-2)**:29-33.
6. Reisner RM, Cohen JR: **Gallstone ileus: a review of 1001 reported cases.** *Am Surg* 1994, **60**:441-446.
7. Berger My, van der Velden JJ, Lijmer JG, de Kort H, Prins A, Bohnen AM: **Abdominal symptoms: do they predict gallstones? A systematic review.** *Scand J Gastroenterol* 2000, **35**:70-76.
8. Ferraina P, Gancedo MC, Elli F, *et al*: **Video-assisted laparoscopic enterolithotomy: new technique in the surgical management of gallstone ileus.** *Surg Laparosc Endosc Percutan Tech* 2003, **13(2)**:36-38.
9. Rigler L, Borman C, Noble J: **Gallstone obstruction: pathogenesis and roentgen manifestation.** *JAMA* 1941, **117**:1753.
10. Lassandro F, Gagliardi N, Scuderi M, *et al*: **Gallstone ileus analysis of radiological findings in 27 patients.** *Eur J Radiol* 2004, **50**:23-29.
11. Ripolles T, Miguel-Dasit A, Errando J, *et al*: **Gallstone ileus. Increased diagnostic sensitivity by combining plain film and ultrasound.** *Abdom imaging* 2001, **26**:401-405.
12. Lasson A, Loren I, Nilsson A, Nirhov N, Nilsson P: **Ultrasonography in gallstone ileus: a diagnostic challenge.** *Eur J Surg* 1995, **161**:259-263.
13. Yu CY, Lin CC, Shyu RY, *et al*: **Value of CT in the diagnosis and management of gallstone ileus.** *WJ Gastroenterol* 2005, **11**:2142-2147.
14. Lobo DN, Jobling JC, Balfour TW: **Gallstone ileus: diagnostic pitfalls and therapeutic successes.** *J Clin Gastroenterol* 2000, **30**:72-76.
15. Sime RG: **Management of gallstone ileus.** *Can J Surg* 1989, **32**:61-64.
16. Lubbers H, Mahlke R, Lankisch PG: **Gallstone ileus: endoscopic removal of a gallstone obstructing the upper jejunum.** *J Inter Med* 1999, **246(6)**:593-597.
17. Zielinski MD, Ferreira LE, Baron TH: **Successful endoscopic treatment of colonic gallstone ileus using electrohydraulic lithotripsy.** *World J Gastroenterol* 2010, **16(12)**:1533-1536, Mar 28.
18. Sarli L, Pietra N, Costi R, Gobbi S: **Gallstone ileus: laparoscopic-assisted enterolithotomy.** *J Am Surg* 1998, **186(3)**:370-371.
19. Pavlidis TE, Atmatzidis KS, Papaziogas BT, *et al*: **Management of gallstone ileus.** *J Hepatobiliary Pancreat Surg* 2003, **10**:299-302.
20. Tan YM, Wong WK, Ooi LL: **A comparison of two surgical strategies for the emergency treatment of gallstone ileus.** *Singapore Med J* 2004, **45**:69-72.
21. Zuegel N, Hehl A, Lindemann F, Witte J: **Advantages of one-stage repair in case of gallstone ileus.** *Hepatogastroenterology* 1997, **44**:59-62.
22. Rodriguez-Sanjuan JC, Casado F, Fernandez MJ, *et al*: **Cholecistectomy and fistula closure versus enterolithotomy alone in gallstone ileus.** *Br J Surg* 1997, **84**:634-637.
23. Muratori R, Cennamo V, Menna M, Cecinato P, Eusebi LH, Mazzella G, Bazzoli F: **Colonic gallstone ileus treated with radiologically guided extracorporeal shock wave lithotripsy followed by endoscopic extraction.** *Endoscopy* 2012, **44(Suppl 2)**, UCTN:E88-9.
24. Allen JW, McCurry T, Rivas H, *et al*: **Totally laparoscopic management of gallstone ileus.** *Surg Endosc* 2003, **17**:352.
25. Qureshi I, Awad ZT: **Predictors of failure of the laparoscopic approach for the management of small bowel obstruction.** *Am Surg* 2010, **76(9)**:947-950, Sep.
26. Zygomalas A, Karamanakos S, Kehagias I: **Totally laparoscopic management of gallstone ileus: technical report and review of the literature.** *J Laparoendosc Adv Surg Tech A* 2012, **22(3)**:265-268, Apr.

Bilio-entero-gastrostomy: prospective assessment of a modified biliary reconstruction with facilitated future endoscopic access

Mostafa A Hamad[1*] and Hussein El-Amin[2]

Abstract

Background: Hepaticojejunostomy (HJ) is the classical reconstruction for benign biliary stricture. Endoscopic management of anastomotic complications after hepaticojejunostomy is extremely difficult. In this work we assess a modified biliary reconstruction in the form of bilio-entero-gastrostomy (BEG) regarding the feasibility of endoscopic access to HJ and management of its stenosis if encountered.

Methods: From October 2008 till February 2011 all patients presented to the authors with benign biliary stricture who needed bilio-enteric shunt were considered. For each patient bilio-entero-gastrostomy (BEG) of either type I, II or III was constructed. In the fourth week postoperatively, endoscopy was performed to explore the possibility to access the biliary anastomosis and perform cholangiography.

Results: BEG shunt was performed for seventeen patients, one of whom, with BEG type I, died due to myocardial infarction leaving sixteen patients with a diagnosis of postcholecystectomy biliary injury (9), inflammatory stricture with or without choledocholithiasis (5) and strictured biliary shunt (2). BEG shunts were either type I (3), type II (3) or type III (10). Endoscopic follow up revealed successful access to the anastomosis in 14 patients (87.5%), while the access failed in one type I and one type II BEG (12.5%). Mean time needed to access the anastomosis was 12.6 min (2-55 min). On a scale from 1–5, mean endoscopic difficulty score was 1.7. One patient (6.25%), with BEG type I, developed anastomotic stricture after 18 months that was successfully treated endoscopically by stenting. These preliminary results showed that, in relation to the other types, type III BEG demonstrated the tendency to be surgically simpler to perform, endoscopicall faster to access, easier and with no failure.

Conclusions: BEG, which is a modified biliary reconstruction, facilitates endoscopic access of the biliary anastomosis, offers management option for its complications, and, therefore, could be considered for biliary reconstruction of benign stricture. BEG type III tend to be surgically simpler and endoscopically faster, easier and more successful than type I and II.

Background

Benign biliary stricture is most commonly caused by operative injury of the common bile duct (CBD) during cholecystectomy or less frequently by inflammatory stenosis with or without stone formation, chronic pancreatitis, primary sclerosing cholangitis, strictured bilioenteric shunt and CBD injury due to penetrating trauma to the porta hepatis or during other operative procedures involving gastric, pancreatic, or hepatic resection [1-3]. Treatment of benign biliary stricture requires multidisciplinary approach including endoscopy, interventional radiology and surgery [4]. Whenever surgery is indicated, the procedure of choice is a Roux-en-Y hepaticojejunostomy (HJ) [3,5-8].

Stricture of the bilioenteric shunt following Roux-en-Y HJ is reported to range from 2% to 25% [2,3,7-10]. This is a major complication which is associated with repeated cholangitis and, if left untreated, with biliary cirrhosis and portal hypertension. Treatment could be by surgery, interventional radiology or endoscopy. Surgical treatment aiming at revision of the reconstruction of

* Correspondence: mostafa_hamad@yahoo.com
[1]Departments of General Surgery, Faculty of Medicine, Assiut University, Assiut, Egypt
Full list of author information is available at the end of the article

bilioenteric shunt is often difficult and represents major challenge to the surgeon [11]. Percutaneous transhepatic interventional therapy could be effective but is invasive especially to the liver which is often the seat of impaired function or overt cirrhosis [12,13].

Endoscopic management is not only the least invasive but also very effective via either balloon dilatation or stenting of the stricture. The main obstacle for endoscopic approach is the extremely difficult access of the endoscope to the bilioenteric shunt due to the altered anatomy of the Roux-en-Y construction. Some authors advocated the use of double [14] or single [15] balloon enterostomy to overcome this difficulty. Still, however, the procedure is difficult and time consuming. Others construct surgical access loop to be used by the endoscopist to reach the HJ stoma. These access loops could be jejunocutaneous either superficial [16] or subfacial [17], jejunal loop interposition [18], jejunoduodenostomy [19] or gastric access loop [20-22].

This study is a consecutive case series in which we prospectively assess bilio-entero-gastrostomy (BEG), which is a modified bilioenteric shunt with gastric access loop, regarding the feasibility of endoscopic access to HJ and management of its stricture if encountered. Additionally, we compare three different construction techniques of BEG in this regard.

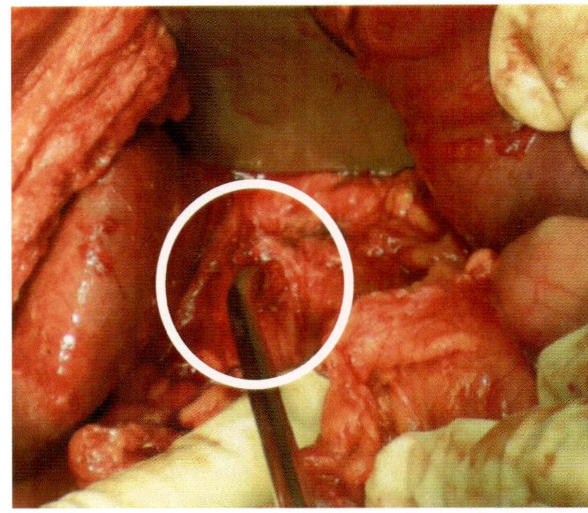

Figure 1 Preparation of the proximal CBD stoma.

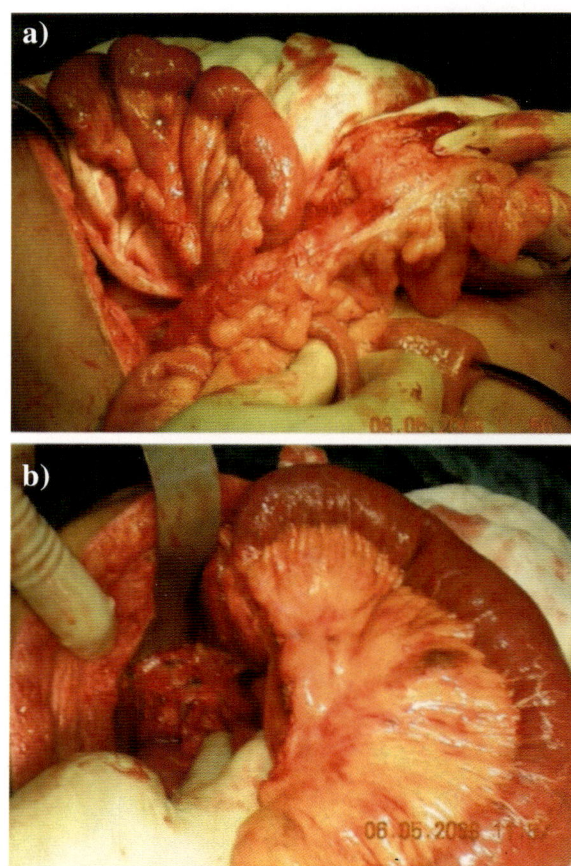

Figure 2 a) Preparation of the Roux jejunal loop after lengthening of the mesentery. b) Passing the loop retrocolic.

Methods

This is a prospective study, in the form of consecutive case series, the protocol of which was approved by the ethical committee of Assiut Faculty of Medicine. Included in the study are all patients presenting to the authors with a diagnosis of benign biliary stricture for which surgical correction is indicated in the period from October 2008 till February 2011. For those patients other therapeutic options as percutaneous transhepatic cholangiography (PTC) or endoscopic retrograde cholangiopancreatography (ERCP) dilatation or stenting were either not applicable or not successful.

For all patients, full medical history, clinical examination, laboratory investigations in the form of liver function tests (LFT), prothrombin time and concentration (PTT), complete blood count (CBC) and kidney function tests (KFT) were performed. Imaging studies were also carried out in the form of abdominal ultrasonography (US), computerized tomography scan (CT) of the abdomen and magnetic resonance cholangiography (MRC) if indicated. ERCP and/or PTC were performed, whenever applicable, whether for diagnosis or therapeutic trial. Thorough preoperative medical fitness assessment was done before surgery.

Surgical technique: under general intubation anesthesia after administration of prophylactic antibiotic in the form of third generation cephalosporin, a generous right subcostal incision was performed and could be extended on demand upward to the xyphoid process and/or to the left subcostal area. Thorough dissection and adesiolysis was performed to reach the CBD and prepare the unaffected proximal part for anastomosis (Figure 1). The Roux jejunal loop was prepared with lengthening of the mesentery and then passed retrocolic to reach the porta hepatis (Figure 2). Afterwards, BEG was constructed depending on the type; I, II or III. In all types, the HJ is end to side anastomosis using interrupted sutures of polyglactin 910 of 4–0 size. The level of HJ is dependent on Bismuth classification [10] of the level of the stricture and also on the diameter of CBD and the operative circumstances. If the level was at the carena (Bismuth type III), the HJ could be performed, using the Hepp-Couinaud technique [23], with widening of the stoma by extension through the wall of the left hepatic duct. When the two ducts constituted separate openings (Bismuth type IV), the septum in between, if applicable, could be sutured and cut to transform both ducts into single stoma. The rest of the anastomoses, including the enterogastrostomy (EG), are constructed according to the type of BEG. All JG are anastomosed to the anterior wall of the stomach as near as possible to the pyloric orifice. In BEG type I (Figure 3), a side loop of the Roux jejunum is anastomosed at its apex to the stomach with another side to side enteroenterostomy as a conduit of bile away from the stomach. In BEG type II (Figure 4), the Roux jejunum is transected about 10 to 15 cm from HJ without interference with its mesentery. The distal end is anastomosed to the stomach, while the proximal end is anastomosed to the side of the distal loop as a conduit of bile. In BEG type III (Figure 5), HJ is constructed leaving the distal end of the Roux jejunum long enough to be anastomosed to the side of the stomach. All the enterogastrostomies and enteroenterostomies were in the form of single-layer continuous sutures of polyglactin 910 of 3–0 size. An intraperitoneal drain was left in the hepatorenal pouch before closing the incision.

The choice of the type of BEG was an evolving process. We began with the BEG type I. The endoscopist faced difficulty with this technique due to the presence of more than one lumen at the site of gastroenterostomy making the decision and technique of entery more complex. Consequently, we modified the reconstruction to the BEG type II which appeared to be relatively easier for the endoscopist. However, some difficulty was still present for the endoscopic approach due to the side to end enteroenterostomy needed for this type. Moreover,

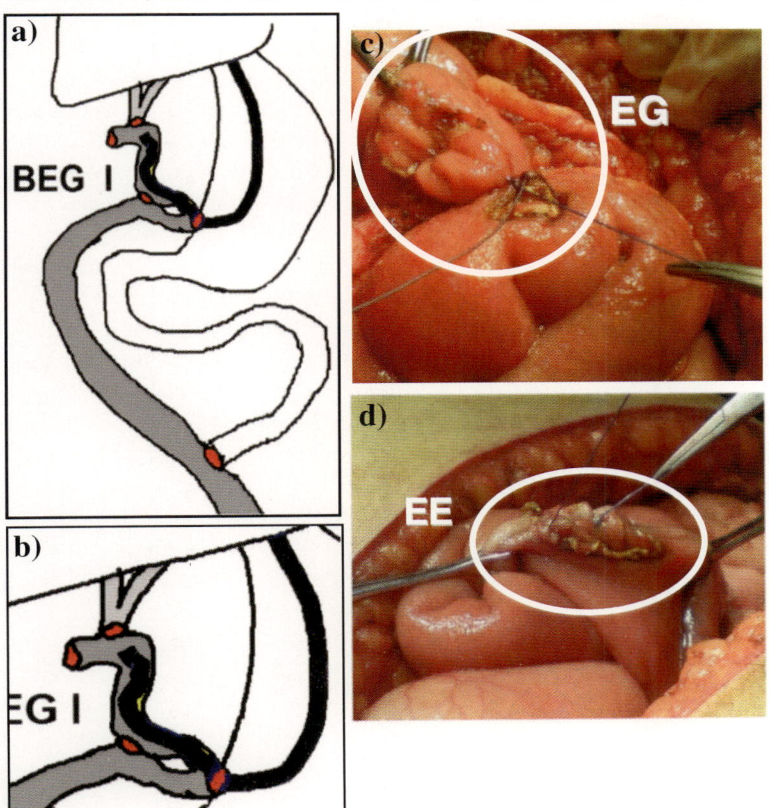

Figure 3 BEG type I. a) and **b**) Diagrams of the construction. **c**) Enterogastrostomy [EG]. **d**) Enteroenterostomy [EE].

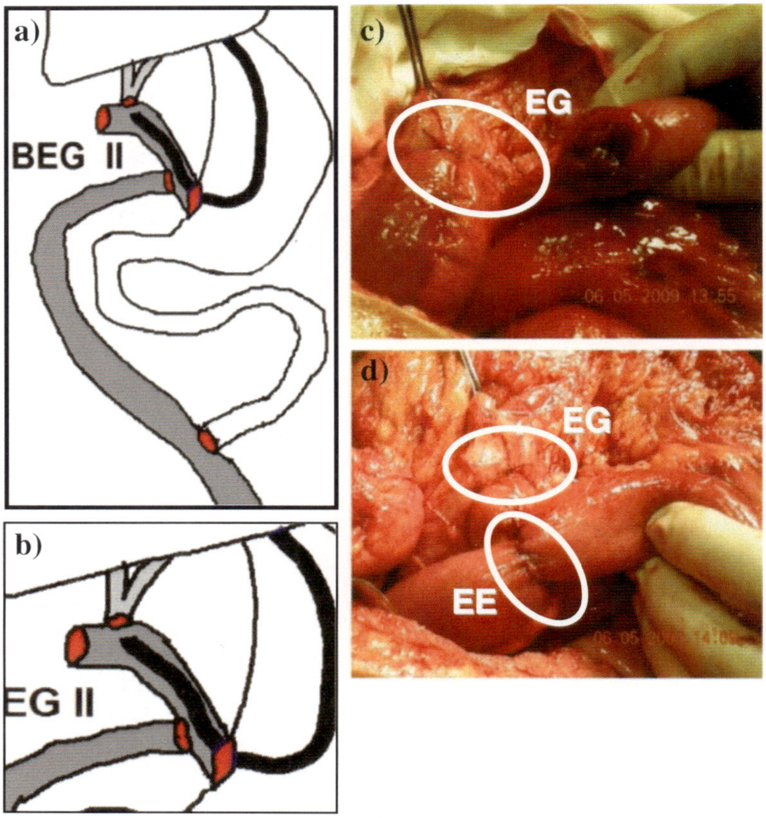

Figure 4 BEG type II. a) and **b**) Diagrams of the construction. **c**) Enterogastrostomy [EG]. **d**) Enteroenterostomy [EE].

BEG type II was more complex to be performed surgically. Consequently the technique was further modified to BEG type III which was not only the simplest to perform surgically but also the easiest for the endoscopist to reach the anastomosis due to the presence of only one lumen at the site of the enterogastrostomy. This may explain the sequence of cases in relation to the type of BEG, the increased number of BEG type III and the concentration of the cases with this type toward the later period of the study. Consequently, toward the end of the study, we decided to perform all cases using BEG type III.

Postoperatively, antibiotics in the form of third generation cephalosporin were administered twice daily for at least five days. The patients were closely followed up for any bile leak, improvement in the LFT, restoration of gastrointestinal motility and oral feeding. The patients were discharged from the hospitals once they were well mobilized, oral feeding was restored, and LFT were relatively improved.

Follow up visits, after hospital discharge, were scheduled weekly for the first four weeks then monthly for three months then every six months or whenever there were abnormal symptoms. In each visit, the patients underwent clinical assessment specially manifestation of cholangitis and laboratory assessment specially serum bilirubin and alkaline phosphatase levels. In the fourth postoperative week, endoscopic assessment of the BEG shunt with evaluation of the HJ was scheduled for all patients.

Endoscopic technique: within the 4th postoperative week, gastroenteroscopy was performed using end-view gastroduodenoscope (pentax 3440, Tokyo, Japan). The aim was to assess the feasibility to access the HJ stoma and perform cholangiography. With the patient in the left lateral position, monitored anesthesia care (MAC) sedation with propofol was used with an initiation dose of 100–150 mcg/kg/min for a period of 3–5 minutes and a maintenance dose of 25–75 mcg/kg/min which was adjusted to clinical response. The endoscope was introduced through the esophagus to the stomach where we assessed the amount of bile in the stomach on a scale of 0 to 2 where 0 meant no bile, 1 meant minimal amount of bile staining the gastric mucosa, and 2 meant large amount of bile accumulating and needed to be sucked. The gastroenterostomy stoma was assessed as regard to its site, diameter, as well as the difficulties we faced to pass through it. We passed through the gastroenterostomy either directly with the scope or over a guiding catheter. Thereafter, when we

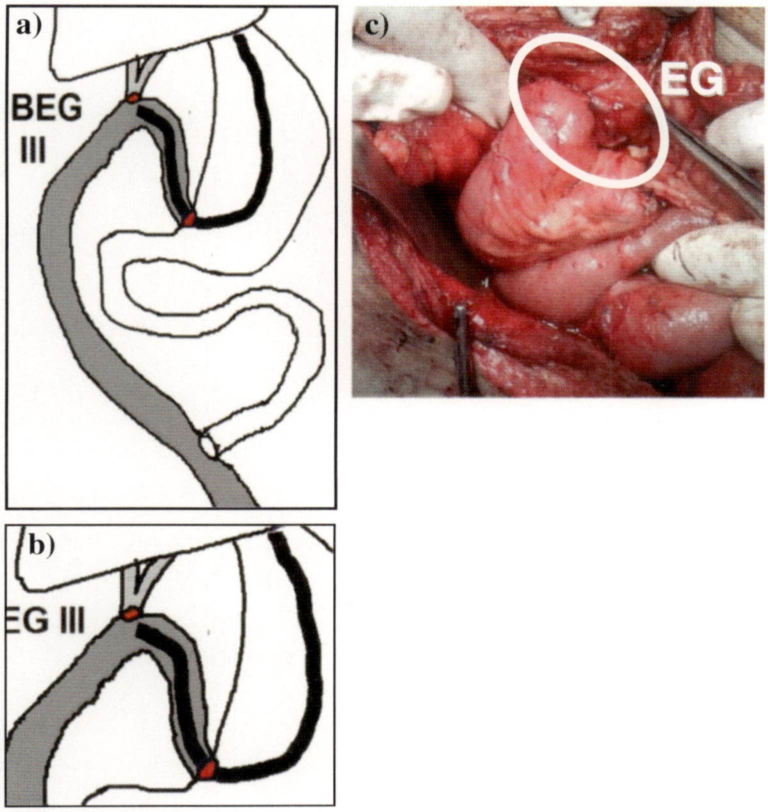

Figure 5 BEG type III. a) and **b**) Diagrams of the construction. **c**) Enterogastrostomy [EG].

reached the HJ stoma, we inject a diluted dye into the cannulated bile ducts using an ERCP catheter to obtain cholangiography. Time to reach the gastroenterostomy as well as time to reach the HJ was reported for each case. Failure of endoscopic access was defined as failure to reach the HJ and perform cholangiography. For failed cases, the cause of failure and the type of BEG performed were reported. After the end of each procedure, the endoscopist was asked to score the difficulty of it on a scale from 1 to 5 where 1 is the easiest and 5 is the most difficult. It is worth mentioning that all endoscopies were performed with the same endoscopist (HE) who has more than fifteen years of experience in gastrointestinal endoscopy including ERCP and therapeutic endoscopies.

During the follow up, if the patient suffered cholangitis that required medical treatment, imaging studies were performed including abdominal US and MRC to exclude the presence of HJ stricture. If stricture did exist, endoscopic diagnosis and therapeutic trial was performed aiming at either balloon dilatation and/or stent placement through the strictured anastomosis. According to Terblanche grading of clinical outcome of HJ (Table 1) [24], the patients were assessed and categorized.

All data were prospectively collected for assessment and for comparing the results of the three different types of BEG.

Table 1 Terblanche clinical grading of long term clinical results of hepaticojejunostomy

Grade I	Excellent	No biliary symptoms
Grade II	Good	Transitory symptoms / No treatment
Grade III	Fair	Biliary symptoms requiring medical therapy
Grade IV	Poor	Biliary symptoms due to recurrent stricture requiring intervention

Results

In the period of the study, seventeen cases of benign biliary stricture were treated by the authors using BEG shunt. One patient, with BEG type one reconstruction, died of myocardial infarction on the second postoperative day and was excluded from the study. This left sixteen patients to be included. Seven patients were males and nine were females. The age ranged from 22 to 72 years with a mean age of 40.9 years.

Tables 2, 3 and 4 show the main preoperative, operative, and postoperative data of the patients respectively. The diameter of the proximal biliary channel above the level of the stricture ranged from 6 mm to 20 mm. One patient (6.26%) with BEG type I developed HJ stricture

Table 2 Preoperative data of the patients

Data	Description		No. (%)		Total
Diagnosis	Post-cholecystectomy CBD injury	Immediate leak	3	9 (56.25%)	16
		Immediate obstruction	3		
		Late Stricture	3		
	Strictured Hepatico-Jejunostomy (after original post-cholecystectomy CBD injury)		2 (12.50%)		
	Inflammatory stricture (cholangitis)	With CBD stones	3	5 (31.25%)	
		Without CBD stones	2		
Bismuth type of stricture	I (>2 cm from the confluence)		5 (31.25%)		16
	III (<2 cm from the confluence)		3 (18.75%)		
	IIII (hilar with preserved confluence)		7 (43.75%)		
	IV (hilar with separate right and left ducts)		1 (6.25%)		
	VI (sectorial right hepatic duct)		0 (0%)		
Liver functions	Total bilirubin (μmol/L)	Elevated	14(87.50%)		16
		Normal	2 (12.50%)		
	Alkaline phosphatase (U/L)	Elevated	16 (100%)		16
		Normal	0 (0.0%)		
Cholangio-graphy	ERCP	Number of procedures	21		16*
		Number of patients	14 (87.50%)		
	MRC	Number of procedures	7		
		Number of patients	7 (43.75%)		

CBD: common bile duct, ERCP: endoscopic retrograde cholangiopancreatography, MRC: magnetic resonance cholangiography, * represents the total number of patients that had cholangiography whatever the type.

about 18 months after the operation. The patient presented with recurrent cholangitis and MRC revealed strictured HJ. Endoscopic cholangiography was performed and the stricture was dilated with placement of a ten-french stent through it (Figure 6). The patient was followed up for eleven months with uneventful course.

Endoscopic data are shown in Table 5. Endoscopic access to the HJ was successful in 14 cases (87.5%) while failed in 2 cases (12.5%). The first failure was in case number two with BEG type I. The enterogastrostomy (EG) was impossible to be entered by the endoscope as it was placed high on the lesser curve of the stomach. Afterwards, all EG anastomoses were placed as near to the pyloric orifice as possible. The second failure was in case number seven with BEG type II. The EG was too narrow to pass the endoscope, however the endoscopist stated that whenever the access is mandatory, the EG could be dilated enough to accommodate the endoscope. In spite of that, we considered this case as a failure to endoscopic access of the HJ.

Table 6 compares between the three types of BEG. It is shown that type III BEG tend to be better than the other

Table 3 Operative data of the patients

Data	Description	No. (%)	Total
Level of bilioenteric shunt from the carena	≥2 cm	5 (31.25%)	16
	<2 cm	3 (18.75%)	
	At the carena (classic technique)	2 (12.50)	
	At the carena (left duct extension-Hepp Couinaud technique)	5 (31.25%)	
	Two separate ducts (septum was sutured and cut to form one stoma)	1 (6.25%)	
Type of BEG	Type I	3 (18.75%)	16
	Type II	3 (18.75%)	
	Type III	10 (62.50%)	
Other procedures	Yes (cholecystectomy)	5 (31.25%)	16
	No	11 (68.75%)	
Operative time (min)Mean (range)	227.5 min (150–350 min)		

BEG: bilioenterogastrostomy.

Table 4 Postoperative data of the patients

Data	Deascription	No. (%)	Total
Clinical improvement	1 week	10 (62.50%)	16
	2 weeks	6 (37.50%)	
	≥3 weeks	0 (0%)	
Laboratory improvement	1 week	3 (18.75%0	16
	2 weeks	7 (43.75%)	
	≥3 weeks	6 (37.50%)	
Hospital stay Mean (range) days	10 (7–20) days		
Long term clinical results (cholangitis)	Grade I (excellent)	12 (75.00%)	16
	Grade II (good)	2 (12.50%)	
	Grade III (fair)	1 (6.25%)	
	Grade IV (poor)	1 (6.25%)	
Follow up period Mean (range) months	23 (7–35) months		
HJ stricture	One case, presented after 18 months	1 (6.25%)	16
	BEG type I, endoscopic stent,		
	Normal after 9 months follow up		
	Patent HJ	15 (93.75%)	

HJ: hepaticojejunostomy.

two types regarding the success rate of access to HJ, time to reach HJ, and difficulty to the endoscopist. Additionally, BEG type III is easier to perform requiring only three anastomoses per case while the other two types require five anastomoses. However, further assessment may be needed due to the small number of cases and the difference in number between the groups.

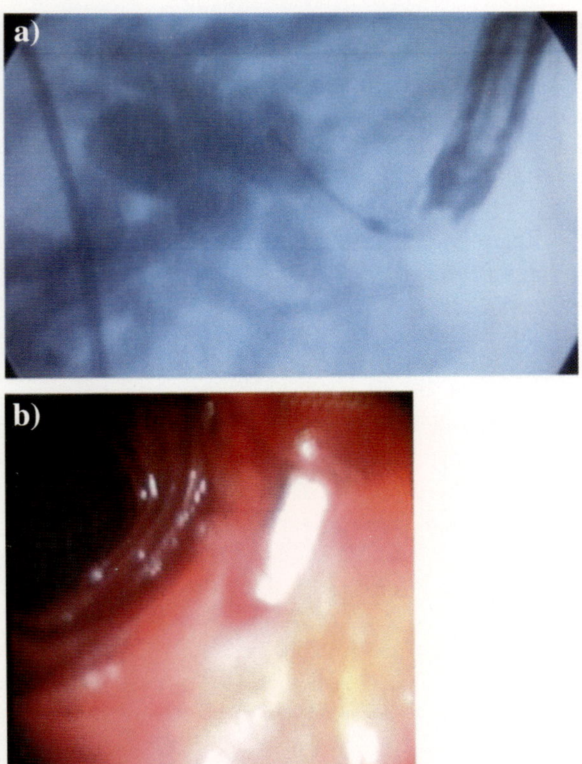

Figure 6 Endoscopic stenting of the case complicated by anastomotic stricture. a) Fluroscopic view of the stent pushed in place over the guide wire. **b**) endoscopic view of the stent in place.

Discussion

Roux-en-Y hepaticojejunostomy is the most commonly used surgical technique for reconstruction of the biliary tract in patients with benign biliary stricture [3,5-8]. In those patients, there is a relatively high incidence of strictured HJ ranging from 2% to 25% [2,3,7-10]. The endoscopic management of these complications seems to be the best option and least invasive compared to interventional radiology or reoperation [11-13]. However, the altered anatomy of the Roux-en-Y construction represents a major difficulty to access the HJ by the endoscope. The use of standard gastroduodenoscope proved to be extremely difficult, time consuming and with high failure rate [14,15].

Several attempts were reported to overcome these difficulties in endoscopic approach to HJ. The use of long enteroscope, whether double balloon or single balloon, was shown to improve the results of endoscopic access. However, these reports are still few with limited number of cases and the availability of the enteroscopes and their assigned accessories are still not universally present in all endoscopy units [14,15].

On the other hand, several modifications of the surgical technique of the HJ have been suggested to

Table 5 Endoscopic data of the patients

No	BEG type	Time to reach JG*	Access to HJ	Time to reach HJ*	Difficulty score (1–5)	Bile in stomach score (0–1)
1	I	3	Succeeded	24	3	1
2	I	2	Failed	Failed	Failed	1
3	II	2	Succeeded	10	2	2
4	I	2	Succeeded	55	4	1
5	II	2	Succeeded	20	3	1
6	III	1	Succeeded	7	1	0
7	II	2	Failed	Failed	Failed	1
8	III	2	Succeeded	12	2	1
9	III	2	Succeeded	10	1	2
10	III	1	Succeeded	8	1	2
11	III	1	Succeeded	12	2	0
12	III	1	Succeeded	2	1	0
13	III	2	Succeeded	7	1	1
14	III	2	Succeeded	6	1	1
15	III	1	Succeeded	2	1	1
16	III	1	Succeeded	2	1	2
Mean		1.6		12.6	1.7	1

*Time is in minutes.

enable access to the shunt either by interventional radiology or endoscopy. Some authors recommended an associated jejonostomy to be used for access for one year postoperatively and closed afterwards [16]. However, other authors tried to overcome the inconvenience of the stoma to the patient in addition to the possibility of delayed shunt problems later than the suggested one year period by making perminant jejunostomy subcutaneously and open it under local anesthesia whenever the access is needed then close it again [17]. Another approach is to construct an interpositioned jejunal loop to act as a conduit between the CBD and the duodenum [18]. It was found that a jejunal loop less than 20 cm in length will help the endoscope pass through but a loop more than 40 cm will prevent recurrent ascending cholangitis; a controversy that is difficult to solve [18,25]. Other authors recommended the use of duodenal access through side jejunoduodenostomy [19] or gastric access through enterogastrostomy [20-22].

To our knowledge, there are three series of gastric access loop in the literature that will be discussed in view of the available data. Sitaram et al. [20] reported the first series in ten patients. They succeeded to enter the enterogastrostomy in five patients only. In another study, Selvakumar et al. [21] reported eleven patients with gastric access loop with 73% success rate of endoscopic access of the HJ stoma. The failed three cases were due to strictured enterogastrostomy. Their follow up period was relatively long (mean 51 months). They encountered one strictured HJ (9%) which did not benefit from the access loop. The patients did not have clinical or endoscopic evidence of bile gastritis. In the third study, Jayasundara et al. [22] reported 27 patients who had bilioenteric shunt with gastric access loop. Three patients (11%) developed strictured HJ that were successfully managed endoscopically through the access loop. During the follow up period of about two and half years, they did not discover gastric access related morbidity using the dyspepsia disability score. In our series with 16 cases, we assessed different construction of gastric access loop in the form of bilioenterogastrostomy (BEG) type I, II and III regarding endoscopic access of the HJ. We found that the overall success rate of endoscopic access to the HJ

Table 6 Comparison between the three types of BEG

Type	No. of cases	No. of Anast. per case	Success of Endoscopic access to HJ	Time to reach HJ (min)	Difficulty score (mean score)	Bile in Stomach (mean score)
BEG I	3	5	2 (66%)	39.5	3.5	1
BEG II	3	5	2 (66%)	15	2.5	1.3
BEG III	10	3	10 (100%)	6.8	1.2	1

BEG: bilioenterogastrostomy, HJ: hepaticojejunostomy, Anast.: anastomoses.

through the three types of BEG was 87.5%, while it was 100% for BEG type III, which is a construction similar to the three series that were discussed previously [20-22]. These success rates compared favorably with other similar series [20,21] except Jayasundara et al. [22]. In spite of having bile in the stomach in most of the cases, the patients did not show any clinical manifestations of biliary gastritis which is similar to the results of other authors [20-22]. The endoscopist considered the procedure easy with a mean score of 1.7 and 1.2 for the whole series and for BEG type III respectively on a scale from 1 to 5. The mean procedure time was convenient reaching 12.6 minutes for the whole series and 6.8 minutes for BEG type III. Our cases were a mixture of different indications for BEG including two difficult cases of revision of strictured HJ. Also, different levels of HJ were reported from Bismuth type I to type IV. We think that these wide varieties constitute a good assessment of the BEG technique. We had a follow up period with a mean of 23 months that was comparable to the other similar series [20,22] except for Selvakumar et al. [21] who reported a mean of 51 months follow up. We think that our follow up period would better be extended to have long term results that can better reflect the real comlication rate. We had one strictured HJ (6.25%) which compared favorably with the other series [20-22]. This case was successfully treated endoscopically by stenting which proved the efficacy of BEG construction in facilitating endoscopic management of complicated bilioenteric shunt as was previously shown by other authors [22].

Regarding the three types of BEG, type I and II were more complex in construction with five anastomoses per case and meant to prevent bile reflux in the stomach in relation to type III. These two types, however, did not improve the bile reflux. Additionally, we found that BEG type III, which was easier to perform with only three anastomoses per case, was more successful in accessing HJ, required shorter time to reach it, was easier for the endoscopist. This explains why, from the middle of the series, we preferred to use BEG type III and abandoned the other two types.

Conclusions

In conclusion, bilioenterogastrostomy (BEG), which is a modified biliary reconstruction using a gastric access loop, facilitates endoscopic access of the biliary anastomosis, offers management option for its future complications, and, therefore, could be considered as an advantageous option for reconstruction of benign biliary stricture. BEG type III tend to be surgically simpler and endoscopically faster, easier and more successful than type I and II.

Competing interests
The authors declare that they have no competing interests.

Author details
[1]Departments of General Surgery, Faculty of Medicine, Assiut University, Assiut, Egypt. [2]Departments of Medicine, Faculty of Medicine, Assiut University, Assiut, Egypt.

Authors' contributions
MAH conceived the idea and design the operative protocol. He was also the main operator for all cases. In addition, the participated in drafting the manuscript. HE designed the endoscopic protocol, was the endoscopist of all cases, and revised the manuscript. All authors read and approved the final manuscript.

References

1. He ZP, Hou WL, Bie P, Dong JH, Wang SG, Han BL, Cai JX, Li ZH, Chen P, Ma KS, Zheng SG: **Etiology and surgical treatment of hilar bile duct stricture.** *Hepatobiliary Pancreat Dis Int* 2003, **2**:587–593.
2. Lillemoe KD, Melton GB, Cameron JL, Pitt HA, Campbell KA, Talamini MA, Sauter PA, Coleman J, Yeo CJ: **Postoperative bile duct strictures: management and outcome in the 1990s.** *Ann Surg* 2000, **232**:430–441.
3. Tocchi A, Costa G, Lepre L, Liotta G, Mazzoni G, Sita A: **The long-term outcome of hepaticojejunostomy in the treatment of benign bile duct strictures.** *Ann Surg* 1996, **224**:162–167.
4. Costamagna G, Familiari P, Tringali A, Mutignani M: **Multidisciplinary approach to benign biliary strictures.** *Curr Treat Options Gastroenterol* 2007, **10**:90–101.
5. Jabłońska B, Lampe P: **Iatrogenic bile duct injuries: etiology, diagnosis and management.** *World J Gastroenterol* 2009, **15**:4097–4104.
6. Tocchi A, Mazzoni G, Liotta G, Costa G, Lepre L, Miccini M, De Masi E, Lamazza MA, Fiori E: **Management of benign biliary strictures: biliary enteric anastomosis vs endoscopic stenting.** *Arch Surg* 2000, **135**:153–157.
7. Machado NO: **Biliary complications postlaparoscopic cholecystectomy: mechanism, preventive measures, and approach to management: a review.** *Diagn Ther Endosc* 2011, **967017**:. Epub 2011 Jun 12.
8. Csendes A, Navarrete C, Burdiles P, Yarmuch J: **Treatment of common bile duct injuries during laparoscopic cholecystectomy: endoscopic and surgical management.** *World J Surg* 2001, **25**:1346–1351.
9. Pellegrini CA, Thomas MJ, Way LW: **Recurrent biliary stricture. Patterns of recurrence and outcome of surgical therapy.** *Am J Surg* 1984, **147**:175–180.
10. Bismuth H, Majno PE: **Biliary strictures: classification based on the principles of surgical treatment.** *World J Surg* 2001, **25**:1241–1244.
11. Yan JQ, Peng CH, Ding JZ, Yang WP, Zhou GW, Chen YJ, Tao ZY, Li HW: **Surgical management in biliary restricture after Roux-en-Y hepaticojejunostomy for bile duct injury.** *World J Gastroenterol* 2007, **13**:6598–6602.
12. Halpenny DF, Torreggiani WC: **The infectious complications of interventional radiology based procedures in gastroenterology and hepatology.** *J Gastrointestin Liver Dis* 2011, **20**:71–75.
13. Draganov PV: **Endoscopic management of biliary stricture after liver transplantation.** *World J Gastroenterol* 2009, **15**:3725–3733.
14. Koornstra JJ: **Double balloon enteroscopy for endoscopic retrograde cholangiopancreatography after Roux-en-Y construction: case series and review of the literature.** *Neth J Med* 2008, **66**:275–279.
15. Itoi T, Ishii K, Sofuni A, Itokawa F, Tsuchiya T, Kurihara T, Tsuji S, Ikeuchi N, Umeda J, Moriyasu F: **Single-balloon enteroscopy-assisted ERCP in patients with Billroth II gastrectomy or Roux-en-Y anastomosis (with video).** *Am J Gastroenterol* 2010, **105**:93–99.
16. Barker EM, Winkler M: **Permanent-access hepaticojejunostomy.** *Br J Surg* 1984, **71**:188–191.
17. Al-Ghnaniem R, Benjamin IS: **Long-term outcome of hepaticojejunostomy with routine access loop formation following iatrogenic bile duct injury.** *Br J Surg* 2002, **89**:1118–1124.
18. Moellmann B, Ruhnke M, Kremer B: **Cholangio-duodenal interposition of an isolated jejunal segment after central resection.** *Hepatobiliary Pancreat Dis Int* 2004, **3**:259–264.

19. Prakash K, Ramesh H, Jacob G, Venugopal A, Lekha V, Varma D, Ramesh GN, Augustine P: **Multidisciplinary approach in the long-term management of intrahepatic stones: Indian experience.** *Indian J Gastroenterol* 2004, **23**:209–213.
20. Sitaram V, Perakath B, Chacko A, Ramakrishna BS, Kurian G, Khanduri P: **Gastric access loop in hepaticojejunostomy.** *Br J Surg* 1998, **85**:110.
21. Selvakumar E, Rajendran S, Balachandar TG, Kannan DG, Jeswanth S, Ravichandran P, Surendran R: **Long-term outcome of gastric access loop in hepaticojejunostomy.** *Hepatobiliary Pancreat Dis Int* 2008, **7**:152–155.
22. Jayasundara JASB, De Silva WMM, Pathirana AA: **Therapeutic value and outcome of gastric acces loops created during hepaticojejunosytomy for iatrogenic bile duct injuries.** *Surgeon* 2010, **8**:325–329.
23. Hepp J: **Hepaticojejunostomy using the left biliary trunk for iatrogenic biliary lesions: the Frensh connection.** *World J Surg* 1985, **9**:507–511.
24. Terblanche J, Worthley CS, Spence RAJ, Krige JAJ: **High or low hepaticojejunostomy for bile duct strictures.** *Surgery* 1990, **108**:828–834.
25. Pappalardo G, Correnti S, Mobarhan S, Trentino P, Pietropaolo A, Frattaroli F, Castrini G: **Long-term results of Roux-en-Y hepaticojejunostomy and hepaticojejunoduodenostomy.** *Ann Surg* 1982, **196**:149–152.

15

Post-operative depletion of platelet count is associated with anastomotic insufficiency following intrahepatic cholangiojejunostomy: a case–control study from the results of 220 cases of intrahepatic cholangiojejunostomy

Takehiro Noji*, Takahiro Tsuchikawa, Yuma Ebihara, Toru Nakamura, Kentaro Kato, Joe Matsumoto, Eiichi Tanaka, Toshiaki Shichinohe and Satoshi Hirano

Abstract

Background: Post-operative anastomotic insufficiency following major hepato-biliary surgery has significant impacts on the post-operative course. Recent reports have revealed that platelets play an important role in liver regeneration and wound healing. From these experimental and clinical results on platelet function, we hypothesized that post-operative platelet depletion (to $<10 \times 10^4/\mu L$) would be associated with delayed liver regeneration as well as anastomotic insufficiency of intrahepatic cholangiojejunostomy. However, little information is available regarding correlations between platelet count and these complications. The purposes of the present study were, firstly, to evaluate the incidence of anastomotic insufficiency following intrahepatic cholangiojejunostomy and, secondly, to evaluate whether platelet depletion represents a risk factor for anastomotic insufficiency in intrahepatic cholangiojejunostomy.

Methods: Participants in this study comprised 220 consecutive patients who underwent intrahepatic cholangiojejunostomy following hepato-biliary resection for biliary malignancies between September 1998 and December 2010. Anastomotic insufficiency was confirmed by cholangiographic demonstration of leakage from the anastomosis using contrast medium introduced via a biliary drainage tube or prophylactic drain placed during surgery.

Results: Anastomotic insufficiency of the intrahepatic cholangiojejunostomy occurred in 13 of 220 patients (6%). Thirteen of the 220 patients, including one with anastomotic insufficiency, died during the study. Uni- and multivariate analyses both revealed that platelet depletion on post-operative day 1 ($<10 \times 10^4/\mu L$) correlated with anastomotic insufficiency.

Conclusion: Post-operative platelet depletion was closely associated with anastomotic insufficiency following intrahepatic cholangiojejunostomy. This correlation has been established, but the underlying mechanisms have not.

Keywords: Biliary reconstruction, Intrahepatic cholangiojejunostomy, Platelet depletion, Liver regeneration

* Correspondence: drnoji@med.hokudai.ac.jp
Department of Gastroenterological Surgery II, Graduate School of Medicine, Hokkaido University, N15W7, Kita-ku, Sapporo Hokkaido 060-8638, Japan

Background

Liver resection with intrahepatic cholangiojejunostomy for biliary malignancies is one of the most demanding surgeries and is associated with a high morbidity rate. Recent reports have revealed post-operative morbidity rates ranging from 42% to 59% [1-6]. Morbidity is high because the operations comprise various difficult and highly technical procedures. We have previously reported that the most frequent post-operative complications are organ/space surgical-site infection (SSI), liver failure, respiratory complications, and anastomotic insufficiency of the intrahepatic cholangiojejunostomy [7].

In general, intrahepatic cholangiojejunostomy is thought to be more technically demanding than hepaticojejunostomy. Previous reports have therefore shown that the incidence of anastomotic insufficiency after intrahepatic cholangiojejunostomy (6.8-50%) is higher than that after hepaticojejunostomy (0.4-8%) [4,8-12]. Several studies have reported on bile leakage after intrahepatic cholangiojejunostomy, but those did not clearly specify whether the bile leak arose from the liver stump or from the site of anastomosis for the hepaticojejunostomy, as Nagino et al. suggested in their previous report [9]. Precise determination of the incidence of, and risk factors for, anastomotic insufficiency after intrahepatic cholangiojejunostomy remains difficult.

Recent experimental studies have suggested that blood platelets play a pivotal role in liver regeneration after partial liver resection [13-16]. A depleted platelet count severely suppresses liver regeneration, whereas induction of thrombocytosis by administration of thrombopoietin or splenectomy has been shown to accelerate liver regeneration [14-16]. Some evidence also suggests that platelet-derived serotonin plays an essential role in platelet-mediated liver regeneration [16]. In addition, several clinical studies have revealed that platelet counts below $10 \times 10^4/\mu L$ pre-operatively and immediately post-operatively are associated with an increased risk of mortality and delayed recovery of liver function after partial liver resection [17-19]. Experimental evidence has also shown that bile duct cells regenerate along with other hepatocytes [20]. Other recent experimental studies have concluded that platelets play important roles in not only liver regeneration, but also tissue repair [21,22]. Given these results regarding platelet functions, we hypothesized that post-operative platelet depletion (to $<10 \times 10^4/\mu L$) would be associated with delayed liver regeneration and anastomotic insufficiency after intrahepatic cholangiojejunostomy. However, data for this hypothesis are lacking. The purpose of this study was therefore to evaluate whether post-operative depletion of platelets was associated with anastomotic insufficiency following intrahepatic cholangiojejunostomy. The primary outcome parameter was incidence of anastomotic insufficiency with intrahepatic cholangiojejunostomy. We performed uni- and multivariate analyses to identify both clinical variables associated with anastomotic insufficiency and clinical factors correlated with platelet depletion in the post-operative period.

Methods

Study participants

Participants comprised 220 consecutive patients who underwent intrahepatic cholangiojejunostomy following hepato-biliary resection for biliary malignancies from September 1998 and December 2010.

Pre-operative biliary drainage

All hepatectomies were performed after the total bilirubin concentration had decreased to below 2 mg/dL. Pre-operative biliary decompression was performed to reduce serum bilirubin concentration to below 2 mg/dL for all patients with jaundice, and to control segmental cholangitis.

Pre-operative portal vein embolization (PE)

Pre-operative PE of the liver was performed when right trisegmentectomy, right hepatectomy, or left trisegmentectomy was planned. Indications and procedures for PE have been described previously [23].

Surgery

Hepatectomies were classified according to the Brisbane 2000 Terminology [24]. Hepatoduodenal ligament skeletonization, lymphadenectomy, and various hepatectomies with *en bloc* resection of the caudate lobe and extrahepatic bile duct were performed. Details of these procedures have been described previously [7].

Our procedure for bilioenteric anastomosis using the Roux-en-Y jejunal limb has been described previously with video [25]. Briefly, the jejunal limb was brought to the hepatic ducts via the standard retrocolic-anteduodenal route. In the case of hepatic pancreatoduodenectomy, reconstruction was performed according to Child's method with an end-to-side pancreaticojejunostomy. All cholangiojejunostomies were performed by anastomosing the mucosal layers of the bile duct and intestine. Transanastomotic stents were placed in all patients, usually introduced via a trans-jejunal route or occasionally a transhepatic route. Although most bile ducts to be anastomosed were drained by percutaneous transhepatic biliary drainage, a trans-jejunal route rather than a transhepatic route was preferred because the sinus tract between the liver and abdominal wall was usually broken at laparotomy.

Drains were placed prophylactically near the anastomosis and the cut surface of the liver. Until the end of 2004, Penrose drains were used along the hepatic stump.

From 2005, 10-mm capillary silicone drains were placed in the same spaces.

Definitions of post-operative complications

Post-operative complications were graded according to the Clavien-Dindo classification [26]. Anastomotic insufficiency of intrahepatic cholangiojejunostomy was identified by cholangiographic demonstration of leakage from the anastomosis using contrast medium introduced via a biliary drainage tube or prophylactic drain placed during surgery [9]. This procedure allowed us to differentiate between an anastomotic leak and bile leaking from the liver stump.

Organ/space SSI was defined as follows: with intra-abdominal collections; drain/s left in place for more than 3 weeks; patients with severe complications such as sepsis requiring admission to the intensive care unit; hemorrhage needing interventional radiology; or repeat laparotomy. In this group, pancreatic- or bile-related infectious complications were also included. Patients with organ/space SSI did not include those with anastomotic insufficiency. Post-operative liver failure was defined as International Study Group of Liver Surgery (ISGLS) liver failure grade B/C [27].

Statistical analysis

Statistical analyses were performed using the Mann–Whitney U test, a χ^2 test, or Fisher's exact test and the Kruskal-Wallis test. Values of $p < 0.05$ were considered statistically significant. All variables reaching a p-value of less than 0.1 in univariate analysis were included in a multivariate analysis using a logistic step-by-step regression model. Results are presented as odds ratios (ORs) with 95% confidence intervals (CIs).

Informed consent

The need to obtain informed consent for participation in this retrospective study was waived by the institutional review board.

Statements

We confirm that all study protocols were approved by ethics committee of Hokkaido University Hospital.

Results

A total of 220 patients (146 men, 74 women) were enrolled, comprising 140 with extra-hepatic bile duct cancer, 45 with intrahepatic cholangiocarcinoma, and 35 with gallbladder carcinoma. Median age was 68 years (range, 41–81 years).

Pre- and post-operative patient characteristics are presented in Table 1. Median operation time was 647 min (range, 415–1180 min) and median estimated blood loss was 1783 mL (range, 510–24,520 mL). The median number of reconstructed bile ducts was 3 (range, 1–5).

Table 1 Subject characteristics

Subject characteristics		Number of subjects
Age (years) median: 68	>68	126
Sex	Male/Female	146/74
Preoperative diagnosis	BDC	140
	GBC	35
	ICC	45
Body mass index; median: 22	<22	105
Diabetes mellitus	Positive	39
ICGR15 > 10%	Yes	129
ICGR15 > 15%	Yes	37
Preoperative biliary drainage	ENBD/PTBD	64/111
Preoperative albumin (g/dL); median: 3.8	<3.9	112
Preoperative portal vein embolism	Yes	114
Type of hepatectomy	Right	118
	Left	79
	Trisegmentectomy: Right/Left	10/11
	Other	2
Operative blood loss (mL); median: 1783	>1700	108
Operation time (min); median: 647	>660	154
Pancreaticoduodenectomy	Yes	30
Vascular combined resection	Hepatic artery	24
	Portal vein	118
Number of bile duct reconstructions; median: 3	≥3	139
Blood transfusion	Yes	84
Post-operative max AST (IU); median: 443	>440	110
Post-operative max ALT (IU); median: 372	>370	110
Platelet count (pre-operative period)	$<12 \times 10^4/\mu L$	6
Platelet count (post-operative day 1)	$<10 \times 10^4/\mu L$	30

BDC: extrahepatic cholangiocarcinoma, GBC: gallbladder cancer, ICC: intrahepatic cholangiocarcinoma, ICGR15: indocyanine green retention rate at 15 min, ENBD: endoscopic nasobiliary drainage, PTBD: percutaneous transhepatic biliary drainage, Right: right extended hepatectomy, Left: left extended hepatectomy, max: maximum, AST: aspartate aminotransferase, ALT: alanine aminotransferase.

Anastomotic insufficiency of the intrahepatic cholangiojejunostomy occurred in 13 (6%) of the 220 patients. Other post-operative complications are shown in Table 2. All instances of anastomotic leakage were treated conservatively, by maintenance of a drain that had been placed prophylactically near the cholangiojejunostomy during surgery. One patient died due to post-operative liver failure following anastomotic insufficiency.

Table 2 Postoperative complications

Postoperative complication	Number of subjects
Clavien-Dindo classification IIIa	74
IIIb	5
IVa	8
IVb	0
V	13
Liver failure	28
Anastomotic insufficiency of intrahepatic cholangiojejunostomy	13
Organ/space surgical-site infection	72
Vascular thrombosis	7
Liver abscess	7
Respiratory complications	2
Postoperative bleeding	15

Next, we investigated whether platelet depletion (to $<10 \times 10^4/\mu L$ on post-operative day (POD)1) was associated with anastomotic insufficiency. According to univariate analysis, platelet depletion was associated with anastomotic insufficiency ($p < 0.01$), but post-operative liver failure was not. Multivariate analyses revealed that platelet count $<10 \times 10^4/\mu L$ on POD1 was a significant predictor of anastomotic insufficiency. Vascular combined resection (portal vein and/or hepatic artery) was not associated with anastomotic insufficiency (Table 3).

Finally, we examined clinical factors correlated with platelet count $<10 \times 10^4/\mu L$ on POD1. According to univariate analysis, platelet counts $<10 \times 10^4/\mu L$ on POD1 were closely associated with pre-operative platelet count $<12 \times 10^4/\mu L$ (below the institutional lower limit of normal), operative blood loss >1700 mL, activated partial thromboplastin time (APTT) on POD1 > 40 s, and post-operative organ/space SSI. Among these clinical factors, pre-operative platelet count, operative blood loss, and APTT on POD1 were significant independent predictors of platelet count $<10 \times 10^4/\mu L$ on POD1 in multivariate analysis (Table 4).

We verified that patients with pre-operative platelet depletion did not show any significant differences in pre-operative liver functions (prothrombin time-international normalized ratio (PT-INR) or indocyanine green retention rate at 15 min (ICGR-15)). No patients with severe sepsis and platelet depletion underwent hepatectomy.

Discussion

This study found a 6% incidence of anastomotic insufficiency following intrahepatic cholangiojejunostomy and also revealed that post-operative platelet depletion (to $<10 \times 10^4/\mu L$ on POD1) might be associated with increased risk of anastomotic insufficiency.

The incidence of anastomotic insufficiency following intrahepatic cholangiojejunostomy is thought to be higher than that with hepaticojejunostomy. Nagino et al. proposed that this was because the bile duct is small and fragile, and multiple anastomoses are often necessary. However, their surgical results for intrahepatic cholangiojejunostomy were suitable, with an anastomotic insufficiency rate of 6.4% (3.6% in the later period with increased experience) [9]. Our operative results with intrahepatic cholangiojejunostomy (anastomotic insufficiency rate, 6%) also appear suitable. Furthermore, Nagino et al. suggested that intra-operative massive hemorrhage or patient age were more closely associated with anastomotic insufficiency than the number of bile ducts reconstructed [9].

The present study identified a different risk factor for anastomotic insufficiency: post-operative platelet depletion. Our data showed operative blood loss >1700 mL was associated with post-operative platelet depletion on univariate analysis (Table 4). Previous results from Nagino et al. that intra-operative massive hemorrhage was associated with anastomotic insufficiency might thus be explained by post-operative platelet depletion [9].

A potentially important determinant of anastomotic insufficiency due to poor wound healing is blood supply, which for the bile ducts are accomplished mainly by the arterial system. We hypothesize that concomitant hepatic artery resection and reconstruction might have been associated with anastomotic insufficiency of intrahepatic cholangiojejunostomy, because these cases had risk factors for thrombosis. Our series included no cases with hepatic artery obstruction in the post-operative period, and our data showed no correlation with hepatic artery combined resection or anastomotic insufficiency (Table 4).

Recent clinical studies have revealed that platelet depletion in the pre- and post-operative periods is associated with delayed liver regeneration [17], and the present data support this.

Alkozai et al. noted that patients with a low immediate post-operative platelet count ($<10 \times 10^4/\mu L$) displayed worse post-operative liver function. A low platelet count immediately post-operatively was identified as an independent risk factor for delayed post-operative recovery of liver function [17]. Liver regeneration means not only regeneration of hepatocytes, but also endothelial cells, Kupffer cells, and bile duct cells. Indeed, experimental evidence has suggested that bile duct cells regenerate along with other hepatocytes [20]. Post-operative platelet count may thus be directly related to recovery at the anastomotic site after intrahepatic cholangiojejunostomy.

The mechanism by which platelets participate in liver regeneration may work as follows: contact between platelets and hepatocytes initiates signal transduction involved in growth factor activation. Hepatocyte growth factor (HGF), vascular endothelial growth factor (VEGF), and insulin-like

Table 3 Possible risk factors for anastomotic insufficiency following intrahepatic cholangiojejunostomy

			Univariate analysis	Multivariate analysis		
Subject characteristics		**Anastomotic insufficiency (n =13)**	***P***	**Odds ratio**	**95% CI**	***P***
Age (years)	68 > (n =102)	7	*1*			
Sex	Male (n =146)	9	*1*			
	Female (n =74)	4				
BMI	<22 (n =109)	3	*0.083*			*NS*
	>25 (n =33)	1	*0.697*			
Diabetes mellitus	Positive (n =39)	2	*1*			
ICGR15 (%); median: 10	>10 (n =129)	8	*1*			
	>15 (n =38)	3	*0.475*			
Preoperative biliary drainage	ENBD (n =110)	4	*0.262*			
	PTBD (n =64)	6				
	None (n =46)	3				
Preoperative portal vein embolism	Yes (n = 114)	5	*0.396*			
Preoperative PT-INR; median: 1.1	>1.1 (n =75)	4	*1*			
Preoperative albumin (mg/dL)	<3.9 (n = 112)	7	*1*			
Type of hepatectomy	Left lobectomy (n =79)	6	*0.389*			
	Right lobectomy/ trisegmentectomy (n =139)	7				
	Other (n =2)	0				
PD	Yes (n =30)	0	*0.224*			
Operative blood loss (mL)	>1700 (n =108)	7	*0.781*			
	>3000 (n =34)	3	*0.429*			
	>5000 (n =13)	2	*0.174*			
Operation time (min)	>660 (n =103)	6	*1*			
Vascular combined resection	Hepatic artery (n =24)	2	*0.639*			
	PV (n =118)	7	*1*			
Number of bile duct reconstructions	≥3 (n =139)	9	*0.772*			
Postoperative max AST (IU)	>440 (n =110)	9	*0.251*			
Postoperative max ALT (IU)	>370 (n =110)	8	*0.569*			
Platelet count (POD1)	<10 x 10^4/μL (n =30)	5	*0.020*	3.63	1.15-13.01	*0.029*
PT-INR (POD1); median: 1.8	>1.8 (n =105)	5	*0.769*			
APTT (POD1); median: 40	>40 (n =107)	6	*1*			
Postoperative liver failure	Yes (n =28)	3	*0.198*			

BMI: body mass index, DM: diabetes mellitus, ENBD: endoscopic nasobiliary drainage, PTBD: percutaneous transhepatic biliary drainage, PT-INR: prothrombin time-international normalized ratio, PV: portal vein, ICGR: indocyanine green retention rate at 15 min, PD: pancreaticoduodenectomy, AST: aspartate amino transferase, ALT: alanine aminotransferase, POD: postoperative day, N.S: no statistically significant difference.

growth factor-1 were also found to contribute to hepatocyte proliferation [2].

Other recent experimental studies have concluded that platelets play an important role in not only liver regeneration, but also tissue repair mechanisms [21,22]. At least 60 different biologically active substances in platelets are involved in tissue-repair mechanisms such as chemotaxis, cell proliferation and differentiation, angiogenesis, intracellular matrix deposition, immune modulation, anti-micro-bial activity, and remodeling. Among these, growth factors (epidermal growth factor, platelet-derived growth factor, transforming growth factor alpha, and transforming growth factor beta) are thought to be the most important [22]. Platelet-rich plasma (PRP) has long been used as a source of platelet-related growth factors [21,22]. Several studies using animal models have shown that PRP

Table 4 Correlation between platelet depletion on POD1 and clinical characteristics

Subject characteristics		Platelet count (POD 1) <10 × 10^4/μL N =30	Univariate analysis *P*	Multivariate analysis Odds ratio	95% CI	*P*
Age (years)	>68	19	*0.553*			
BMI	<22	10	*0.116*			
Diabetes mellitus	Yes	8	*0.197*			
ICGR-15	>10%	21	*0.231*			
	>15%	7	*0.430*			
Pre-operative albumin (mg/dL)	<3.9	16	*0.845*			
Pre-operative platelet count	<12 × 10^4/μL	5	*<0.01*	34.7	3.16-380.2	*<0.01*
Preoperative Portal vein embolism	Yes	20	*0.716*			
Type of hepatectomy	Right/trisegmen-tectomy	21	*0.542*			
PD	Yes	3	*0.775*			
Operative blood loss (mL)	>1700	24	*<0.01*	5.24	1.69-16.2	*<0.01*
Operation time (min)	>660	21	*1*			
Concomitant resection	Hepatic artery	5	*0.339*			
	PV	12	*0.432*			
Number of bile duct reconstructions	>3	14	*0.065*	-	-	*N.S*
Postoperative AST (IU)	>370	15	*1*			
Postoperative ALT (IU)	>440	16	*0.844*			
PT-INR (POD1)	>1.8	18	*0.171*			
APTT (POD1)	>40	26	*<0.01*	5.31	1.71-16.46	*<0.01*
Organ/space SSI (n =30)	Yes	9	*<0.01*	-	-	*N.S*

POD1: post-operative day 1, BMI: body mass index, ICGR-15: indocyanine green retention rate at 15 min), PV: portal vein, Right: right extended hepatectomy, PD: pancreaticoduodenectomy, AST: aspartate amino transferase, ALT: alanine aminotransferase, PT-INR: prothrombin time-international normalized ratio, APTT: activated partial thromboplastin time, SSI: surgical-site infection, N.S: no statistically significant difference.

exerts positive effects on inflammation, remodeling, and increased vascularity after intestinal or bronchial anastomosis [28,29].

The above experimental evidence, along with clinical data (including the present findings), supports the hypothesis that post-operative platelet depletion is closely associated with anastomotic insufficiency following intrahepatic cholangiojejunostomy. Various mechanisms have been thought to be associated with post-operative platelet depletion. Post-operative platelet depletion was commonly attributed to severe systemic infection with disseminated intravascular coagulation or massive hemorrhage. Our data showed that infectious complications were not associated with post-operative platelet depletion (on multivariate analysis), and none of our patients showed sepsis during the early post-operative period (data not shown). Our data do not rule out the possibility that post-operative platelet depletion is associated with intra-operative hemorrhage.

A few limitations to this study must be considered when interpreting our findings. One problem was the limited number of patients with anastomotic insufficiency (n = 13), which rules out identification of strong correlations with any risk factor. A multi-institutional database would allow further discussion of the risk factors for anastomotic insufficiency after hepatic resection for cholangiocarcinoma. However, the present findings represent a first step toward such a multi-institutional study to clarify the risk factors for anastomotic insufficiency following intrahepatic cholangiojejunostomy.

Another problem was that our present study was limited by its retrospective design. We also cannot fully exclude the possibility that patients with a low platelet count on POD1 were simply in a worse general condition, and therefore showed delayed recovery of liver regeneration or a greater incidence of anastomotic insufficiency than patients with normal platelet counts. However, we could not identify any significant differences between patients with and without pre-operative platelet depletion in terms of pre-operative liver function (PT-INR or ICGR-15). The reasons for the association between pre-operative platelet depletion and anastomotic insufficiency following intrahepatic cholangiojejunostomy thus remain unclear. The point clearly identified by our data was that pre-operative platelet depletion and intra-operative massive hemorrhage were both closely associated with post-operative platelet depletion, and post-operative platelet depletion was a significant cause of anastomotic insufficiency following intrahepatic cholangiojejunostomy.

If platelet depletion was a significant cause of anastomotic insufficiency following intrahepatic cholangiojejunostomy, one potential strategy could be to deliberately increase the platelet count during the early post-operative period. However, the current findings should not be seen as a recommendation for more liberal use of platelet concentrates from blood donors, as several studies have shown that platelet transfusion is associated with increased risks of post-operative morbidity and mortality [30-32]. In contrast to endogenous platelets, platelets from blood donors are frequently in an activated state and may induce a range of inflammatory reactions and unwanted side effects [33,34]. New strategies for increasing platelet count safely or for the use of growth factors associated with wound healing and liver regeneration are thus needed. One possible strategy is the use of PRP to decrease anastomotic insufficiency. However, before clinical applications can be seriously contemplated, further investigation is needed to clarify whether PRP is useful for reducing the incidence of anastomotic insufficiency following intrahepatic cholangiojejunostomy. Given our findings and the results from Nagino et al., minimizing intra-operative hemorrhage is important [9].

Conclusion

The incidence of anastomotic insufficiency following intrahepatic cholangiojejunostomy was 6% in this single, high-volume center experience.

Post-operative platelet depletion (to $<10 \times 10^4/\mu L$ on POD1) was associated with anastomotic insufficiency following intrahepatic cholangiojejunostomy, but further experimental and clinical studies are needed to elucidate the underlying mechanisms and clarify correlations between platelet count and intrahepatic cho langiojejunostomy.

Competing interests

The authors declare that they have no competing interests.

Authors' contribution

TN and TT participated in the design of the study, performed the statistical analysis, and wrote all parts of the manuscript. YE, TN, KK, JM, and TS participated in coordination and helped to draft the manuscript. ET and SH performed most of the surgery in this series, participated in the design, and also helped to draft the manuscript. All authors read and approved the final manuscript.

Acknowledgement

The authors wish to thank all the members of Gastroenterological Surgery II, Hokkaido University Hospital for their clinical assistance.

References

1. Hasegawa S, Ikai I, Fujii H, Hatano E, Shimahara Y: Surgical resection of hilar cholangiocarcinoma: analysis of survival and postoperative complications. *World J Surg* 2007, **31**(6):1256–1263.
2. Matsuo K, Rocha FG, Ito K, D'Angelica MI, Allen PJ, Fong Y, Dematteo RP, Gonen M, Endo I, Jarnagin WR: The Blumgart preoperative staging system for hilar cholangiocarcinoma: analysis of resectability and outcomes in 380 patients. *J Am Coll Surg* 2012, **215**(3):343–355.
3. Igami T, Nishio H, Ebata T, Yokoyama Y, Sugawara G, Nimura Y, Nagino M: Surgical treatment of hilar cholangiocarcinoma in the "new era": the Nagoya University experience. *J Hepatobiliary Pancreat Sci* 2010, **17**(4):449–454.
4. Otani K, Chijiiwa K, Kai M, Ohuchida J, Nagano M, Tsuchiya K, Kondo K: Outcome of surgical treatment of hilar cholangiocarcinoma. *J Gastrointest Surg* 2008, **12**(6):1033–1040.
5. Silva MA, Tekin K, Aytekin F, Bramhall SR, Buckels JA, Mirza DF: Surgery for hilar cholangiocarcinoma; a 10 year experience of a tertiary referral centre in the UK. *Eur J Surg Oncol* 2005, **31**(5):533–539.
6. Ohtsuka M, Ito H, Kimura F, Shimizu H, Togawa A, Yoshidome H, Shimamura F, Shimizu Y, Miyazaki M: Extended hepatic resection and outcomes in intrahepatic cholangiocarcinoma. *J Hepatobiliary Pancreat Surg* 2003, **10**(4):259–264.
7. Hirano S, Kondo S, Tanaka E, Shichinohe T, Tsuchikawa T, Kato K, Matsumoto J, Kawasaki R: Outcome of surgical treatment of hilar cholangiocarcinoma: a special reference to postoperative morbidity and mortality. *J Hepatobiliary Pancreat Sci* 2010, **17**(4):455–462.
8. Antolovic D, Koch M, Galindo L, Wolff S, Music E, Kienle P, Schemmer P, Friess H, Schmidt J, Buchler MW, Weitz J: Hepaticojejunostomy–analysis of risk factors for postoperative bile leaks and surgical complications. *J Gastrointest Surg* 2007, **11**(5):555–561.
9. Nagino M, Nishio H, Ebata T, Yokoyama Y, Igami T, Nimura Y: Intrahepatic cholangiojejunostomy following hepatobiliary resection. *Br J Surg* 2007, **94**(1):70–77.
10. Miyazaki M, Ito H, Nakagawa K, Ambiru S, Shimizu H, Shimizu Y, Kato A, Nakamura S, Omoto H, Nakajima N, Kimura F, Suwa T: Aggressive surgical approaches to hilar cholangiocarcinoma: hepatic or local resection? *Surgery* 1998, **123**(2):131–136.
11. Ferrero A, Russolillo N, Vigano L, Sgotto E, Lo Tesoriere R, Amisano M, Capussotti L: Safety of conservative management of bile leakage after hepatectomy with biliary reconstruction. *J Gastrointest Surg* 2008, **12**(12):2204–2211.
12. de Castro SM, Kuhlmann KF, Busch OR, van Delden OM, Lameris JS, van Gulik TM, Obertop H, Gouma DJ: Incidence and management of biliary leakage after hepaticojejunostomy. *J Gastrointest Surg* 2005, **9**(8):1163–1171. discussion 1171–1163.
13. Murata S, Hashimoto I, Nakano Y, Myronovych A, Watanabe M, Ohkohchi N: Single administration of thrombopoietin prevents progression of liver fibrosis and promotes liver regeneration after partial hepatectomy in cirrhotic rats. *Ann Surg* 2008, **248**(5):821–828.
14. Murata S, Matsuo R, Ikeda O, Myronovych A, Watanabe M, Hisakura K, Nakano Y, Hashimoto I, Ohkohchi N: Platelets promote liver regeneration under conditions of Kupffer cell depletion after hepatectomy in mice. *World J Surg* 2008, **32**(6):1088–1096.
15. Tomikawa M, Hashizume M, Highashi H, Ohta M, Sugimachi K: The role of the spleen, platelets, and plasma hepatocyte growth factor activity on hepatic regeneration in rats. *J Am Coll Surg* 1996, **182**(1):12–16.
16. Lesurtel M, Graf R, Aleil B, Walther DJ, Tian Y, Jochum W, Gachet C, Bader M, Clavien PA: Platelet-derived serotonin mediates liver regeneration. *Science* 2006, **312**(5770):104–107.
17. Alkozai EM, Nijsten MW, de Jong KP, de Boer MT, Peeters PM, Slooff MJ, Porte RJ, Lisman T: Immediate postoperative low platelet count is associated with delayed liver function recovery after partial liver resection. *Ann Surg* 2010, **251**(2):300–306.
18. Taketomi A, Kitagawa D, Itoh S, Harimoto N, Yamashita Y, Gion T, Shirabe K, Shimada M, Maehara Y: Trends in morbidity and mortality after hepatic resection for hepatocellular carcinoma: an institute's experience with 625 patients. *J Am Coll Surg* 2007, **204**(4):580–587.
19. Poon RT, Fan ST, Lo CM, Liu CL, Lam CM, Yuen WK, Yeung C, Wong J: Improving perioperative outcome expands the role of hepatectomy in management of benign and malignant hepatobiliary diseases: analysis

of 1222 consecutive patients from a prospective database. *Ann Surg* 2004, **240**(4):698–708. discussion 708–610.
20. Clavien PA, Petrowsky H, DeOliveira ML, Graf R: **Strategies for safer liver surgery and partial liver transplantation.** *N Engl J Med* 2007, **356**(15):1545–1559.
21. Anitua E, Andia I, Ardanza B, Nurden P, Nurden AT: **Autologous platelets as a source of proteins for healing and tissue regeneration.** *Thromb Haemost* 2004, **91**(1):4–15.
22. Rozman P, Bolta Z: **Use of platelet growth factors in treating wounds and soft-tissue injuries.** *Acta Dermatovenerol Alp Panonica Adriat* 2007, **16**(4):156–165.
23. Hasegawa Y, Abo D, Sakuhara Y, Kato F, Kamishimma T, Shimizu T, Ito YM, Terae S, Shirato H: **Usefulness of portography and contrast-enhanced computed tomography to predict the embolized area in percutaneous transhepatic portal vein embolization with absolute ethanol under temporary balloon occlusion.** *Jpn J Radiol* 2012, **30**(1):53–61.
24. Ttcot IHPBA: **The Brisbane 2000 terminology of hepatic anatomy and resections.** *HPB Surgery* 2000, **2**:333–339.
25. Hirano S, Tanaka E, Tsuchikawa T, Matsumoto J, Shichinohe T, Kato K: **Techniques of biliary reconstruction following bile duct resection (with video).** *J Hepatobiliary Pancreat Sci* 2012, **19**(3):203–209.
26. Dindo D, Demartines N, Clavien PA: **Classification of surgical complications: a new proposal with evaluation in a cohort of 6336 patients and results of a survey.** *Ann Surg* 2004, **240**(2):205–213.
27. Rahbari NN, Garden OJ, Padbury R, Brooke-Smith M, Crawford M, Adam R, Koch M, Makuuchi M, Dematteo RP, Christophi C, Banting S, Usatoff V, Nagino M, Maddern G, Hugh TJ, Vauthey JN, Greig P, Rees M, Yokoyama Y, Fan ST, Nimura Y, Figueras J, Capussotti L, Büchler MW, Weitz J: **Posthepatectomy liver failure: a definition and grading by the International Study Group of Liver Surgery (ISGLS).** *Surgery* 2011, **149**(5):713–724.
28. Yol S, Tekin A, Yilmaz H, Kucukkartallar T, Esen H, Caglayan O, Tatkan Y: **Effects of platelet rich plasma on colonic anastomosis.** *J Surg Res* 2008, **146**(2):190–194.
29. Gomez-Caro A, Ausin P, Boada M: **Platelet rich plasma improves the healing process after airway anastomosis.** *Interact Cardiovasc Thorac Surg* 2011, **13**(6):552–556.
30. de Boer MT, Christensen MC, Asmussen M, van der Hilst CS, Hendriks HG, Slooff MJ, Porte RJ: **The impact of intraoperative transfusion of platelets and red blood cells on survival after liver transplantation.** *Anesth Analg* 2008, **106**(1):32–44. table of contents.
31. Spiess BD: **Transfusion of blood products affects outcome in cardiac surgery.** *Semin Cardiothorac Vasc Anesth* 2004, **8**(4):267–281.
32. Pereboom IT, Lisman T, Porte RJ: **Platelets in liver transplantation: friend or foe?** *Liver Transpl* 2008, **14**(7):923–931.
33. Cognasse F, Boussoulade F, Chavarin P, Acquart S, Fabrigli P, Lamy B, Garraud O: **Release of potential immunomodulatory factors during platelet storage.** *Transfusion* 2006, **46**(7):1184–1189.
34. Khan SY, Kelher MR, Heal JM, Blumberg N, Boshkov LK, Phipps R, Gettings KF, McLaughlin NJ, Silliman CC: **Soluble CD40 ligand accumulates in stored blood components, primes neutrophils through CD40, and is a potential cofactor in the development of transfusion-related acute lung injury.** *Blood* 2006, **108**(7):2455–2462.

16

The effect of ursodeoxycholic acid in liver functional restoration of patients with obstructive jaundice after endoscopic treatment

Enver Fekaj[1*], Arben Gjata[2] and Mehmet Maxhuni[1]

Abstract

Background: In patients with obstructive jaundice, multi-organ dysfunction may develop.

Methods/Design: This trial is a prospective, open-label, randomized, and controlled study with the objective to evaluate the effect of ursodeoxycholic acid in liver functional restoration in patients with obstructive jaundice after endoscopic treatment. The aim of this study is to evaluate the effect of ursodeoxycholic acid in liver functional restoration of patients with obstructive jaundice after endoscopic treatment. The hypothesis of this trial is that patients with obstructive jaundice, in which will be administered UDCA, in the early phase after endoscopic intervention will have better and faster functional restoration of the liver than patients in the control group. Patients with obstructive jaundice, randomly, will be divided into two groups: (A) test group in which will be administered ursodeoxycholic acid twenty-four hours after endoscopic procedure and will last fourteen days, and (B) control group.
Serum-testing will include determination of bilirubin, alanine transaminase, aspartate transaminase, gama-glutamil transpeptidase, alkaline phosphatase, albumin, and cholesterol levels. These parameters will be determined one day prior endoscopic procedure, and on the third, fifth, seventh, tenth, twelfth and fourteenth days after endoscopic intervention.

Discussion: This trial is a prospective, open-label, randomized, and controlled study to asses the effect of ursodeoxycholic acid in liver functional restoration of patients with obstructive jaundice in the early phase after endoscopic treatment.

Keywords: Obstructive jaundice, Ursodeoxycholic acid, Treatment with ursodeoxycholic acid

Background

The most common causes of obstructive jaundice are choledocholithiasis, strictures of the biliary tract, cholangiocarcinoma, carcinoma of pancreas, and pancreatitis.

First-line serum testing in a patient with obstructive jaundice should include determination of bilirubin (total and direct fractions), aspartate transaminase (AST), alanine transaminase (ALT), gama-glutamil transpeptidase, and alkaline phosphatase levels [1].

In a prolonged obstruction, multi-organ dysfunction including renal failure, cardiac dysfunction, pulmonary dysfunction, poor hepatic metabolism and hemostasis impairment may develop [2].

It is the conventional concept that the high level of serum bilirubin may cause multisystemic damage in patients with obstructive jaundice. Current pathophysiological studies on obstructive jaundice have shown that the damage to the liver, kidney, and immune system of the patients are closely related to endotoxemia. The key

* Correspondence: enverfekaj@hotmail.com
[1]Department of Abdominal Surgery, University Clinical Centre of Kosovo, Rrethi i Spitalit, str: p.n., Pristina 10000, Republic of Kosovo
Full list of author information is available at the end of the article

event in the pathophysiology of obstructive jaundice-associated complications is endotoxemia of gut origin because of intestinal barriere failure.

Biliary tract obstruction can cause damage to liver cells and Kupffer cell function. In obstructive jaundice hyper secretion of TNF (tumour necrosis factor) by Kupffer cells may support the production of systemic cytokine and be responsible for significant complications [3-5].

Patients with obstructive jaundice frequently suffer haemodynamic and body fluid disturbances. Acute renal failure is a relevant complication in obstructive jaundice. The extra cellular water volume depletion and myocardial dysfunction affects haemodynamic and renal disturbance in patients with obstructive jaundice [6].

Experimental and clinical studies have suggested that a period of at least four to six weeks is needed for the restoration of normal major synthetic and clearance functions of the liver, as well as mucosal intestinal barrier functions [7].

Even though there is a general assumption about the increased bleeding tendency in obstructive jaundiced patients, it was demonstrated tendency for hyper coagulation independent of increased prothrombin times. The most probable cause of this effect is the increased activity of fibrin polymers on platelet membrane [8].

It is important to emphasize that the most patients with obstructive jaundice require appropriate endoscopic and surgical procedures for their treatment [1].

There are a many studies, where ursodeoxycholic acid (UDCA) was administrated in patients with cholestatic liver diseases.

UDCA was discovered, by Hammerstein in 1902, as the principal bile acid in the polar bear [9].

It is used for the dissolution of cholesterol-rich gallstones in patients with functioning gallbladders, and in the treatment of primary biliary cirrhosis [10,11].

Mechanisms underlying the beneficial therapeutic effects of UDCA on cholestatic liver diseases include: 1) protection of injured cholangiocytes against toxic effects of bile acids, 2) stimulation of impaired biliary secretion, 3) protection of hepatocytes against bile acid-induced apoptosis, 4) immunomodulatory properties with reduce immune-related liver damage [12-15].

In current literature, there are no a randomized, controlled trials testing the effect of UDCA in liver functional restoration of patients with obstructive jaundice after endoscopic treatment.

Hypothesis

The hypothesis of this trial is that patients with obstructive jaundice, in which will be administered UDCA, in the early phase after endoscopic intervention will have better and faster functional restoration of the liver than patients in the control group.

Aim and purpose of the research

General aim

The aim of this study is to evaluate the effect of UDCA in liver functional restoration of patients with obstructive jaundice in the early period after endoscopic intervention.

Specific aims

Specific aims are:

- To evaluate the effect of UDCA in relation to the aetiology of obstructive jaundice.
- To assess that in which functional parameters of the liver, treatment with UDCA will have greater impact.

Methods/Design

Study objectives

This trial will be a prospective, open-label, randomized, and controlled study. The objective will be to evaluate the effect of ursodeoxycholic acid (UDCA) in the functional restoration of the liver in patients with obstructive jaundice in the early post-endoscopic phase.

Study design

After diagnosis, patients with obstructive jaundice will be divided into two groups: (A) the test group in which will be administered UDCA in the early phase after endoscopic treatment, and (B) control group, in which no treatment will be applied with UDCA.

Diagnostic methods will be biochemical findings, ultrasound examination, endoscopic retrograde cholangio pancreatography (ERCP), CT-scan and magnetic resonance cholangio pancreatography (MRCP).

Serum-testing in patients with obstructive jaundice will include determination of bilirubin (total and direct fractions), alanine transaminase (ALT), aspartate transaminase (AST), gama-glutamil transpeptidase (GGT), alkaline phosphatase, albumin, and cholesterol levels. These parameters will be determined one day prior endoscopic intervention, and on the third, fifth, seventh, tenth, twelfth and fourteenth days after endoscopic intervention.

Endoscope procedure that will end with the internal derivation of bile shall be named as the internal bile drainage.

Inclusion criteria are:

- Patients with obstructive jaundice
- Serum bilirubin level higher than 50 μmol/l
- 19+ years of age
- Written informed consent

Exclusion criteria are:

- Cholangitis
- Acute pancreatitis
- Pregnant women
- Women during the breastfeeding
- Suspected or proven primary liver diseases
- My family members
- Patients who are unable to understand our study purpose

During our trial, from the study will be excluded patients who show signs of serious side effects and allergic reactions after treatment with UDCA.

UDCA administration

UDCA administration will begin twenty-four hours after endoscopic procedure and will last fourteen days. UDCA dose will be administered at 750 mg/day, divided into three doses.

Power of the study

A clinically relevant improvement of liver functional tests is defined as an improvement of 70% of liver functional tests in test group, and an improvement only 40% in control group. In our study, to have an 80% chance of detecting about a 40% difference (70% vs. 40%) between two groups on improvement of liver functional tests at an alpha level of 0.05, the power calculation indicates that each of the two groups should have at least 48 patients.

Data sources and search strategy

An electronic search was performed on PubMed (from 1 January 1985 to 1 February 2012). A combination of keywords and MeSH terms where: 'ursodeoxycholic acid' AND 'obstructive jaundice', 'obstructive jaundice' AND 'liver function tests', 'obstructive jaundice' AND 'acute renal failure'. I have used, also, limits: Type of article (selection was- clinical trial, meta-analyses), Species (selection was- human, animals), Text options (selection was- links to free full text, abstract), Languages (English), Sex (male, female), Age (all adult 19+ years), Field (all fields).

Outcomes

The primary outcome measure in this trial is liver functional restoration. The secondary outcome is assessment liver functional parameters in which, treatment with UDCA, will have greater impact. Follow-up measures will be collected one day prior endoscopic intervention, and on the third, fifth, seventh, tenth, twelfth and fourteenth days after endoscopic intervention.

Randomisation

Patients have to sign an informed consent for the involving in the trial a day before endoscopic procedure. Randomisation will be performed at the time of transfer to the endoscope room by using random number generator at http://www.stattrek.com.

Ethics

This study will be conducted in accordance with the principles of the Declaration of Helsinki. The study protocol has been approved by Ethics and Professional Committee at University Clinical Centre of Kosovo. Informed consent will be obtained from all participants.

Data collection and statistical analyses

Data including serum-test results will be collected in a computer secured study platform. These data will be collected continuously, for each patient, starting one day before endoscopic procedure until the last data fourteen days after intervention.

X^2-analysis or Fisher exact test will perform to test the differences in proportions of qualitative variables between groups. Mann Whitney U test and Kruskal Wallis test will use for testing the difference between quantitative variables when distribution is not normal and Student t-test or ANOVA test when distribution is normal. The level $P < 0.05$ will consider as the cut-off value for significance.

Discussion

In many studies, it was shown the positive effect of UDCA administration in patient with cholestatic liver desease.

UDCA exerts anti-apoptic effects in experimental in vivo models as well as in vitro in primary human hepatocytes. This anti-apoptic effect may contribute to the alleviation of liver injury during UDCA treatment [16].

After UDCA administration in patients with non-alcoholic fatty liver disease, the results show that UDCA is able to reduce serum levels of hepatic enzymes, but this effect is not related to modifications in liver fat content [17].

The study by Willot S, demonstrates the beneficial effect of UDCA on liver function in children after successful surgery for biliary atresia [18].

UDCA in a dose of 13–15 mg\kg\day should be considered in all patients with primary biliary cirrhosis who have abnormal liver enzymes [19].

Long-term high-dose UDCA therapy is associated with improvement in serum liver tests in primary sclerosing cholangitis, but does not improve survival and was associated with higher rates of serious adverse events [20].

UDCA administration can be considered in cases of nodular regenerative hyperplasia of the liver associated with abnormalities of liver enzymes [21].

It seems that combined therapy with UDCA and polyunsaturated phosphatidylcholine could be considered in obstetric cholestasis [22].

It was demonstrated that ciprofloxacin and UDCA have a synergic effect on prevention of bacterial translocation in obstructive jaundiced patients [23].

This trial is a prospective, open-label, randomized, and controlled study with the objective to evaluate the effect of ursodeoxycholic acid in liver functional restoration in patients with obstructive jaundice after endoscopic treatment. The hypothesis of this trial is that patients with obstructive jaundice, in which will be administered UDCA, in the early phase after endoscopic intervention will have better and faster functional restoration of the liver than patients in the control group.

Abbreviations

TNF: Tumour necrosis factor; UDCA: Ursodeoxycholic acid; ERCP: Endoscopic retrograde cholang o pancreatography; CT: Computerized tomography; MRCP: Magnetic resonance cholangio pancreatography; ALT: Alanine transaminase; AST: Aspartate transaminase; GGT: Gama-glutamil transpeptidase; HCV: Hepatitis C virus.

Competing interests

The authors declare that they have no competing interests. This study has not received external funding.

Authors' contributions

EF wrote the manuscript and designed the study. AGJ revised the manuscript and co-authored the writing of the manuscript. MM revised the manuscript. All authors have read and approved the final manuscript.

Acknowledgements

We thank Sanie Gashi for her contribution to design the section "Data collection and statistical analyses".

Author details

[1]Department of Abdominal Surgery, University Clinical Centre of Kosovo, Rrethi i Spitalit, str: p.n., Pristina 10000, Republic of Kosovo. [2]Department of Surgery, University Clinical Centre, "Nene Tereza", Rruga Dibres 370, Tirana, Albania.

References

1. Roche SP, Kobos R: **Jaundice in the adult patient.** *Am Fam Physician* 2004, **69**(2):299–304.
2. Rerknimitr R, Kullavanijaya P: **Operable malignant jaundice: To stent or not to stent before the operation?** *World J Gastrointest Endosc* 2010, **2**(1):10–14.
3. Yi-Jun Y, Jing-Sen SH, Shu-Min X, De-Ting ZH, Bing-Sheng C: **Effects of different drainage procedures on levels of serum endotoxin and tumor necrosis factor in patients with malignant obstructive jaundice.** *HBPD Int* 2003, **2**:426–430.
4. Scott-Conner CE, Grogan JB: **The pathophysiology of biliary obstruction and its effect on phagocytic and immune function.** *J Surg Res* 1994, **57**(2):316–336.
5. Assimakopoulos SF, Scopa CD, Vaginos CE: **Pathophysiology of increased intestinal permeability in obstructive jaundice.** *World J Gastroenterol* 2007, **13**(48):6458–6464.
6. Naranjo A, Cruz A, Lopez P, Chicano M, Martin-Malo A, Sitger-Serra A, Muntane J, Padillo J: **Renal function after dopamine and fluid administration in patients with malignant obstructive jaundice. A prospective randomized study.** *J Gastrointestin Liver Dis* 2011, **20**(2):161–167.
7. Van der Gaag NA, Rauws EAJ, Van Eijek CHJ, Maro JB, Van der Harst E, Kubben FJ, Gerritsen JJ, Greve JW, Gerhards MF, de Hingh IH, Klinkenbijl JH, Nio CY, de Castro SM, Busch OR, van Gulik TM, Bossuyt PM, Gouma DJ: **Preoperative biliary drainage for cancer of the head of the pancreas.** *N Engl J Med* 2010, **362**:129–137.
8. Cakir T, Cingi A, Yegen C: **Coagulation dynamics and platelet functions in obstructive jaundiced patients.** *J Gastroenterol Hepatol* 2009, **24**(5):748–751.
9. Fromm H: **Gallstone dissolution and the cholesterol-bile acid-lipoprotein axis: Propitious effects of ursodeoxycholic acid.** *Gastroenterology* 1984, **87**:229–233.
10. Bachrach WH, Hofmann AF: **Ursodeoxycholic acid in the treatment of cholesterol cholelithiasis.** *Part II Dig Dis Sci* 1982, **27**:833–856.
11. Parfitt K: *MARTINDALE, The complete drug reference*, Volume 32. London: Pharmaceutical Press; 1999. p. 1642.
12. Paumgartner G, Beuers U: **Mechanisms of action and therapeutic efficacy of ursodeoxycholic acid in cholestatic liver disease.** *Clin Liver Dis* 2004, **8**:67–81.
13. Kowdley KV: **Ursodeoxycholic acid therapy in hepatobiliary disease.** *Am J Med* 2000, **108**:481–486.
14. Hempfling W, Dilger K, Beuers U: **Systematic review: ursodeoxycholic acid—adverse effects and drug interactions.** *Aliment Pharmacol Ther* 2003, **18**(10):963–972.
15. Copaci I, Micu L, Iliescu L, Voiculesku M: **New therapeutical indications of ursodeoxycholic acid.** *Roman J Gastroenterol* 2005, **14**(3):259–266.
16. Hohenester S, Ronald PJ, Elferink O, Beuers U: **Primary biliary cirrhosis.** *Semin Immunopathol* 2009, **31**(3):283–307.
17. Santos VN, Lanzoni VP, Szejnfeld J, Shigueoka D, Parise ER: **A randomized double-blind study of the short-time treatment of obese patients with nonalcoholic fatty liver disease with ursodeoxycholic acid.** *Braz J Med Biol Res* 2003, **36**(6):723–729.
18. Willot S, Uhlen S, Michaud L, Briand G, Bonnevalle M, Sfeir R, Gottrand F: **Effect of ursodeoxycholic acid on liver function in children after successful surgery for biliary atresia.** *Pediatrics* 2008, **122**(6):1236–1241.
19. Abbas G, Lindor KD: **Pharmacological treatment of biliary cirrhosis with ursodeoxycholic acid.** *Expert Opin Pharmacother* 2010, **11**(3):387–392.
20. Lindor KD, Kowdley KV, Luketic VA, Harrison ME, McCashland T, Befeler AS, Harnois D, Jorgensen R, Petz J, Keach J, Mooney J, Sargeant C, Braaten J, Bernard T, King D, Miceli E, Schmoll J, Hoskin T, Thapa P, Enders F: **High dose ursodeoxycholic acid for the treatment of primary sclerosing cholangitis.** *Hepatology* 2009, **50**(3):808–814.
21. Ranucci G, Cirillo F, Corte CD, Vecchione R, Vallone G, Iorio R: **Successful use of ursodeoxycholic acid in nodular regenerative hyperplasia of the liver.** *Ann Pharmacother* 2011, **45**(4):20.
22. Marciniak B, Kimber-Trojnar Z, Leszezynska-Gorzelak B, Patro-Malysza J, Trojnar M, Oleszezuk J: **Treatment of obstetric cholestasis with polyunsaturated phosphatidylcholine and ursodeoxycholic acid.** *Ginekol Pol* 2011, **82**(1):26–31.
23. Kaya O, Ozdemir F, Atli M, Aslan V, Cagatay M, Anlar M, Alper M: **The effects of ciprofloxacine and ursodeoxycholic acid on bacterial translocation in obstructive jaundice.** *Turk J Gastroenterol* 2009, **20**(3):186–191.

17

Surgical anatomy of the right hepatic artery in Rouviere's sulcus evaluated by preoperative multidetector-row CT images

Shuichi Aoki[1], Masamichi Mizuma[1*], Hiroki Hayashi[1], Kei Nakagawa[1], Takanori Morikawa[1], Fuyuhiko Motoi[1], Takeshi Naitoh[1], Shinichi Egawa[2] and Michiaki Unno[1]

Abstract

Background: Lymph node dissection in Rouviere's sulcus (RS) is essential during left-sided hepatectomy and caudate lobectomy for hilar cholangiocarcinoma. However, the small segmental or subsegmental arteries (SA/SSA) are often encountered in RS and must be preserved to prevent critical complications, such as liver infarction or liver failure. The aim of this study is to elucidate the anatomy of SA/SSA around RS, which should be understood preoperatively.

Methods: Between January 2008 and April 2013 from a total of 124 consecutive patients with hilar cholangiocarcinoma, preoperative multidetector-row computed tomography (MDCT) images were obtained at our institution and evaluated. The bifurcation patterns of the SA/SSA, the courses of the posterior SA/SSA and the bifurcation site of the SA/SSA were investigated using MDCT images.

Results: The typical form, in which right hepatic artery (RHA) bifurcated into the anterior (Aant) and posterior (Apost) hepatic artery and thereafter, Aant/Apost bifurcated into the SA and SSA, was observed in 75 patients (60.5 %). On the other hand, the atypical forms, in which the SA/SSA were independently branched off from RHA before the main bifurcation of the Aant and Apost, were observed in 43 patients (34.7 %). The prior branched arteries supplied the whole or ventral area of segment VI (A6 or A6a) in 11 patients (8.9 %), which was most commonly observed in the atypical form. 15 patients (34.9 %) of the 43 patients with atypical form had partially supraportal posterior branches, that showed early-bifurcated posterior SA/SAA following supraportal course, while the other posterior SA/SSA followed infraportal course. The SA/SSA were extrahepatically bifurcated in 82 patients (66.1 %), comprised of all 43 atypical form and 39 of typical form, while the SA/SSA were intrahepatically bifurcated in remaining 36 patients of typical forms (29.0 %).

Conclusion: The extrahepatic bifurcation of the SA/SSA from RHA was relatively common. The early-bifurcated SA/SSA was often observed (34.7 % of total cohort) and, in 34.8 % of those atypical forms, posterior SA/SSA from RHA followed a supraportal course. The detailed preoperative knowledge of the anatomy, including SA/SSA, is crucial for left-sided hepatectomy for hilar cholangiocarcinoma.

Keywords: Right hepatic arteries, Cholangiocarcinoma, Postoperative complications

* Correspondence: masamichi@surg1.med.tohoku.ac.jp
[1]Department of Surgery, Tohoku University Graduate School of Medicine, Aobaku, Sendai, Japan
Full list of author information is available at the end of the article

Background

Left-sided hepatectomy with caudate lobectomy is ordinarily applied for patients with Bismuth type IIIb hilar cholangiocarcinoma. In recent years, even if a Bismuth type IIIb tumor extends to the right-side hilum involving the right hepatic artery (RHA), long-term survival after left hepatectomy or trisectionectomy with concomitant arterial resection and reconstruction has been reported [1–3]. However, this surgical technique is still extremely difficult and has a high risk for postoperative complications. To understand thoroughly the surgical anatomy around Rouviere's sulcus (RS) is pivotal for lymph node dissection and arterial reconstruction in left-sided hepatectomy for hilar cholangiocarcinoma.

In RS, located at the boundary between the caudate lobe and the right hepatic lobe, the branches from the right hepatic artery, right portal vein and right hepatic bile duct run into the liver parenchyma. In general, RHA is bifurcated from the proper hepatic artery (primary bifurcation) and, thereafter, bifurcates into the anterior (Aant) and posterior (Apost) hepatic artery immediately before entering into the liver parenchyma (secondary bifurcation). Then, segmental (SA) or subsegmental arteries (SSA) from Aant or Apost are bifurcated within the liver parenchyma (tertiary bifurcation). However, SA or SSA is often atypically branched off from the RHA. In addition, the posterior SA or SSA occasionally run cranially to the right portal vein (RPV) (supraportal course), although Apost typically runs caudally to RPV (infraportal course) [4]. Thus, the branching form of the arteries around RS is complicated. The preoperative understanding of anatomical variation of the SA/SSA branches and course variations of the arterial posterior branches around RS, especially the supraportal/infraportal posterior SA/SSA, is crucial in left-sided hepatectomy for hilar cholangiocarcinoma in order to avoid critical surgical complications, such as intraoperative arterial injury, hepatic infarction and hepatic failure. However, there have been few reports that provide a detailed discussion about the anatomical variation of SA/SSA in RS from the standpoint of surgical resection.

The objective of this study is to elucidate the bifurcation patterns of the SA/SSA using multidetector-row computed tomography (MDCT). We clarified the incidence of early-bifurcated SA/SSA around RS, the variations in the courses they followed. The findings of this study should be helpful for left-sided hepatectomy for hilar cholangiocarcinoma.

Methods

Patients

Between January 2008 and April 2013, 124 consecutive patients with hilar cholangiocarcinoma who underwent preoperative MDCT and received surgical resection at our institution were examined. The bifurcation pattern and the course of SA/SSA from RHA around RS were evaluated using preoperative MDCT. This study was approved by the institutional review board of Tohoku University, which waived the need for consent because this study was a retrospective study using enhanced CT images obtained during usual clinical examinations under written consent from all of the patients.

MDCT imaging

MDCT is the gold standard for imaging the anatomy of the hilar vessels and assessment of the cancer progression. The 64-row MDCT (Toshiba) was performed in all patients except for those allergic to iodine contrast medium prior to the biliary drainage. In cases in which the patients had already received biliary intervention at another institution, MDCT imaging was evaluated at our institution immediately after referral. Images were taken prior to injection and at 20 s (early arterial phase); 40 s (late arterial phase); 70 s (portal phase); and 120 s (delayed phase) after injection of a nonionic contrast agent (300 mg/ml) at a rate of 4 ml/h. In addition to axial images, multi planar reformation (MPR) images were routinely obtained using OsiriX® medical imaging software (open source software, http://www.osirix-viewer.com/). Three-dimensional (3D) images of the arteries and portal vein were prepared by a volume-rendering method to improve understanding of vascular relationships.

Bifurcation pattern of the SA/SSA from RHA

RHA typically bifurcates into Aant and Apost and, thereafter, Aant/Apost bifurcates into the SA and SSA, defined as the typical form. SA/SSA, such as the artery to segment VI (A6) or the artery to the ventral area of VI (A6a), often branch off separately before the main bifurcation into the Aant and Apost, classified as the atypical form (Figs. 1 and 2). The bifurcation patterns of the SA/SSA from RHA, comprised of typical and atypical forms, were evaluated. Moreover, the course patterns of the posterior SA/SSA around the RPV, namely supraportal or infraportal [4], were investigated.

To examine whether SA/SSA bifurcated inside or outside the liver, the cohort was separated into the two groups, "extrahepatic type" and "intrahepatic type" (Figs. 3 and 4). "Extrahepatic type" was defined as a bifurcation of the SA/SSA that showed no direct contact with the hepatic parenchyma in MDCT. On the other hand, contact between the bifurcation and the hepatic parenchyma or the bifurcation inside the hepatic parenchyma was designated as the "intrahepatic type". The

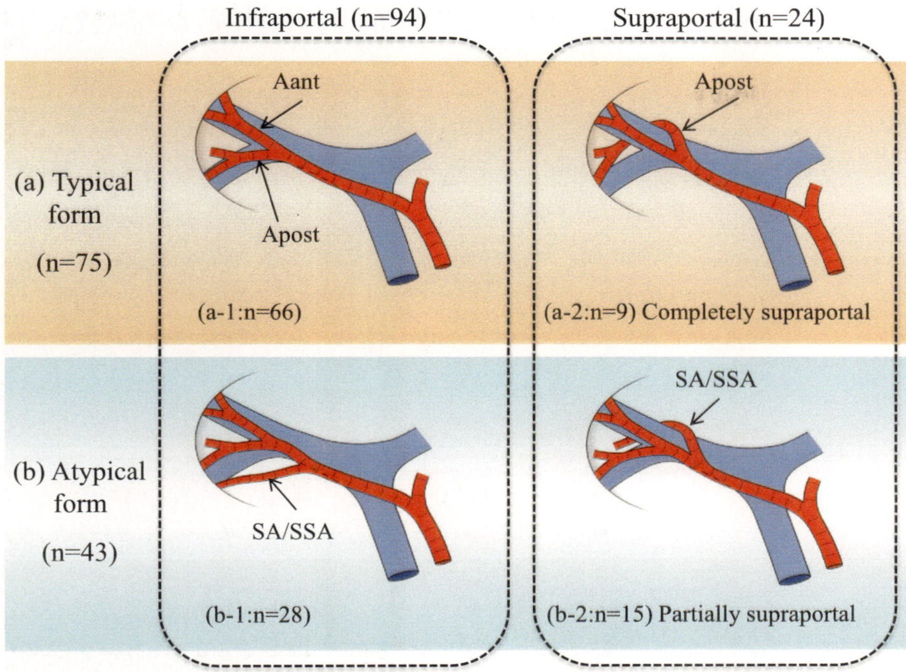

Fig. 1 Arterial anatomy of SA/SSA from RHA around the RS. **a** typical form: RHA bifurcates into Aant and Apost, and then ramifies into the SA/SSA as a tertiary bifurcation. **b** atypical form: SA/SSA branched off independently before the main bifurcation of Aant and Apost. *(a-1/b-1)* infraportal course: Apost runs caudally to RPV. *(a-2/b-2)* supraportal course: Apost, including posterior SA/SSA, run cranially to RPV. The atypical form was observed in 43 cases. 15 cases of atypical form showed prior branched posterior SA/SSA following a supraportal type, while the other posterior branches were the infraportal type, defined as "partially supraportal type" *(b-2)*

frequency and anatomical characteristics of the extrahepatic and intrahepatic types were investigated.

Permission was granted by the patients for the publication of Figs. 2 and 4.

Results

Patient characteristics and surgical procedures

Of 124 patients (median age: 69 y.o.), 80 men and 44 women received surgical resection. Left hepatectomy, left trisectionectomy, right hepatectomy and right trisectionectomy with caudate lobectomy were performed in 50 patients (40.3 %), 9 patients (7.3 %), 60 patients (48.3 %) and 3 patients (2.3 %), respectively (Table 1). 2 patients (1.6 %) underwent biliary resection with no hepatectomy. Patients with concomitant resection and reconstruction of the portal vein and the hepatic artery were 34 (27.4 %) and 6 (4.8 %), respectively. Hepatectomy combined with pancreaticoduodenectomy was done in 22 patients (17.7 %).

Bifurcation pattern of RHA (typical or atypical form)

The typical form was observed in 75 patients (60.5 %) (Table 2 and Fig. 1). On the other hand, the atypical form was seen in 43 patients (34.7 %), 24 patients (19.4 %) of whom showed SA/SSA branching off separately before the bifurcation of the Aant and Apost. These separately branched arteries supplied the whole or ventral area of segment VI (A6 or A6a) in 11 patients (8.9 %), which was most commonly observed in the atypical type. Trifurcation of RHA was revealed in 18 patients (14.5 %), and indicated Aant + A6 + A7 in 9 patients (7.3 %). One patient (0.8 %) showed a RHA that diverged into four branches, designated as A6 + A7 + A8a (arteries to the ventral region of segment VIII) + A8c (arterial branches to the posterior region of segment VIII). The bifurcation pattern could not be identified in six patients (4.8 %) due to tumor infiltration.

The course of the posterior SA/SSA in relation to RPV

The posterior segmental arteries including their branches followed an infraportal course or a supraportal course in 94 patients (75.8 %) or 24 patients (19.4 %), respectively (Table 3). Of 24 patients with supraportal courses, 9 patients (7.3 %) showed a completely supraportal course without any infraportal branches, while 15 patients (12.1 %) showed a partially supraportal course with infraportal branches (Fig. 1). Of the 15 partially supraportal cases, 4 patients (3.2 %) had infraportal A6 and supraportal A7 (Fig. 2). In the

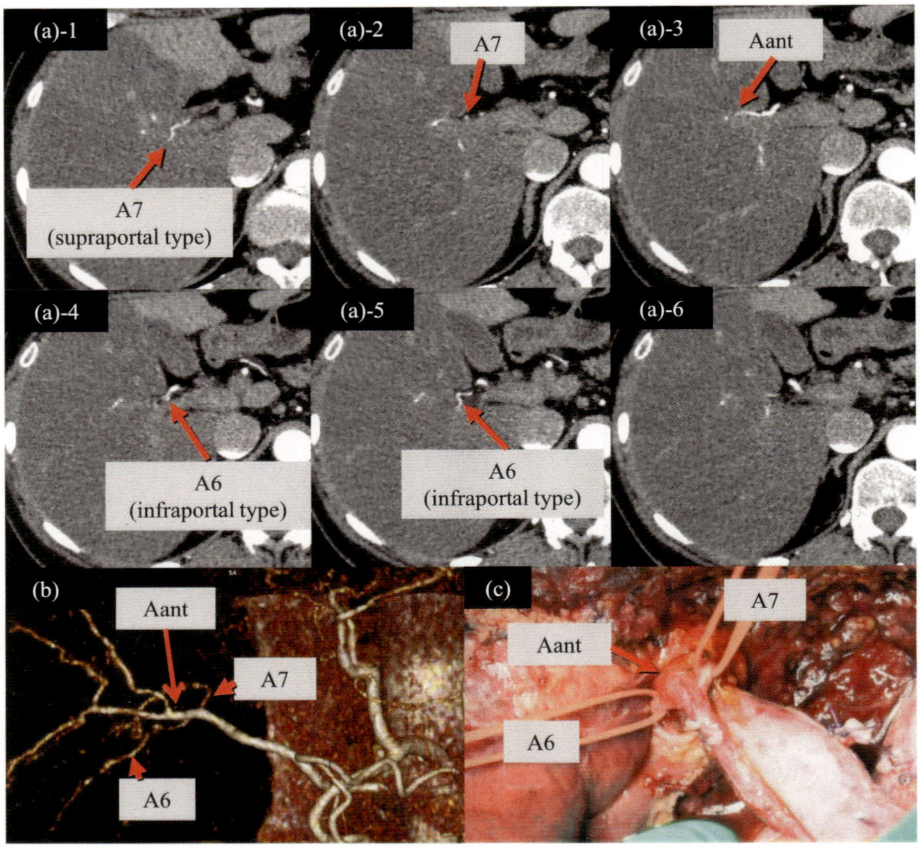

Fig. 2 A representative case of the partially supraportal type. **a** Transverse MDCT images in early arterial phase and **b** three-dimensional arteriogram obtained in a 57-year-old woman with hilar cholangiocarcinoma. **c** Intraoperative photograph after left hepatectomy and caudate lobectomy with hilar lymph node dissection. RHA branched off A7 of the supraportal type before the bifurcation of A6 of the infraportal type and Aant. A6 and 7 supplied segment VI and VII, respectively

remaining 11 patients (8.9 %), A6a followed an infraportal course and the other posterior segmental arteries (A6bc7) followed a supraportal course. All of the partially supraportal cases, in whom the supraportal posterior branches were early bifurcated from the RHA, were classified as the atypical form. On the other hand, 15 cases (34.9 %) of the 43 atypical form cases showed early-bifurcated posterior SA/SAA with partially supraportal course (Fig. 1).

Site of SA/SSA bifurcation (extrahepatic/intrahepatic type)

Extrahepatic bifurcation of the SA/SSA branches was revealed in 82 patients (66.1 %), consisting of 39 with the typical form and all 43 with the atypical form (Table 4 and Figs. 3 and 4). The remaining 36 patients with the typical form (29.0 %) were the intrahepatic type.

Discussion

Lymph node dissection in RS is essential in left-sided hepatectomy for hilar cholangiocarcinoma. In recent years, left-sided hepatectomy with concomitant resection and reconstruction of RHA may offer a better chance of long-term survival in patients with the Bismuth type IIIb cholangiocarcinoma involving RHA [1–3]. However, small SA/SSA, which early bifurcate from the RHA and separately enter the hepatic parenchyma, are often found in RS during lymph node dissection. Therefore, a detail preoperative examination of these vascular bifurcation patterns around RS is more crucial in en block arterial resection with left-sided hepatectomy for hilar cholangiocarcinoma to avoid postoperative complications, such as hepatic infarction and subsequent hepatic failure. The present study clarified the various anatomical patterns of SA/SSA around the RS from three viewpoints, bifurcation patterns of the SA/SSA (typical or atypical form), course of the posterior SA/SSA for the RPV (supraportal or infraportal course) and bifurcation site of the SA/SSA (extrahepatic or intrahepatic bifurcations).

The ramification variant of RHA, bifurcated from the superior mesenteric artery or the celiac trunk, has

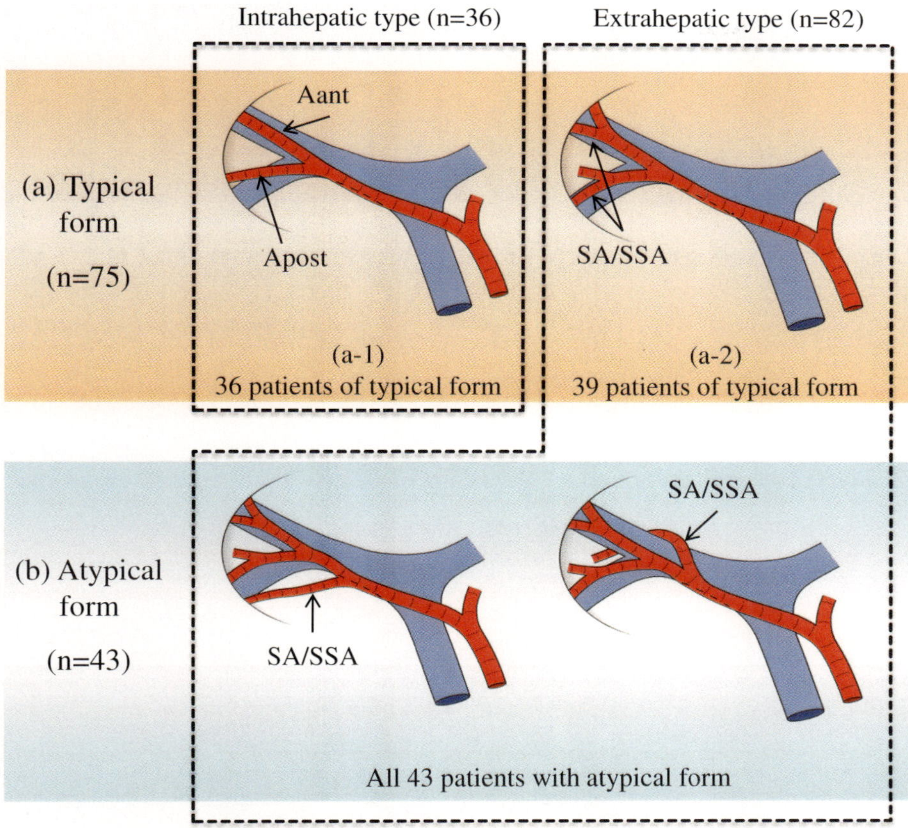

Fig. 3 Bifurcation site of the SA/SSA (intrahepatic/extrahepatic type). **a** typical form, **b** atypical form. Intrahepatic type: The SA/SSA branches were intrahepatically bifurcated from Aant or Apost in 36 patients with the typical form (29.0 % of total cohort)*(a-1)*. Extrahepatic type: Extrahepatic bifurcation of the SA/SSA branches was revealed in 82 patients (66.1 % of total cohort), consisting of 39 with the typical form (*a-2*) and all 43 with the atypical form (*b*)

already been reported [5]. On the other hand, there have been few detailed reports on anatomical variants of the SA or SSA around the RS. In this study, atypical SA or SSA (A6 or A6a and so on), which bifurcated independently prior to the main bifurcation of Aant and Apost, were observed in 34.7 % of the hilar cholangiocarcnioma patients. Furthermore, in cases with the atypical form, the early-bifurcated posterior SA/SSA following supraportal course, which is called as "partially supraportal type", was seen in more than 30 %. In total cohort of our study, the frequency of supraportal posterior branches was 19.5 %, similar to that in a previous report [4]. In Bismuth type IIIb patients with supraportal posterior branches, the risk of intraoperative arterial injury during left-sided hepatectomy is increased. Particularly, during left trisectionectomy for patients with partially supraportal branches, meticulous attention is needed to avoid mistaking partially suprapotal branches (A7 and so on) for the anterior ones. Misidentification of the supraportal posterior branches can result in severe postoperative complications, such as hepatic infarction and hepatic failure [4]. Additionaly, in *en bloc* resection and reconstruction of RHA with cancer invasion, the uninvolved distal arterial branch should be identified around RS before hepatic transection. However, in cases of supraportal Apost, it is difficult to find uninvolved distal Apost. Since supraportal Apost runs behind portal pedicles, distal Apost is usually exposed on the cutting surface during or after hepatic transection, increasing the risk of arterial injury. Therefore, preoperative examination of the bifurcation pattern of SA/SSA and the course of the posterior SA/SSA (supraportal or partially supraportal) using MDCT is mandatory for left-sided hepatectomy, especially left trisectionectomy.

Anatomical variations of an artery, portal vein or bile duct commonly arise around the hepatic hilum before forming Glisson's triad. Since Glisson's triad is formed with an intimate fixation in the liver parenchyma, abnormal ramification of these vessels is rare in the liver parenchyma [6]. In this study, the SA/SSA were bifurcated

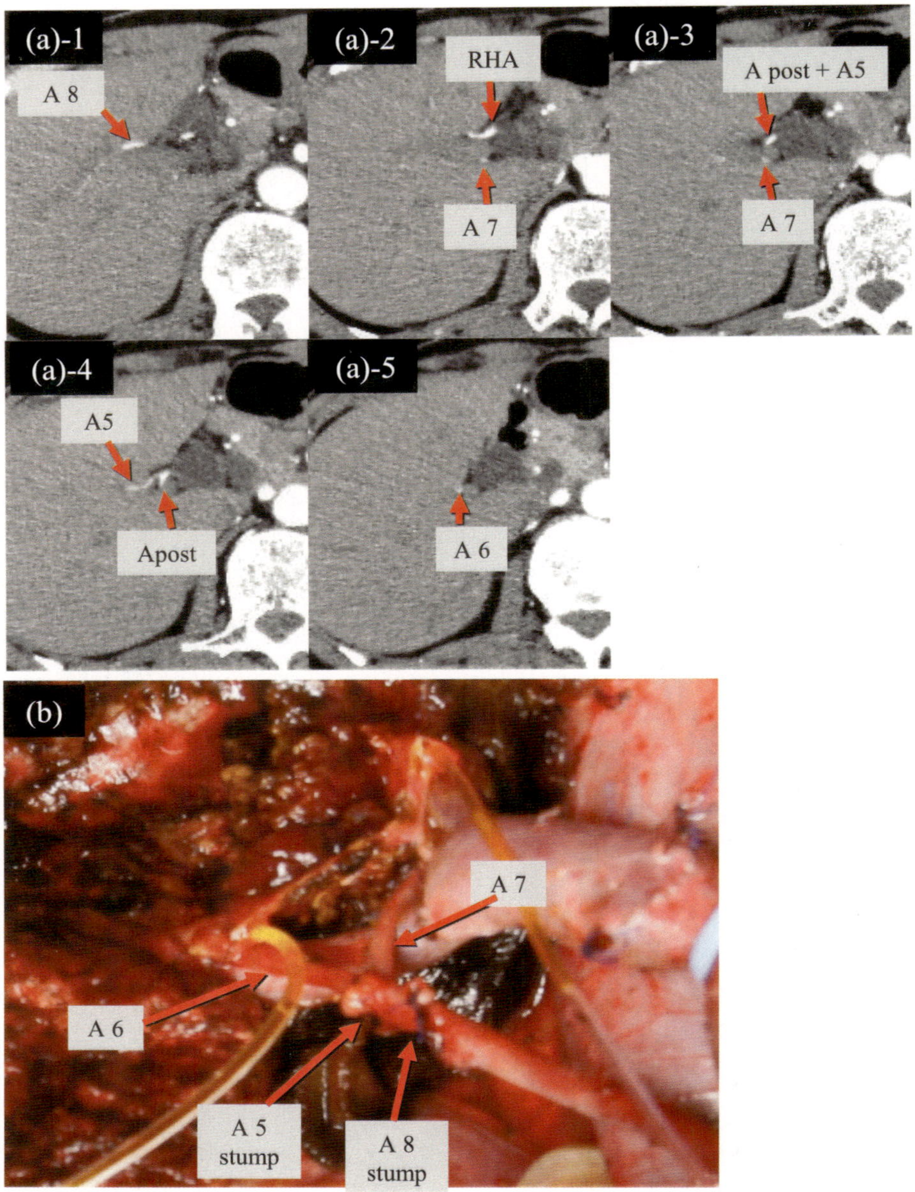

Fig. 4 A representative case of the extrahepatic type. **a** Transverse MDCT images in early arterial phase obtained in a 57-year-old man with hilar cholangiocarcinoma. RHA bifurcated into A8 and Apost + A5 (common trunk of Apost and A5), thereafter Apost + A5 bifurcated into Apost and A5. A8 and A5 extrahepatically branched off from RHA. A8 and 5 supply segment VIII and V, respectively. **b** Intraoperative photograph after left trisectionectomy with caudate lobectomy and hilar lymph node dissection. Stumps of A5 and A8 are shown. During hilar lymph node dissection, A5 and A8 were exposed and cut

extrahepatically (extrahepatic type) in 82 (66.1 %) of total cohort, all 43 atypical forms and in 39 of 75 typical forms. Even in typical forms, the extrahepatic bifurcation of SA/SSA was observed in 52 %. There is a limitation in our classification of the two types, the extrahepatic or intrahepatic types, due to the difficulty in identifying the starting point of Glisson's sheath using MDCT. In other words, these types do not necessarily correspond to an anatomical boundary between the outside and inside of the liver. However, based on the CT criteria of the present study, a bifurcation of the SA/SSA determined to be the extrahepatic type is usually exposed during lymph node dissection for RS. Furthermore, even in some patients classified as the intrahepatic type, the bifurcation of the SA/SSA might be exposed at the extrahepatic area in cases of left trisectionectomy or soft

Table 1 Patients characteristics and surgical procedures

Gender	Male		80
	Female		44
Age	Median		69
	Range		41–82
Surgical procedure	Hepatectomy[a]		
		S1,2,3,4,5,8,	9
		S1,2,3,4,	50
		S1,5,6,7,8,	60
		S1,4,5,6,7,8,	3
		Bile duct resection	2
	Other combined resection		
		Portal vein reconstruction	34
		Hepatic artery reconstruction	6
		Pancreaticoduodenectomy	22

[a]Resection area of the liver is described as Couinaud's hepatic segment(s)

hepatic parenchyma, enabling the RS to be opened easily. Our results showed that the extrahepatic type occurred with a high incidence (66.1 %).

In this study, arterial variation around the RS evaluated with preoperative MDCT was not confirmed intraoperatively in all cases because we included cases of right-sided hepatectomy. However, imagining of the vascular 3D structure has been dramatically improved due to advances in the spatial resolution of volume-rendered multidetector CT angiography. Consequently, homology between the preoperative anatomical imaging and intraoperative findings has been reported [4]. Meanwhile, in recent years, the advent of imaging analysis software such as SYNAPSE Vincent® (Fuji Film) has enabled 3D visualization of the vascular structure and liver volumetry of perfused regions, and is expected to be applied for intraoperative navigation [7, 8]. Nevertheless, there are limitations in the automated vascular analysis of these kinds of software. A thin and complex vessel configuration is not necessarily delineated by the software, such as branches of the SA/SSA in RS. Surgical procedures in which injury to the SA/SSA has a critical impact on the residual hepatic function still need a conventional detailed investigation using MDCT to obtain 3D imaging of the anatomical structure.

Table 2 The bifurcation pattern of SA/SSA from RHA

Typical form		75 (60.5 %)
Atypical form		43 (34.7 %)
SA/SSA separately branched off before main bifurcation of Aant and Apost		24 (19.4 %)
	A5	2
	A6 or A6a	11
	A7	4
	A8 or A8a or A8c	7
Trifurcarion of RHA		18 (14.5 %)
	A5 + A8 + Apost	4
	A8a + A8c + Apost	5
	Aant + A6 + A7	9
Simultaneous ramification of RHA to four branches		1 (0.8 %)
	A6 + A7 + A8a + A8c	1
Unclear form (because of cancer invasion)		6 (4.8 %)

SA/SSA segmental or subsegmental arteries, *RHA* right hepatic artery, *Aant and Apost* anterior and posterior hepatic artery, *SA/SSA* segmental or subsegmental arteries, *A5, 6, 7 and 8* segmental artery supplying segment V, VI, VII and VIII, respectively, *A6a, A8a and A8c* subsegmental artery suppling ventral segment VI, ventral segment VIII and dorsal segment VIII, respectively

Table 3 The courses of the posterior SA/SSA in relation to RPV

Infraportal form	94 (75.8 %)
Supraportal form	24 (19.4 %)
Completely supraportal	9 (7.3 %)
Partially supraportal	15 (12.1 %)
A6a of infraportal course and A6bc7 of supraportal course	11 (8.9 %)
A6 of infraportal course and A7 of supraportal course	4 (3.2 %)
Unclear form (because of cancer invasion)	6 (4.8 %)

SA/SSA segmental or subsegmental arteries, *RPV* right portal vein, *A6 and 7* segmental artery supplying segment VI and VII, respectively, *A6a* subsegmental artery suppling ventral segment VI, *A6bc7* subsegmental arteries suppling lateral and dorsal segment VI and segment VII

Conclusion

Extrahepatic bifurcation of the SA/SSA from RHA is relatively common (66.1 %). In particular, more than 30 % of the early-branched posterior SA/SSA from RHA (atypical form) often follow a supraportal course. Although the anatomical variation of arterial branches around the RS is complex, detailed preoperative knowledge of the anatomy, including SA/SSA, is crucial for left-sided hepatectomy for hilar cholangiocarcinoma.

Table 4 The bifurcation site of the SA/SSA (intrahepatic/extrahepatic type)

Intrahepatic type	36 (29.0 %)
Extrahepatic type	82 (66.1 %)
Branched off before main bifurcation of Aant and Apost (atypical form)	43
Branched off after main bifurcation of Aant and Apost (typical form)	39
Unclear (because of cancer invasion)	6 (4.9 %)

SA/SSA segmental or subsegmental arteries, *Aant and Apost* anterior and posterior hepatic artery

Abbreviations

3D images, three-dimensional images; Aant, anterior hepatic artery; Apost, posterior hepatic artery; MDCT, multidetector-row computed tomography; MPR, multi planar reformation; RHA, right hepatic artery; RPV, right portal vein; RS, Rouviere's sulcus; SA, segmental artery; SSA, subsegmental arteries

Acknowledgements

The authors thank Yu Katayose (Tohoku Rosai Hospital, Sendai, Japan), Hiroshi Yoshida (Iwaki Kyoritsu Hospital, Iwaki, Japan) and the other surgeons in the division of Hepato-Biliary Pancreatic Surgery, Tohoku University Hospital. The authors also thank all radiologists and technologists in the department of diagnostic radiology, Tohoku University Hospital.

Funding

Michiaki Unno: Management Expenses Grants from the Government of Japan to national university corporations supplied every fiscal year.

Authors' contributions

SA designed and performed the research. MM supported this research and SA and MM wrote the paper. HH, KN, TM, FM, TN, SE and MU reviewed the manuscript and revised it critically for important intellectual content. MM integrated the entire study. All authors read and approved the final manuscript.

Competing interests

The authors declare that they have no competing interests.

Author details

[1]Department of Surgery, Tohoku University Graduate School of Medicine, Aobaku, Sendai, Japan. [2]Division of International Cooperation for Disaster Medicine, Tohoku University, 1-1 Seiryomachi, Aobaku, Sendai 980-8574, Japan.

References

1. Nagino M, Nimura Y, Nishio H, Ebata T, Igami T, Matsushita M, et al. Hepatectomy with simultaneous resection of the portal vein and hepatic artery for advanced perihilar cholangiocarcinoma: an audit of 50 consecutive cases. Ann Surg. 2010;252(1):115–23. doi:10.1097/SLA.0b013e3181e463a7.
2. Sakamoto Y, Sano T, Shimada K, Kosuge T, Kimata Y, Sakuraba M, et al. Clinical significance of reconstruction of the right hepatic artery for biliary malignancy. Langenbecks Arch Surg. 2006;391(3):203–8. doi:10.1007/s00423-006-0026-8.
3. Shimada H, Endo I, Sugita M, Masunari H, Fujii Y, Tanaka K, et al. Hepatic resection combined with portal vein or hepatic artery reconstruction for advanced carcinoma of the hilar bile duct and gallbladder. World J Surg. 2003;27(10):1137–42. doi:10.1007/s00268-003-6801-6.
4. Yoshioka Y, Ebata T, Yokoyama Y, Igami T, Sugawara G, Nagino M. "Supraportal" right posterior hepatic artery: an anatomic trap in hepatobiliary and transplant surgery. World J Surg. 2011;35(6):1340–4. doi:10.1007/s00268-011-1075-x.
5. Hiatt JR, Gabbay J, Busuttil RW. Surgical anatomy of the hepatic arteries in 1000 cases. Ann Surg. 1994;220(1):50–2.
6. Couinaud C. Surgical anatomy of the liver. Several new aspects. Chirurgie memoires de l'Academie de chirurgie. 1986;112(5):337–42.
7. Ohshima S. Volume analyzer SYNAPSE VINCENT for liver analysis. J Hepatobiliary Pancreat Sci. 2014;21(4):235–8. doi:10.1002/jhbp.81.
8. Sakai H, Okuda K, Yasunaga M, Kinoshita H, Aoyagi S. Reliability of hepatic artery configuration in 3D CT angiography compared with conventional angiography–special reference to living-related liver transplant donors. Transpl Int. 2005;18(5):499–505. doi:10.1111/j.1432-2277.2004.00009.x.

Preoperative evaluation of accessory hepatic ducts by drip infusion cholangiography with CT

Hiromichi Ishii*, Akinori Noguchi, Tomoyuki Fukami, Riho Sugimoto, Hiroyuki Tada, Hiroki Takeshita, Seiji Umehara, Hiroyuki Izumi, Naoki Tani, Masahide Yamaguchi and Tetsuro Yamane

Abstract

Background: This retrospective study aimed to investigate the incidence of each type of accessory hepatic duct by drip infusion cholangiography with CT (DIC-CT).

Methods: Five hundred sixty nine patients who underwent preoperative DIC-CT and laparoscopic cholecystectomy were reviewed. Accessory hepatic ducts were classified as follows: type I (accessory hepatic ducts that merged with the common hepatic duct between the confluence of the right and left hepatic ducts and the cystic duct confluence), type II (those that merged with the common hepatic duct at the same site as the cystic duct), type III (those that merged with the common bile duct distal to the cystic duct confluence), type IV (the cystic duct merged with the accessory hepatic duct), and type V (accessory hepatic ducts that merged with the common hepatic or bile duct on the left side).

Results: Accessory hepatic ducts were observed in 50 patients. Type I, II, III, IV, and V accessory hepatic ducts were detected in 32, 3, 1, 11, and 3 patients, respectively. Based on their drainage areas, the accessory hepatic ducts were also classified as follows: a posterior branch in 22 patients, an anterior branch in 9 patients, a combination of posterior and anterior branches in 16 patients, a left-sided branch in 2 patients, and a caudate branch in 1 patient. None of the patients with accessory hepatic ducts suffered bile duct injuries.

Conclusion: There are a number of variants of the accessory hepatic duct. DIC-CT is useful to detect the accessory hepatic duct.

Keywords: Accessory hepatic duct, Drip infusion cholangiography with CT, Laparoscopic cholecystectomy, Bile duct injury

Background

Laparoscopic cholecystectomy (LC) has become the gold standard procedure for patients with cholecystolithiasis or gallbladder polyps; however, the incidence of bile duct injuries during LC has been reported to be about 0.5–1.7% [1, 2]. Anatomical anomalies of the biliary tree are considered to be a risk factor for bile duct injuries, and it was previously reported that the frequency of bile duct injuries is higher in patients with bile duct anomalies than in patients without them [3]. Therefore, it is important to evaluate the anatomy of the biliary tree, especially those of the cystic duct and any accessory hepatic ducts, preoperatively. Usually, drip infusion cholangiography with computed tomography (DIC-CT) or magnetic resonance cholangiopancreatography (MRCP) is performed to evaluate choledocholithiasis and the anatomy of the biliary tree before LC in Japan.

It was reported that accessory hepatic ducts exhibit an incidence rate of 2–11% [1, 4–7]; however, there are few reports about the drainage areas of accessory hepatic ducts.

The aims of this retrospective study are to investigate the incidence, type, and drainage area of accessory hepatic ducts using DIC-CT.

* Correspondence: ishii.hiromichi@jp.panasonic.com
Department of Surgery, Matsushita Memorial Hospital, 5-55 Sotojima-cho, Moriguchi city, Osaka 570-8540, Japan

Methods

Patients

In total, 738 consecutive patients were scheduled to undergo LC for cholecystolithiasis, cholecystitis or gallbladder polyps at Matsushita Memorial Hospital between January 2004 and December 2015. DIC-CT was performed prior to elective LC for cholecystolithiasis, chronic cholecystitis or gallbladder polyps. Of these 738 patients, we investigated retrospectively the 569 consecutive patients who underwent preoperative DIC-CT in this study.

DIC-CT examinations

One hundred milliliters of meglumine iotroxate (Biliscopin; BAYER, Osaka, Japan) were infused intravenously over a period of 30 min, and multidetector CT (Light Speed Ultra; GE Healthcare, Waukesha, USA) was performed 45 min later. Three-dimensional images were reconstructed using a surface-rendering method.

Analysis of DIC-CT images

The bile ducts and cystic duct were evaluated using both two-dimensional and three-dimensional images. The bile duct located on the duodenal side of the bifurcation of the main portal vein was defined as the "main" extrahepatic bile duct, and intrahepatic bile ducts that joined the "main" extrahepatic bile duct were defined as accessory hepatic ducts. The drainage area of each accessory hepatic duct was evaluated using two-dimensional DIC-CT images. Patients involving poor visualization of the secondary branches of the intrahepatic bile ducts and/or the cystic duct were included in the poor study group.

Accessory hepatic ducts were classified according to the method described in previous reports [1]: type I (accessory hepatic ducts that merged with the common hepatic duct between the confluence of the right and left hepatic ducts and the cystic duct confluence), type II (those that merged with the common hepatic duct at the same site as the cystic duct), type III (those that merged with the common bile duct distal to the cystic duct confluence), type IV (cases in which the cystic duct merged with the accessory hepatic duct), and type V (accessory hepatic ducts that merged with the common hepatic or bile duct on the left side). Accessory hepatic ducts that merged with the gallbladder and cases involving two accessory hepatic ducts were classified as "others" (Fig. 1). The accessory hepatic ducts were also classified according to their drainage areas as follows: the posterior branch type (accessory hepatic ducts that drained all or part of the right posterior section), the anterior branch type (those that drained all or part of the right anterior section), the combined posterior and anterior branch type (those that drained all or part of the right posterior section and all or part of the right anterior section), the left-sided branch type (those that drained part of the left hemiliver), and the caudate branch type (those that drained part of the caudate lobe).

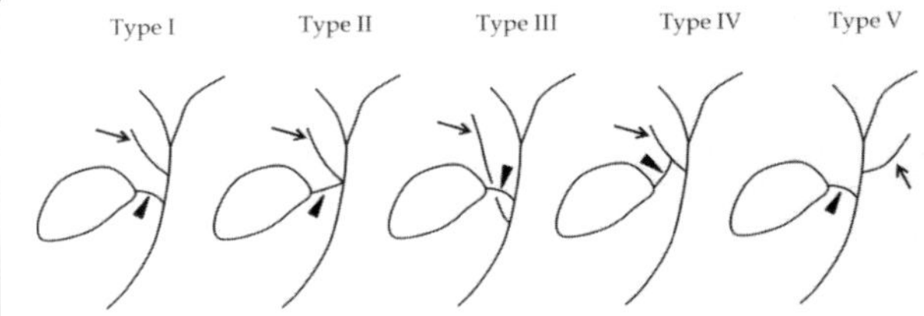

Fig. 1 Classification of accessory hepatic ducts. The *arrow* indicates the accessory hepatic duct, and the *arrow head* shows the cystic duct

Surgical technique

LC was performed using four surgical trocars, and the critical view of safety technique is adopted for almost all patients. Intraoperative cholangiography was not carried out routinely. LC was converted to open cholecystectomy in cases involving severe adhesion around the gallbladder, bile duct injuries, or uncontrolled bleeding.

Results

Of a total of 738 consecutive patients who underwent LC, DIC-CT was performed in 569 patients, MRCP was conducted in 94 patients, endoscopic retrograde cholangiography was carried out in 34 patients, cholangiography was performed using a percutaneous transhepatic gallbladder drainage tube in 3 patients, and no examination of the biliary tree was conducted in 38 patients. Of the 569 patients that underwent DIC-CT, 11 belonged to the poor study group.

Fifty (9%) of the 558 patients that did not belong to the poor study group had accessory hepatic ducts (Table 1). Type I, II, III, IV, and V accessory hepatic ducts were observed in 32 (64%) (Fig. 2), 3 (6%) (Fig. 3), 1 (2%) (Fig. 4), 11 (22%) (Fig. 5), and 3 patients (6%) (Figs. 6, 7), respectively. The accessory hepatic ducts were classified as the posterior branch type in 22 patients (44%) (Figs. 3, 5), the anterior branch type in 9 patients (18%) (Fig. 4), the combined posterior and anterior branch type in 16 patients (32%) (Fig. 2), the left-sided branch type in 2 patients (4%) (Fig. 6), and the caudate branch type in 1 patient (2%) (Fig. 7). Following the separation of the gallbladder from the liver bed, the cystic duct was clipped and divided to prevent bile duct injuries in the patients with type IV accessory hepatic ducts.

Although bile duct injuries occurred in 4 (0.7%) of the 569 patients that underwent LC, none of the patients with accessory hepatic ducts suffered bile duct injuries. All of the bile duct injuries were noticed during the operation, and primary repair of the injuries was performed via conversion to open laparotomy. Two patients underwent

Table 1 Variations in the types and drainage areas of accessory hepatic ducts

	Type I	Type II	Type III	Type IV	Type V	Others	Total
Posterior branch	16	1	0	5	0	0	22
Anterior branch	6	0	1	2	0	0	9
Combined branch	10	2	0	4	0	0	16
Left-sided branch	0	0	0	0	2	0	2
Caudate branch	0	0	0	0	1	0	1
Total	32	3	1	11	3	0	50

cholangioduodenostomy, and two patients underwent simple closure of their bile duct injuries. LC was converted to open cholecystectomy in 23 patients (4%) due to severe adhesion in 15 patients, bile duct injuries in 4 patients, uncontrolled bleeding in one patient, and other reasons in 3 patients. Conversion to open cholecystectomy was necessary in one of the 50 patients with accessory hepatic ducts due to severe adhesion.

Discussion

DIC-CT or MRCP is usually performed preoperatively in patients who undergo cholecystectomy to evaluate choledocholithiasis and the anatomy of the biliary tree in Japan. Although MRCP is the most widely used noninvasive means of evaluating biliary disease, DIC-CT depicts small bile ducts (e.g., accessory hepatic ducts, the cystic duct, or the caudate branch) than MRCP [7, 8]. Because only 11 patients (1.9%) were classified in the poor study group in this study, DIC-CT is successful in assessing the biliary tree anatomy. Therefore, DIC-CT is performed routinely at our institution except in patients who exhibit adverse reactions to contrast media or severe thyroid disease. We consider that the radiation during DIC-CT does not affect the patient's health because the radiation dose during DIC-CT is about 8 mGy. The side effects of meglumine iotroxate have been reported, however, severe side effects such as anaphylactic shock did not occur in this study.

The incidence of accessory hepatic ducts was reported to range from 2 to 11% in previous studies [1, 4–7], whereas it was 9% in this study. The incidence rates of type I, II, III, IV, and V accessory hepatic ducts were previously reported to range from 35 to 66.7%, 2–19%, 0–21.6%, 13–25%, and 0–7.7%, respectively [1, 4–7]. In this study, type I accessory hepatic ducts exhibited the highest frequency, followed by type IV ducts. Types II, III, and V were less common, as was found in previous studies. On the other hand, there have been few reports about the drainage areas of accessory hepatic ducts. It was reported that most accessory hepatic ducts (86.7–100%) are right posterior bile ducts [1, 6]. Hirao et al. [7] found that of 13 patients with accessory hepatic ducts 9 (69%) had posterior ducts, two had anterior

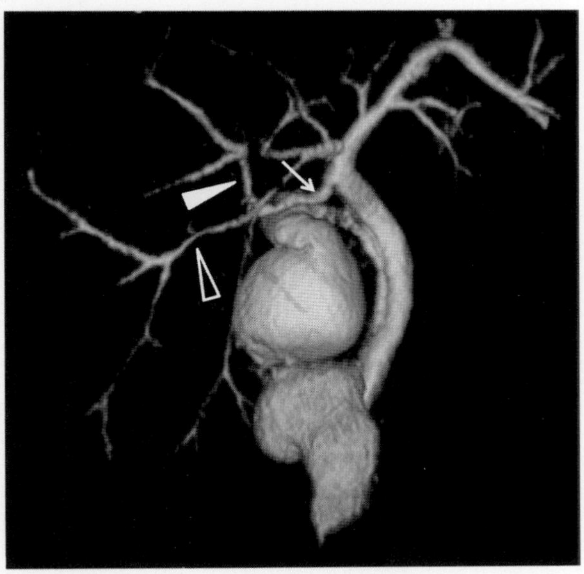

Fig. 2 Three-dimensional DIC-CT (right ventral view) showing a type I accessory hepatic duct. The accessory hepatic duct (*arrow*) drained both the dorsal area of the right anterior section (*white arrow head*) and the right posterior section (*black arrow head*) and was classified into the combined posterior and anterior branch type

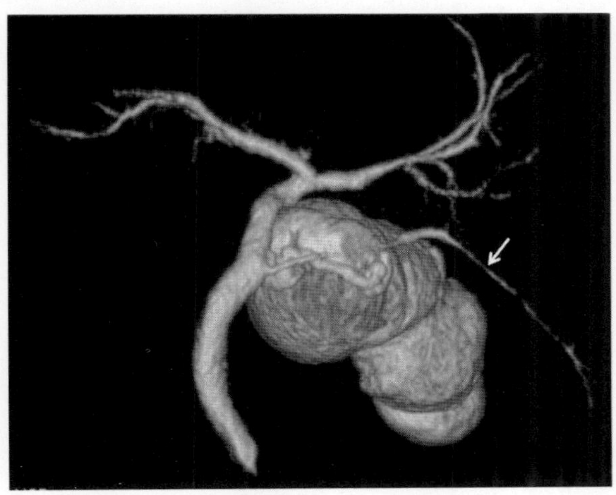

Fig. 3 Three-dimensional DIC-CT image (dorsal view) showing a type II accessory hepatic duct. The accessory hepatic duct drained segment 6 (*arrow*) and was classified as belonging to the posterior branch type

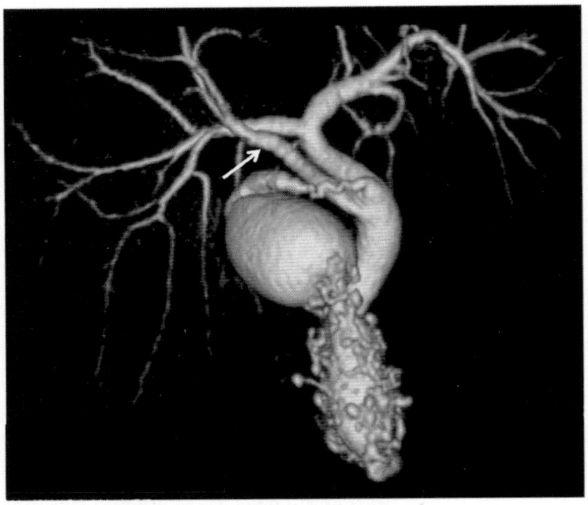

Fig. 4 Three-dimensional DIC-CT image (ventral view) showing a type III accessory hepatic duct. The accessory hepatic duct drained the right anterior section (*arrow*) and was classified as belonging to the anterior branch type

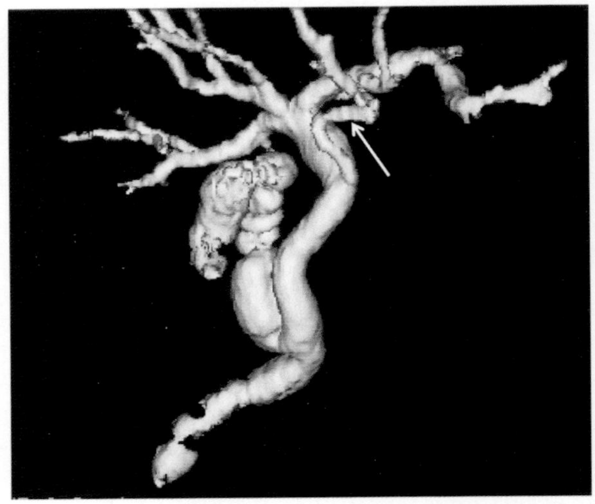

Fig. 6 Three-dimensional DIC-CT image (ventral view) showing the type V accessory hepatic duct. The accessory hepatic duct drained segment 4 (*arrow*) and was classified into the left-sided branch type

ducts (15%), one had an anteroinferior branch (8%), and a caudate branch was seen in the remaining patient (8%). In our study, we investigated the drainage areas of accessory hepatic ducts in detail. Although the posterior branch type exhibited the highest incidence (44%), several other types of accessory hepatic ducts, such as the combined posterior and anterior branch type (32%), anterior branch type (18%), left-sided branch type (4%), and caudate branch type (2%) were also seen. This information is important not only for cholecystectomy, but also for surgery for cholangiocarcinoma [9, 10], pancreatic head tumors [11] and for transplant procedures involving living liver donors [12–14].

The causes of bile duct injuries during LC can be divided into anatomical [3, 15], inflammatory [16], and technical factors. The critical view of safety [17] is the important technique for preventing bile duct injuries during LC. Several authors have reported that intraoperative cholangiography reduces bile duct injury [18, 19], on the other hand, it has been done that intraoperative cholangiography does not reduce bile duct injury [20],

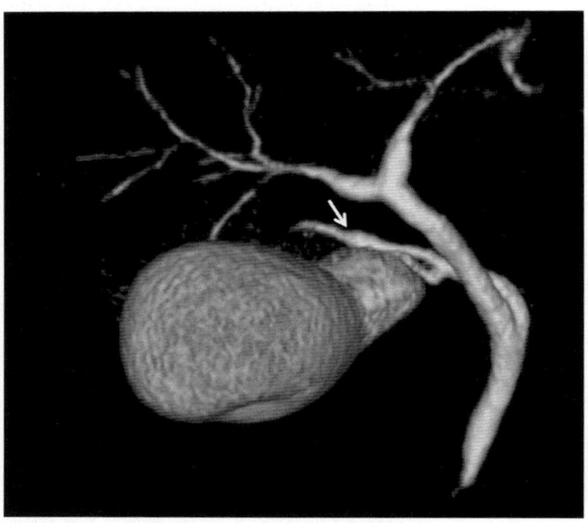

Fig. 5 Three-dimensional DIC-CT image (ventral view) showing a type IV accessory hepatic duct. The accessory hepatic duct drained the right posterior section (*arrow*) and was classified as belonging to the posterior branch type

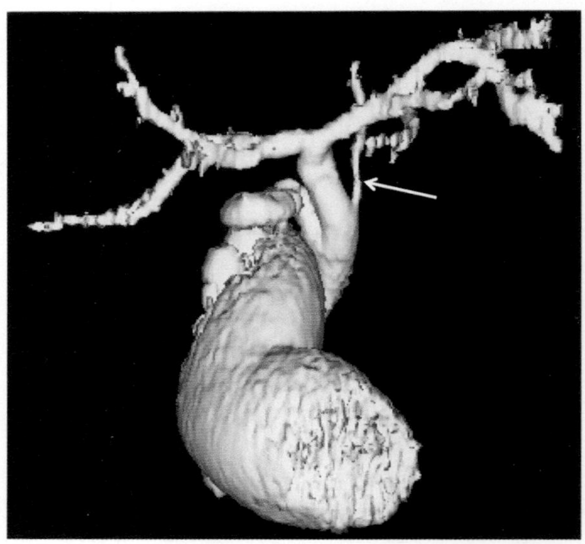

Fig. 7 Three-dimensional DIC-CT image (ventral view) showing a type V accessory hepatic duct. The accessory hepatic duct drained the Spiegel lobe (*arrow*) and was classified into the caudate branch type

and that injuries to accessory hepatic ducts or anomalous cystic ducts cannot be prevented by intraoperative cholangiography because anomalous bile ducts sometimes cannot be found with intraoperative cholangiography [4]. It has been reported that fluorescence cholangiography is a safe and effective procedure that enables real-time visualization of the biliary tree, and this novel procedure may become standard practice in order to prevent bile duct injury [21]. In our study, all of the bile duct injuries occurred in patients with severe inflammatory adhesion due to chronic cholecystitis. Thus, even in patients with accessory hepatic ducts, precise preoperative diagnosis and the meticulous performance of surgical procedures might prevent bile duct injuries. Of the various types of accessory hepatic ducts, type I, II, III, and IV ducts, which were observed in 32 (5.7%), 3 (0.5%), 1 (0.2%), and 11 patients (2.0%), respectively in this study, are at risk of bile duct injuries during the Calot triangle dissection. Especially, type IV ducts carry the greatest risk of bile duct injuries [1, 5, 6]. Noji et al. [4] suggested that the installation of an endoscopic nasobiliary drainage tube prior to LC in cases involving predictable bile duct anomalies might reduce the incidence of complications, and Kurata et al. [6] did that bile duct injuries can be avoided by using a surgical technique that exposes the inner layer of the subserosal layer of the gallbladder wall. We consider that intraoperative fluorescence cholangiography may be useful procedure to avoid bile duct injuries when patients with type I, II, III, or IV accessory hepatic ducts have severe inflammatory adhesion due to chronic cholecystitis. Furthermore, we recommend the dome down technique, in which the cystic duct is divided following the separation of the gallbladder from the liver bed, to prevent bile duct injuries in patients with type IV accessory hepatic ducts. Type V accessory hepatic ducts do not usually cause problem during LC; however, surgeons should take special care to prevent injuries to accessory hepatic ducts in segment 2 (type V) in patients with true left-sided gallbladders [22].

Conclusions

There are a number of variants of the accessory hepatic duct. Surgeons should pay special attention to accessory hepatic ducts to prevent bile duct injuries during LC. Furthermore, the knowledge of the variations in accessory hepatic ducts is important for hepatobiliarypancreatic surgery.

Abbreviations

DIC-CT: Drip infusion cholangiography with computed tomography; LC: Laparoscopic cholecystectomy; MRCP: Magnetic resonance cholangiopancreatography

Acknowledgements

None.

Funding

None.

Authors' contributions

HI collected the data and wrote the paper. AN and NT revised the paper. HI, AN, TF, HT, HT, SU, NT, and TY performed operations. All authors read and approved the final manuscript.

Competing interests

The authors declared that they have no competing interests.

References

1. Uchiyama K, Tani M, Kawai M, Ueno T, Hama T, Yamaue H. Preoperative evaluation of the extrahepatic bile duct structure for laparoscopic cholecystectomy. Surg Endosc. 2006;20:1119–23.
2. Nijssen MA, Schreinemakers JM, Meyer Z, van der Schelling GP, Crolla RM, Rijken AM. Complication after laparoscopic cholecystectomy: a video evaluation study of whether the critical view of safety was reached. World J Surg. 2015;39:1798–803.
3. Hugh TB. New strategies to prevent laparoscopic bile duct injury: surgeons can learn from pilots. Surgery. 2002;132:826–35.
4. Noji T, Nakamura F, Nakamura T, Kato K, Suzuki O, Ambo Y, et al. ENBD tube placement prior to laparoscopic cholecystectomy may reduce the rate of complications in cases with predictably complicating biliary anomalies. J Gastroenterol. 2011;46:73–7.
5. Ochiai T, Yamazaki S, Ohta K, Takahashi M, Iwai T, Irie T, et al. Is drip infusion cholecystocholangiography (DIC) an acceptable modality at cholecystectomy for cholecystolithiasis, considering the frequency of bile duct maljunction and intraoperative bile duct injury? J Hepato-Biliary-Pancreat Surg. 2004;11:135–9.
6. Kurata M, Honda G, Okuda Y, Kobayashi S, Sakamoto K, Iwasaki S, et al. Preoperative detection and handling of aberrant right posterior sectoral hepatic duct during laparoscopic cholecystectomy. J Hepatobiliary Pancreat Sci. 2015;22:558–62.
7. Hirao K, Miyazaki A, Fujimoto T, Isomoto I, Hayashi K. Evaluation of aberrant bile ducts before laparoscopic cholecystectomy: helical CT cholangiography versus MR cholangiography. Am J Roentgenol. 2000;175:713–20.
8. Hyodo T, Kumano S, Kushihata F, Okada M, Hirata M, Tsuda T, et al. CT and MR cholangiography: advantages and pitfalls in perioperative evaluation of biliary tree. Br J Radiol. 2012;85:887–96.
9. Sugiura T, Nagino M, Kamiya J, Nishio H, Ebata T, Yokoyama Y, et al. Infraportal bile duct of the caudate lobe: a troublesome anatomic variation in right-sided hepatectomy for perihilar cholangiocarcinoma. Ann Surg. 2007;246:794–8.
10. Miyamoto R, Oshiro Y, Hashimoto S, Kohno K, Fukunaga K, Oda T, et al. Three-dimensional imaging identified the accessory bile duct in a patient with cholangiocarcinoma. World J Gastroenterol. 2014;20:11451–5.
11. Ajay HB, Ashok DB, Girish DB, Vikas S. Right posterior branch draining into intra-pancreatic common duct: the triple duct sign. Updat Surg. 2010;62: 199–202.
12. Takeishi K, Shirabe K, Yoshida Y, Tsutsui Y, Kurihara T, Kimura K, et al. Correlation between portal vein anatomy and bile duct variation in 407 living liver donors. Am J Transplant. 2015;15:155–60.
13. Mc Sweeney SE, Kim TK, Jang HJ, Khalili K. Biliary anatomy in potential right hepatic lobe living donor liver transplantation (LDLT): the utility of CT cholangiography in the setting of inconclusive MRCP. Eur J Radiol. 2012;81:6–12.
14. Varotti G, Gondolesi GE, Goldman J, Wayne M, Florman SS, Schwartz ME, et al. Anatomic variations in right liver living donors. J Am Coll Surg. 2004;198: 577–82.
15. Chung YH, Kim DJ, Kim IG, Kim HJ, Chon SE, Jeon JY, et al. Relationship between the risk of bile duct injury during laparoscopic cholecystectomy and the types of preoperative magnetic resonance cholangiopancreaticography (MRCP). Korean J Hepatobiliary Pancreat Surg. 2012;16:17–23.
16. Soderlund C, Frozanpol F, Linder S. Bile duct injuries at laparoscopic cholecystectomy: a single-institution prospective study. Acute cholecystitis indicates an increased risk. World J Surg. 2005;29:987–93.
17. Strasberg SM, Hertl M, Soper NJ. An analysis of the problem of biliary injury during laparoscopic cholecystectomy. J Am Coll Surg. 1995;180:101–25.
18. Debru E, Dawson A, Leibman S, Richardson M, Glen L, Hollinshead J, et al. Does routine intraoperative cholangiography prevent bile duct transection? Surg Endosc. 2005;19:589–93.

19. Halawani HM, Tamim H, Khalifeh F, Mailhac A, Jamali FR. Impact of intraoperative cholangiography on postoperative morbidity and readmission: analysis of the NSQIP database. Surg Endosc. 2016;30:5395–403.
20. Ding GQ, Cai W, Qin MF. Is intraoperative cholangiography necessary during laparoscopic cholecystectomy for cholelithiasis? World J Gastroenterol. 2015; 21:2147–51.
21. Pesce A, Piccolo G, Greca GL, Puleo S. Utility of fluorescent cholangiography during laparoscopic cholecystectomy: a systematic review. World J Gastroenterol. 2015;21:7877–83.
22. Ishii H, Noguchi A, Onishi M, Takao K, Maruyama T, Taiyoh H, et al. True left-sided gallbladder with variations of bile duct and cholecystic vein. World J Gastroenterol. 2015;21:6754–8.

19

Good outcome following liver transplantation using pericardial-peritoneum window for hepato-atrial anastomosis to overcome advanced hepatic alveolar echinococcosis and secondary Budd-Chiari Syndrome

Konrad Kobryń[1*], Rafał Paluszkiewicz[1], Krzysztof Dudek[1], Urszula Ołdakowska-Jedynak[2], Michał Korba[1], Joanna Raszeja-Wyszomirska[2], Piotr Remiszewski[1], Michał Grąt[1], Piotr Milkiewicz[2], Waldemar Patkowski[1] and Marek Krawczyk[1]

Abstract

Background: This report presents a case of a 57- year old female with advanced Hepatic Alveolar Echinococcosis causing a secondary Budd-Chiari Syndrome due to infiltration of the suprahepatic inferior vena cava treated successfully by liver transplantation.

Case presentation: A temporary veno-venous bypass was introduced, but a typical end to end cavo-caval anastomosis wasn't possible in this case. In order to access a disease free part of the inferior vena cava, an oval window of the diaphragm was excised, providing communication between the peritoneum and pericardium. A vascular clamp was placed onto the right atrium which allowed for an atrial-caval anastomosis. The remainder of hepatectomy was performed in a conventional manner. In the post-operative period and during the 18 month follow-up there were no complications. The patient remains in good general condition with optimal graft function.

Conclusions: A hepato-atrial anastomosis with a pericardial-peritoneum window during liver transplantation is feasible and extends the curability potential for patients with advanced Hepatic Alveolar Echinococcosis considered for liver transplantation.

Keywords: Atrium–IVC anastomosis, Budd-Chiari Syndrome, Hepatic alveolar Echinococcosis, Liver transplantation, Pericardial-peritoneum window, Case report

* Correspondence: konradkobryn@gmail.com
[1]Department of General, Transplant and Liver Surgery, Medical University of Warsaw, Poland. Banacha Street 1a, 02-097 Warsaw, Poland
Full list of author information is available at the end of the article

Background

Advanced hepatic alveococcosis due to its volume may interfere with the hepatic veins and inferior vena cava (IVC) causing Budd-Chiari syndrome (BCS) which is an indication for liver transplantation (LTx). The thrombosis and stricture may be found at any point, ranging from the hepatic veins to the right atrium along the IVC [1, 2]. When this is the case, hepatectomy of the diseased liver requires supra hepatic IVC clamping at the right atrium, with later end-to-end anastomosis with the donor liver IVC cuff [3–5]. Our report presents a rare approach during hepatectomy, perioperative management and excellent postoperative results of the patient.

Case presentation

A 57 year old female patient was qualified for LTx due to BCS caused by an advanced *Echinococcus multilocularis* infection. The patient received Albendazole treatment for several years which was terminated two years prior to transplantation due to a developed post-drug pancytopenia. No other anthelminthic drugs were administered until LTx. Furthermore, portal hypertension, esophageal and gastric varices, portal hypertensive gastropathy, and ascites were present at time of transplant qualification. Celiac disease, gastro-esophageal reflux disease (GERD), and L1 vertebral fracture were associating commorbidities.

The size of the alveolar lesion in segments III–VIII was 110 × 75 × 70 mm (Fig. 1a) and involved the hepatic vein confluence, causing narrowing of the IVC lumen with mild but disturbed blood flow. The intrahepatic IVC was free of abnormalities. The lesion occluded the left and middle hepatic veins, extending towards the confluence of the right hepatic vein with the IVC (Fig. 1b). The lumen was narrowed, with an organized thrombus visible on ultrasound, but blood flow was maintained.

The donor liver was retrieved from a 43 year old dead brain donor (DBD) matching the recipient's blood type and similar weight and height values. The LTx began on the 16th September, 2014 with the use of an extracorporeal veno-venous bypass. The portal vein and hepatoduodenal ligament was difficult to dissect as it was embodied in post-inflammatory scar tissue. The suprahepatic IVC along with the surrounding diaphragm was involved in the alveolar lesion. A 10 × 10 cm window of the diaphragm was excised creating an opening of the right pleural cavity and pericardium (Fig. 2). Thus, with the exposure of the pericardial part of the IVC, the vascular clamp was placed on the atrium because the whole IVC was infiltrated by the lesion. The infrahepatic part of the IVC was clamped in a standard procedure. Both ends of the IVC were then cut, and the liver was explanted along with its intrahepatic IVC (Fig. 3a). The clamping of the right atrium caused cardiac arrhythmia and the electrocardiogram showed signs of myocardial ischemia. This was managed by the anesthesiologist and hemodynamic stability was achieved throughout the operation.

Two 24 fr pleural drains were placed into the apex and base of the right pleural space. The supra hepatic IVC of the donor graft was sutured directly to the right atrium using an end-to-end anastomosis. The excised window in the diaphragm was minimized by suturing its free ends together without the use of a Prolene patch, and without complete closure of the diaphragm in order to avoid stenosis of the IVC–atrium anastomosis. Communication between the pericardium and right pleural cavity was intentionally sustained to allow for fluid drainage. After completion of the portal anastomosis clamps from the IVC and portal vein were removed. A

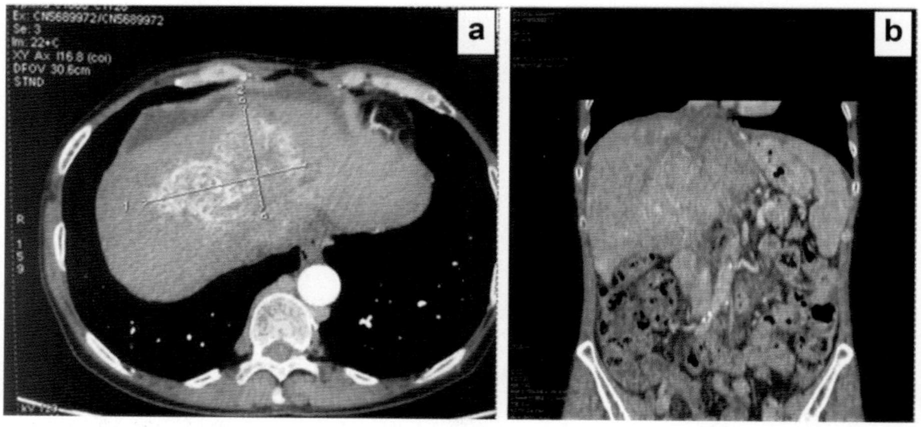

Fig. 1 Pre-Transplant CT-scans presenting: **a** Computed Tomography of a 110 × 75 × 70 mm hepatic alveolar echinoccocal cyst located in segments III–VIII; **b** Hepatic vein thrombosis – Budd-Chiari Syndrome

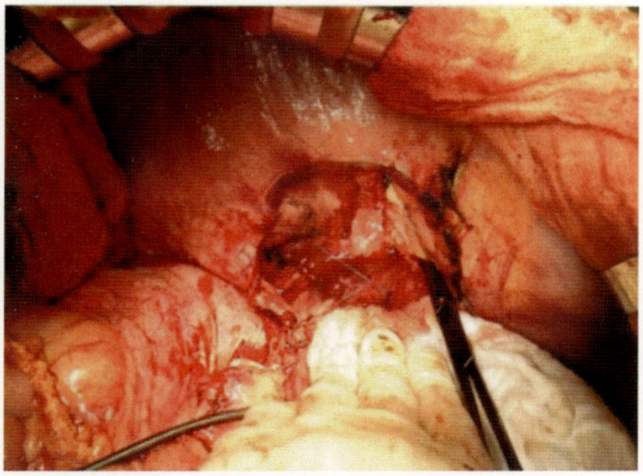

Fig. 2 Clamp applied to the right atrium and positioning of the sutures

mild, 1-min reperfusion syndrome with a systolic pressure of 60 mmHg was observed after 8 h 6 min of cold ischemia. At that point, pleural drainage was enabled. Further steps during transplantation were performed in a standard procedure. Intraoperative blood loss was estimated at 1000 ml; thus, 2 units of red blood concentrate and 4 units of fresh frozen plasma were transfused. The anhepatic phase was 136 min. Total operation time was 6.5 h.

An abdominal ultrasound was performed on the first post-operative day (POD), showing good vascular flow. An echocardiography performed on the second POD found no abnormalities. The pleural drain was removed on the third POD and a chest X-ray confirmed no signs of pneumothorax or effusion in the right pleural space. Time in the intensive transplant care unit was 3.5 days. The immunosuppressive regimen consisted of tacrolimus 0.05 mg/kg × 2 and prednisolone 20 mg × 1. The patient's liver tests recovered gradually. Computed tomography showed satisfactory and functioning hepato-atrial anastomosis (Fig. 4a and b). She was discharged on POD 25 and continued with tacrolimus 7 mg × 2, mycophenolate mofetil 500 mg × 2 and albendazole treatment 400 mg × once daily. Intolerance of the latter drug was not observed during hospitalization. At an 18-month follow-up and recurrence free period, the patient is doing well with good overall outcome and graft function.

Discussion

Hepatic alveolar echinococcosis (HAE) is a parasitic disease that develops slowly. Very often, the first symptoms manifest, as in our case of *E. multilocularis* (Fig. 3b), at a very advanced, mature stage. In the first imaging examinations, HAE can resemble a tumor like hepatocellular carcinoma. Clinical signs, such as mechanical jaundice, repetitive cholangitis, liver abscess, portal hypertension, esophageal varices, and sepsis are secondary to the disease. Additionally, Budd-Chiari Syndrome might be present [3–6].

Surgical resection usually is the main treatment for this disease; however, because alveolar symptoms tend to be absent for a long period of time, the cysts tend to be very advanced at diagnosis. Large lesions without response to drug treatment and with invasion of the vascular tree (Fig. 3c) of the liver will eventually develop BCS, thus should be directly qualified for LTx. This seems to be the only final treatment for HAE, and 90% of patients die within 10 years without surgery [4–7].

LTx due to HAE has been reported to have increased morbidity and mortality. A thorough examination is compulsory with MRI and three-dimensional computed tomography reconstruction in order to minimize intraoperative risk [7]. An early remark on the use of veno-venous bypass allows for better intraoperative preparation and greatly minimizes the risk of bowel congestion, shortens the hepatectomy time and limits the need for excessive maneuvers with the diseased liver, reducing the risk of tissue impairment and excessive bleeding [8–12]. A pericardial-peritoneum window as a procedure has been reported many times, but is performed due to malignant diseases or pericardial effusion and not during LTx [8–10, 12–14].

Several authors state that a pericardial-peritoneum window acts as a collection chamber for pericardial fluid, which is later absorbed through the peritoneum

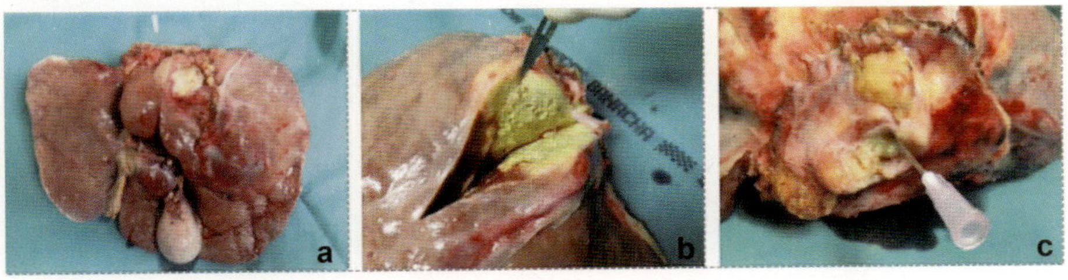

Fig. 3 **a** Explanted diseased liver; **b** Alveolar Cyst with *E. multilocularis* in the explanted liver; **c** Strictured lumen of the supra hepatic inferior vena cava, which was invaded by an alveolar lesion (marked by needle). Dissected diaphragm measured 10 × 10 cm

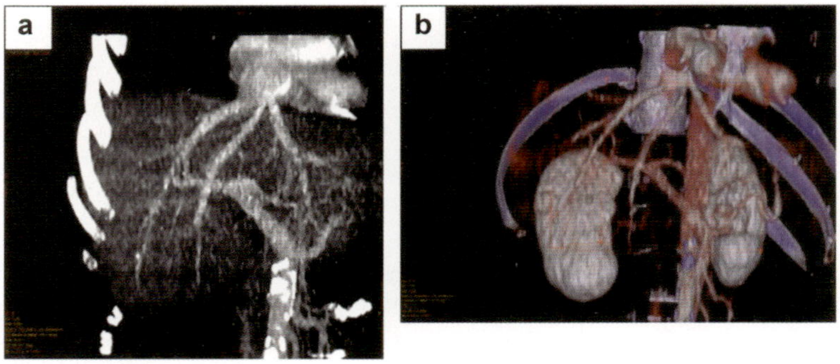

Fig. 4 Post-transplant computed tomography scans: **a** Anterior CT image of hepato-atrial (atrial-caval) anastomosis; **b** 3-Dimensional computed tomography reconstruction of the vascular image presenting the hepato-atrial anastomosis

[9, 10]. In our opinion, the implantation of the donor liver through such a suprahepatic atrium-IVC cuff end-to-end anastomosis allows both lobes of the liver to firmly press against the diaphragm. This creates a continuation of the thoracic-abdominal barrier, simultaneously avoiding future diaphragmatic hernia. Thus, leaving a 20-40-mm opening around the IVC anastomosis avoids its occlusion in the future, provides prompt drainage of fluid, and leaves the diaphragm under less tension. There has been several publications, mainly for initial BCS, presenting different solutions of cavoplasty in order to perform an atrial-caval anastomosis [15, 16]. Though principles are similar, our report presents how to manage a rare case of advanced HAE and in result secondary BCS.

Conclusions

LTx is feasible when performing an IVC hepato-atrial anastomosis. Patient's outcome is not impaired, and the post-operative results, follow up, and quality of life is good. Therefor even advanced cases of HAE may be successfully treated with liver transplantation.

Abbreviations

BCS: Budd-Chiari Syndrome; CD: Celiac Disease; EV: Esophageal Varices; GERD: Gastro-Esophageal Reflux Disease; HAE: Hepatic Alveolar Echinococcosis; IVC: Inferior vena cava; LTx: Liver transplantation; PDPS: Post-drug pancytopenia syndrome; PHG: Portal Hypertensive Gastropathy; POD: Post-operative day

Acknowledgements

Not Applicable.
The authors have adhered to CARE guidelines/methodology.

Funding

There is no funding to be declared for the preparation of this manuscript. The publication fee will be funded by the Medical University of Warsaw.

Authors' contributions

KK designed the report; KK, RP, KD, MKo performed the surgical procedure; PM, JR-W, UO-J post-operatively treated the patient; KK collected the patient's clinical data; KK, RP, JR-W, PR, MG, PM, WP, MKo analyzed the data; KK, RP, PM, MKr wrote and revised the paper. All authors read and approved the final manuscript.

Competing interests

The authors declare that they have no competing interests.

Author details

[1]Department of General, Transplant and Liver Surgery, Medical University of Warsaw, Poland. Banacha Street 1a, 02-097 Warsaw, Poland. [2]Department of Hepatology and Internal Diseases, Medical University of Warsaw, Warsaw, Poland.

References

1. Robles-Medranda C, Lukashok H, Biccas B, et al. Budd-Chiari like syndrome in decompensated alcoholic steatohepatitis and liver cirrhosis. World J Gastroenterol. 2006;12(40):6564–6.
2. Bayraktar UD, Seren S, Bayraktar Y. Hepatic venous outflow obstruction: three similar syndromes. World J Gastroenterol. 2007;13(13):1912–27.
3. Moreno-Gonzalez E, Loinaz Segurola C, Garcia Urena MA, et al. Liver transplantation for echinococcus granulosus hydatid disease. Transplantation. 1994;58:797.
4. Xia D, Yan LN, LI B, et al. Orthotopic liver transplantation for incurable alveolar echinococcosis: report of five cases from west China. Transplant Proc. 2005;37:2181.
5. Chomicz L, Szubert A, Fiedor P, et al. Human cystic and alveolar echinococcosis as indication to liver transplantation. Transplant Proc. 2003; 35:2260.
6. Koch S, Bresson-Hadni S, Miguet JP, et al. Experience of liver transplantation for incurable alveolar echinococcosis: a 45-case European collaborative report. Transplantation. 2003;75:856.
7. Moray G, Shahbazov S, Sevmis S, et al. Liver transplantation in management of alveolar echinococcosis: Two case reports. Transplant Proc. 2009;41:2936.
8. Chen ZY, Yan LN, Zeng Y, et al. Transdiaphragmatic exposure for direct atrioatrial anastomosis in liver transplantation. Chin Med J. 2010;24:3515.
9. Olson JE, Ryan MB, Blumenstock DA. Eleven years' experience with pericardial-peritoneal window in the management of malignant and benign pericardial effusions. Ann Surg Oncol. 1995;2:165–9.
10. Georgen M, Regimbeau JM, Kianmanesh R, et al. Removal of hepatocellular carcinoma extending in right atrium without extracorporeal bypass. J Am Coll Surg. 2002;195:892–4.
11. Facciuto ME, Babu S, Marvin M, et al. Intrapericardial control of the inferior vena cava from the abdominal cavity. J Hepatobiliary Pancreat Surg. 2004; 11:286–9.
12. Chen TW, Tsai CH, Chou SJ, et al. Intrapericardial isolation of inferior vena cava through a transdiaphragmatic pericardial window for tumor resection without sternotomy or thoracotomy. Eur J Surg Oncol. 2007;33:239–42.
13. Nesbitt JC, Soltero ER, Dinney CP, et al. Surgical management of renal cell carcinoma with inferior vena cava tumor thrombus. Ann Thorac Surg. 1997; 63:1592.

20

Management of suspected common bile duct stones on cholangiogram during same-stay cholecystectomy for acute gallstone-related disease

Sandra de Sousa[1*], Olivier Tobler[1], Pouya Iranmanesh[1], Jean-Louis Frossard[2,3], Philippe Morel[1,3] and Christian Toso[1,3]

Abstract

Background: Recent data have suggested that upfront cholecystectomy should be performed even in the presence of moderately abnormal liver function tests (LFTs). As a consequence, more common bile duct (CBD) stones are discovered on intra-operative cholangiogram. We assessed the presentation and management of such patients to refine their management plan.

Methods: Adult patients (>16 years) with an acute gallstone-related disease who had undergone same-stay cholecystectomy from January 2013 to January 2015 were retrospectively assessed. We excluded patients with pre-operative endoscopic CBD exploration.

Results: Among the 612 patients with same-stay cholecystectomy, 399 patients were included in the study, and 213 were excluded because of a pre-operative CBD exploration. Fifty patients (12.5%) presented an image of CBD stone on the intra-operative cholangiogram. Such patients were younger (47 vs. 55 years, $P = .01$) and less likely to present with fever (1 vs. 11.7%, $P = .04$) or signs of cholecystitis on ultrasound (66 vs. 83.7%, $P = .003$). Admission LFTs were higher in patients with an image of a stone. Among the 50 patients with an image on cholangiogram, a stone was confirmed in 26 (52%). Most patients ($n = 32$) underwent post-operative assessment with endoscopic ultrasound (EUS). LFTs did not predict the presence of a confirmed stone. However, the absence of contrast passage into the duodenum was negatively associated with a confirmed stone ($P = .08$), and a filling defect was positively associated with one ($P = .11$). Most confirmed stones were successfully extracted by endoscopic retrograde cholangiopancreatogram (ERCP) (25/26, 96%), except in one patient who needed a per-cutaneous approach because of duodenal diverticuli.

Conclusions: Same-stay cholecystectomy can (and should) be performed even in the presence of moderately abnormal liver function tests. The cholangiogram suspicion of a CBD stone is confirmed in only half of the patients (more often in the presence of a filling defect, and less often with the absence of contrast passage). All stones can be safely treated after surgery (most by ERCP).

Keywords: Suspected common bile duct stone, Same-stay cholecystectomy for acute gallstone-related disease, Filling defect on intra-operative cholangiogram, Trans-cystic drain

* Correspondence: sandra.desousa@hcuge.ch
[1]Division of Abdominal Surgery, Geneva University Hospitals, Faculty of Medicine, Rue Gabrielle-Perret-Gentil 4, 1205, Geneva, Switzerland
Full list of author information is available at the end of the article

Background

Gallstones are common and affect 10–15% of the adult population. Some 4% of these patients become symptomatic each year, with biliary colics, cholecystitis or cholangitis [1, 2]. In addition, 10–15% of the patients with symptoms also present a common bile duct (CBD) stone [3].

The likelihood of an associated CBD stone and its management have been established by the American Society for Gastrointestinal Endoscopy (ASGE) and Society of American Gastrointestinal and Endoscopic Surgeons (SAGES) guidelines [4]. Globally, patients with normal liver function tests (LFTs) are at low risk (<5%) for a CBD stone and should undergo cholecystectomy first. Those with elevated liver function tests (LFTs) are at increased risk, especially those with total bilirubin >70 µmol/l, which carries a risk for a CBD stone >50%. They should undergo a preliminary exploration of the CBD prior to cholecystectomy. We recently demonstrated that intermediate-risk patients with moderately elevated LFTs (including bilirubin <70 µmol/l) are best treated by upfront same-stay cholecystectomy with intra-operative cholangiogram [5]. This strategy is associated with a decreased length of stay and the need for fewer CBD investigations compared with a primary CBD exploration followed by cholecystectomy. The net effect is that more patients are discovered with an intra-operative CBD stone during same-stay cholecystectomy, and a routine intra-operative cholangiogram is needed [4, 5].

The factors predicting the presence of a CBD stone could still be improved. Such factors could be applied prior to or during surgery. However, a perfect split between patients with and without stone will likely never occur due to the heterogeneity of the signs linked to a CBD stone and because some patients present interval migrations (prior to or during cholecystectomy). Finally, many patients show a spontaneous migration to the duodenum [6]; therefore, a cholangiogram image of a stone does not necessarily translate into a stone on the post-operative assessment.

The aims of our study were therefore to (a) explore factors predicting the presence of a CBD stone image during upfront surgery, to (b) define the predictors of a stone on the post-operative assessment in patients with an image of a CBD stone on cholangiogram, and to (c) explore the efficiency of a post-operative EUS/ERCP management in case of intra-operative CBD stone discovery.

Methods

Study design

The study included a retrospective assessment of adult patients (>16 years) with acute gallstone-related disease who had undergone same-stay cholecystectomy from 01.01.2013 to 01.01.2015. Those with a suspected intra-operative CBD stone on cholangiogram were specifically assessed.

Inclusion criteria were: (a) adult patients (>16 years) admitted through the emergency room at the Geneva University Hospitals with a history of acute right upper quadrant pain, (b) radiologically proven gallbladder stone, (c) treatment by cholecystectomy during the same admission, and (d) the absence of CBD investigation prior to cholecystectomy.

Overall, patients presented with (a) prolonged biliary colic, with right upper quadrant pain >6 h, (b) acute cholecystitis with pain, blood signs of inflammation/infection, and a compatible ultrasound assessment, or (c) cholangitis as previously defined [7]. Data were prospectively collected during the hospital stay and analysed at the end of the inclusion period.

Management

Patients could be categorized into three groups according to their risk of presenting a CBD stone following the ASGE/SAGE guidelines [4]. Low-risk patients demonstrated normal LFTs. High-risk patients included those with serum bilirubin ≥ 70 µmol/l, a visible stone on pre-op imaging (ultrasound (US) or computed tomography (CT)), an ascending cholangitis, and those with bilirubin 30–70 µmol/l and CBD diameter >6 mm. Patients at intermediate risk of a CBD stone included those with abnormal LFTs not fulfilling the aforementioned criteria for high risk of a CBD stone. Based on a recent randomized clinical trial, patients at low and intermediate risk of a CBD stone were managed by cholecystectomy first [5] and represented the target population of patients included in the present study. High-risk patients underwent primary CBD endoscopic exploration followed by cholecystectomy and were not included in the present analysis to improve the population homogeneity.

All patients underwent same-stay laparoscopic cholecystectomy with intra-operative cholangiogram (IOC). Of note, the local policy to systematically performed an IOC is based on safety and didactic reasons, and is aiming at better identifying CBD stones. It is not fully supported by the current literature [8–10]. The cholangiogram looked for a filling defect compatible with a stone, the presence/absence of contrast passage into the duodenum, and a potential iatrogenic bile duct lesion. Patients with a suspected CBD stone on the IOC underwent a post-operative CBD exploration, most often based on endoscopic ultrasound (EUS) followed by endoscopic retrograde cholangiopancreatogram (ERCP) in the case of a confirmed stone. According to the clinical situation, and based on the surgeon's decision, some patients could be managed with a trans-cystic drain (Escat CH6 drain, Coloplast, Coloplast Group, Denmark).

Variables of interest

The main outcome of interest was the presence of an image of a CBD stone detected on IOC (filling-defect and/or the absence of contrast passage into the duodenum). We further assessed the patients with a confirmed stone on post-operative EUS.

Studied variables included demographic data (age, gender, body mass index (BMI)), admission data (fever, right upper quadrant pain, signs of cholecystitis on US, admission LFTs), and outcome data (length of hospital stay, conversion rate to a laparotomy, complications according to the Dindo/Clavien classification [11]). In addition, we recorded post-operative LFTs in the patients with an image of a CBD stone on the IOC.

Statistical analysis and ethics

Demographic and admission data were compared between patients with or without the image of a CBD stone on IOC to look for predictors of intra-operative stone. IOC characteristics and post-operative LFTs were compared between patients with or without a confirmed stone on post-operative EUS to identify predictors of a confirmed CBD stone on post-operative EUS. The groups were compared with Student's *t*-test and Chi-squared tests. The standard alpha level of .05 indicated statistical significance. Analyses were conducted using SPSS 18.0 (SPSS, Chicago, IL). Ethical approval was obtained from the Institutional Ethical Review Board under the number GE 15–087.

Results

Predictors of a CBD stone on IOC

During the study period, 612 adult patients were admitted for an acute gallstone-related disease and underwent a cholecystectomy. Among them, 399 patients were included in the study, and 213 were excluded because they underwent a pre-operative CBD assessment. Most of the patients were female (56.1%), with a mean age of 56 ± 19 years and a mean BMI of 28 ± 6 kg/m^2 (Table 1). Only two other patients were admitted during the study period, and were not included because they underwent a delayed cholecystectomy in subsequent hospital stay.

Among the 399 studied patients with upfront cholecystectomy, 50 (12.5%) presented an image of a CBD stone on IOC (Table 1). Such patients were younger (47 vs. 55 years, $P = .01$) than those without an image of a CBD stone on IOC. In addition, they were less likely to present fever on admission (2 vs. 11.7%, $P = .04$) or an associated

Table 1 Demographics and presentation comparing patients with or without a common bile duct stone image on cholangiogram

		Total (*N* = 399)	CBD stone (*N* = 50)	No CBD stone (*N* = 349)	*P* value
Gender	Male, No. (%)	175 (43.9%)	16 (32%)	159 (45.6%)	.07
	Female, No. (%)	224 (56.1%)	34 (68%)	190 (54.4%)	
Age (mean ± SD), years		56 ± 19	47 ± 20	55 ± 18	.01
BMI (mean ± SD), kg/m^2		28 ± 6	29 ± 6	28 ± 5	.58
Clinical presentation	Fever, No. (%)	42 (10.5%)	1 (2%)	41 (11.7%)	.04
	RUQ pain on admission, No. (%)	355 (89%)	42 (84%)	313 (89.7%)	.23
	Associated cholecystitis, No. (%)	325 (81.5%)	33 (66%)	292 (83.7%)	.003
Admission LFTs (mean ± SD)	ASAT, IU/L		167 ± 184	67 ± 146	.001
	ALAT, IU/L		166 ± 197	68 ± 121	.001
	PA, IU/L		123 ± 97	81 ± 48	.005
	GGT, IU/L		245 ± 276	94 ± 139	.001
	Total Bilirubin, µmol/L		26 ± 17	20 ± 12	.01
	Conjugated Bilirubin, µmol/L		18 ± 10	9 ± 7	.002
Abnormal admission LFTs	ASAT (11–42 IU/L), No. (%)	162 (40.6%)	36 (72%)	126 (36.1%)	< .001
	ALAT (9–42 IU/L), No. (%)	163 (40.9%)	34 (68%)	129 (37%)	< .001
	PA (30–125 IU/L), No. (%)	75 (18.8%)	14 (28%)	61 (17.5%)	.07
	GGT (9–35 IU/L), No. (%)	261 (65.4%)	43 (86%)	218 (62.5%)	.001
	Total Bilirubin (7–25 µmol/L), No. (%)	97 (24.3%)	20 (40%)	77 (22.1%)	.006
	Conjugated Bilirubin (2–9 µmol/L), No. (%)	319 (79.9%)	45 (90%)	274 (78.5%)	.06

BMI Body Mass Index, *RUQ* Right Upper Quadrant, *CBD* Common Bile Duct, *LFTs* Liver Function Tests, *SD* Standard Deviation, *ASAT* Aspartate Aminotransferase, *ALAT* Alanine Aminotransferase, *PA* Alkaline Phosphatase, *GGT* Gamma-glutamyl Transferase

cholecystitis on ultrasound (66 vs. 83.7%, $P = .003$). Finally, they demonstrated significantly higher admission LFTs (Table 1). We also assessed similar criteria only looking at patients with intermediate risk of CBD stone (demonstrating similar results as when using the entire cohort) (Additional file 1: Table S1).

In the CBD stone group ($N = 50$), all patients were assessed by IOC. In the No CBD stone group ($N = 349$), the IOC success rate was 81.4% (284/349). In the 65 patients without IOC, the absence of CBD stone was confirmed by MRCP, EUS, ERCP and by following the LFTs until their normalization, and checking the absence of subsequent management for a CBD stone.

Of note the present failure rate is similar to previous ones [9, 10].

Management of patients with a suspected CBD stone on IOC

A total of 50 patients demonstrated an image of a suspected stone on IOC, including 15 (15/50, 30%) with difficult or no contrast passage into the duodenum and 46 (46/50, 92%) with a filling defect compatible with a CBD stone. Among them, 45 patients underwent a post-operative CBD assessment 1.8 ± 1.2 days after surgery (Fig. 1). Among them, 32 underwent post-operative EUS, which confirmed the presence of a CBD stone in 17 patients (53.1%). All but one obtained a successful CBD clearance by ERCP. The only failure was linked to the presence of a duodenal diverticuli, and the stone was extracted by interventional radiology. Seven patients underwent post-operative ERCP without previous EUS. Six of them had a confirmed CBD stone, all successfully extracted. In addition, four patients underwent post-operative magnetic resonance cholangiopancreatography (MRCP), all negative. Two patients were followed with normalized LFT levels, as they refused any further investigation.

One patient underwent intra-operative ERCP with successful stone extraction. Two underwent laparoscopic stone extraction utilizing a Dormia basket. Two patients had a cholangiography through a transcystic drain left during surgery before EUS/ERCP. As this examination was negative, no further endoscopic assessment was performed, and the patients had drain removal a few weeks later.

Linked to the need for added investigation/intervention, patients with an image of a CBD stone on cholangiogram showed a longer length of stay, but the rates of major (stage 3 and 4) complications were not significantly different (6/50, 12% vs. 22/349, 6%, $P = .14$, (Table 2)).

In the CBD stone group, one patient (1/50, 2%) has been converted from laparoscopy to laparotomy because of adhesions and a stomach sero-muscular lesion. In addition, another patient underwent a laparotomy first due to a patent foramen ovale. In the No CBD stone group, 7 patients had a conversion (7/349, 2%), due to adhesions, severe pediculitis, haemorrhage, small bowel perforation, lack of identification of the cystic duct and necrotized gallbladder with peritonitis. In addition, two other patients

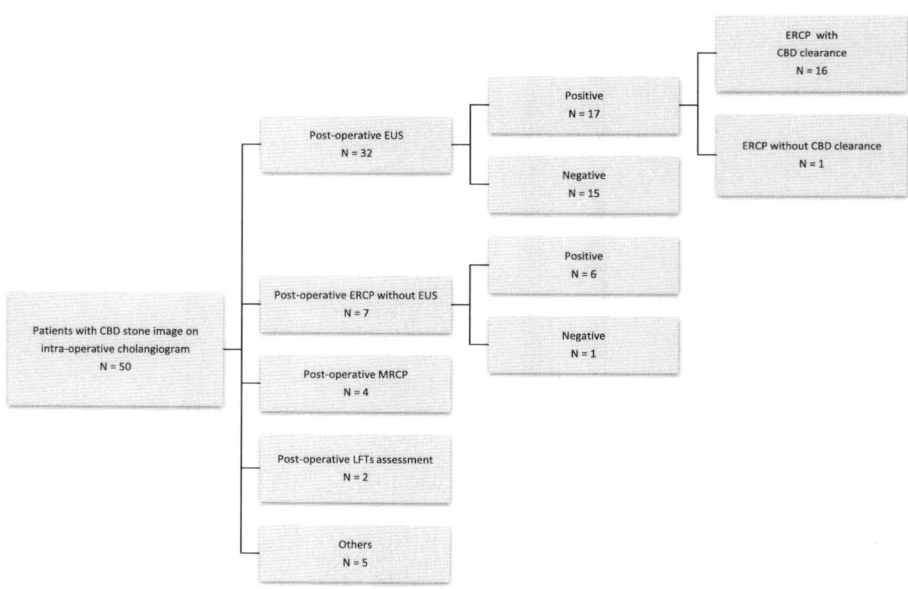

Fig. 1 Management of patients with a CBD stone image on intra-operative cholangiogram. *CBD* Common Bile Duct, *LFTs* Liver Function Tests, *EUS* Endoscopic Ultrasound, *ERCP* Endoscopic Retrograde Cholangiopancreatography, *MRCP* Magnetic Resonance Cholangiopancreatography

Table 2 Outcomes

		Total	CBD stone	No CBD stone	*P* value
		(*N* = 399)	(*N* = 50)	(*N* = 349)	
Conversion from LS to LT, No. (%)		8 (2%)	1 (2%)	7 (2%)	.998
Laparotomy first, No. (%)		3 (0.8%)	1 (2%)	2 (0.6%)	.275
LOS (mean ± SD), days		6.9 ± 4	8.8 ± 4.7	6.6 ± 3.8	.003
Complications (Dindo-Clavien classification)	Grade III, No	21	4	17	.35
	Grade IV, No	7	2	5	.2

LOS Length of Stay, *SD* Standard Deviation, *LS* Laparoscopy, *LT* Laparotomy

underwent a laparotomy first due to severe heart failure and septic shock.

Predictors of a CBD stone on post-operative CBD assessment

To identify predictors of confirmed CBD stones on post-operative EUS (only this group was used for a better homogeneity), the 15 patients with no sign of a remaining stone were compared with the 17 with a confirmed stone. The time between surgery and EUS was similar between the two groups (Table 3). LFTs assessed prior to EUS did not predict the presence of a stone on EUS (Table 3). An image of a filling defect on IOC compatible with a CBD stone tended to predict the presence of a confirmed stone ($P = .11$). Conversely, the absence of contrast passage into the duodenum tended to be associated with an absence of a stone on EUS ($P = .08$).

Impact of a trans-cystic drain

Of the patients described earlier, five (5/50, 10%) were managed with a transcystic drain. Among them, 3 (3/5, 60%) had no contrast passage into the duodenum. The delay between surgery and post-operative CBD investigation was significantly shorter for the group of patients with a transcystic drain than for those without a drain (1 ± 0.4 vs. 2 ± 1.3 days, $P = .003$). There was no significant difference in the length of stay (LOS) (11 ± 8 vs. 9 ± 4 days, $P = .56$). Complication rates were similar, but one patient developed a stage 4 Dindo/Clavien complication due the displacement of the trans-cystic drain (Table 4).

Discussion

The risk of a CBD stone is classically defined by a combination of clinical, biological and radiological parameters [4]. The present study assessed patients without previous CBD exploration and confirmed the value of LFTs, and clinical variables such as fever, as well as signs of cholecystitis on US [12]. In addition, women were more likely to present a stone.

Despite these known risk factors, our local policy is to perform an IOC in all patients undergoing cholecystectomy because models predicting the presence of a stone are not accurate enough [10–12]. Alternatively, IOC appears as efficient as ERCP in predicting the presence of a stone [13, 14]. Additionally, it bears a didactic value, training younger surgeons at approaching the CBD for a potential exploration. Finally, IOC also helps to detect an

Table 3 Comparison of patients with positive versus negative post-operative endoscopic ultrasound

		Positive EUS	Negative EUS	*P* value
		(*N* = 17)	(*N* = 15)	
LFTs before EUS	ASAT, IU/L	119 ± 120	100 ± 87	.62
	ALAT, IU/L	151 ± 194	167 ± 117	.79
	PA, IU/L	128 ± 89	86 ± 43	.18
	GGT, IU/L	290 ± 265	260 ± 233	.76
	Total Bilirubin, μmol/L	24 ± 15	33 ± 28	.28
	Conjugated Bilirubin, μmol/L	21 ± 12	31 ± 21	.34
Pancreatic tests before EUS	Lipase, IU/L	26 ± 9	108 ± 192	.3
Intra-operative cholangiogram	Filling defect present, No.	16	11	.11
	absent, No.	1	4	
	Contrast in duodenum present, No.	14	8	.08
	absent, No.	3	7	
Delay between surgery and post-operative EUS, days		1.8 ± 0.8	1.9 ± 1.4	.81

LFTs Liver Function Tests, *EUS* Endoscopic Ultrasound
ASAT Aspartate Aminotransferase, *ALAT* Alanine Aminotransferase, *PA* Alkaline Phosphatase, *GGT* Gamma-glutamyl Transferase

Table 4 Usefulness and safety of transcystic drainage in patients with an intra-operative suspicion of common bile duct stone

		Patients with transcystic drainage (*N* = 5)	Patients without transcystic drainage (*N* = 45)	*P* value
Duodenal passage of contrast product during IOC	Difficult duodenal passage, No.	2 (40%)	4 (9%)	.04
	No duodenal passage, No.	3 (60%)	4 (9%)	.002
Delay between surgery and post-operative CBD assessment, days		1 ± 0.4	2 ± 1.3	.003
Length of stay (mean ± SD), days		11 ± 8	9 ± 4	.56
Length of transcystic drainage (mean ± SD), days		39 ± 22	0	
Complications (Dindo-Clavien classification)	Grade I, No.	0	7	.34
	Grade II, No.	0	3	.55
	Grade III, No.	0	4	.49
	Grade IV, No.	1	1	.05

IOC Intra-operative Cholangiogram, *CBD* Common Bile Duct, *SD* Standard Deviation

iatrogenic bile duct lesion [15]. We acknowledge, however, that patients with normal LFTs undergoing elective cholecystectomy do not necessarily need an IOC. Conversely, we strongly recommend following the IOC path in patients undergoing cholecystectomy for acute gallstone-related diseases, especially in the case of abnormal LFTs.

Overall, an intra-operative stone was suspected in 12.5% (50/399) of the studied patients, based on IOC abnormalities. The preliminary injection of a limited quantity of contrast agent helps to detect a filling defect, while a stone can be less visible after the injection of a large volume of contrast agent. Of note, manoeuvres such as changing the table position and/or injecting saline help in the differential diagnosis with an air bubble. The second type of abnormality is the lack or a difficult contrast passage into the duodenum, which may be due to a trapped CBD stone, an Oddi's sphincter spasm, or a lesion of the sphincter (neoplasia/inflammation).

Only half of the suspected stones could be confirmed post-operatively. Based on the current data, it remains difficult to predict which patients will finally present a confirmed stone. Post-operative LFTs have no predictive power. LFTs may remain increased because of the previous injection of contrast during IOC or because a liver lesion occurred during the removal of the gallbladder from its bed. Only the presence of a filling defect tends to be predictive of a remaining CBD stone, whereas the absence of contrast passage into the duodenum is not. Most contrast passage alterations are likely linked to spasms. The net results of these observations are that a post-operative CBD assessment is required in all patients with an IOC abnormality and that LFTs do not necessarily need to be repeated after surgery due to their low predictive value.

We favour the use of post-operative EUS (+/-ERCP) in patients with an image of a stone during same-stay cholecystectomy. In fact, EUS accuracy is very high (near 97%) as are the sensitivity (71–100%), specificity (67–100%) and the positive or negative predictive values [16–19].

Such a strategy allowed the extraction of all stones by ERCP (with the exception of one patient treated by interventional radiology). As an alternative, laparoscopic CBD exploration could also be used. However, it can require the use of laparoscopic choledochotomy, with a risk of bile leak up to 15%, especially in patients with non-dilated CBD, and in the presence of inflammation [20]. In addition, the ERCP stone clearance rate appears higher than that after laparoscopic bile duct exploration [21, 22].

Another option would have been to perform ERCP during surgery (with or without rendezvous) [23]. Here again, we have not selected this strategy primarily because half of the patients do not show a confirmed stone on post-operative tests (and would have undergone unnecessary ERCP). Secondarily, emergency intra-operative ERCP is difficult to organize because of endoscopist availability and the positioning of the patient being non-standard for ERCP. The present study is limited by its retrospective nature and its potential for type 2 errors. However, it provides a real-life assessment of the proposed management strategy of patients at risk of CBD stones.

The present study is limited by its retrospective nature and its potential for type 2 errors. However, it provides a real-life assessment of the proposed management strategy of patients at risk of CBD stones.

Conclusion

As a whole, the present study confirms that same-stay cholecystectomy can (and should) be performed even in the presence of moderately abnormal liver function tests. The cholangiogram suspicion of a CBD stone can be confirmed in only half of the patients (more often in the presence of a filling defect, and less often with the absence of contrast passage). All stones can be safely treated after surgery (most by ERCP).

Abbreviations

ALAT: Alanine aminotransferase; ASAT: Aspartate aminotransferase; ASGE: American Society for Gastrointestinal Endoscopy; BMI: Body mass index; CBD: Common bile duct; CT: Computed tomography; ERCP: Endoscopic retrograde cholangiopancreatogram; EUS: Endoscopic ultrasound; GGT: Gamma-glutamyl transferase; IOC: Intra-operative cholangiogram; LFTs: Liver function tests; LOS: Length of stay; LS: Laparoscopy; LT: Laparotomy; MRCP: Magnetic resonance cholangiopancreatography; PA: Alkaline phosphatase; RUQ: Right upper quadrant; SAGES: Society of American Gastrointestinal and Endoscopic Surgeons; SD: Standard deviation; US: Ultrasound

Acknowledgements

CT was supported by the Swiss National Science Foundation (PP00P3_139021).

Funding

Christian Toso, MD, PhD, received salary support from the Swiss National Science Foundation (PP00P3_139021). This grant was not given specifically for the present study and was not used to conduct it.

Authors' contributions

All authors read and approved the final manuscript. The specific contributions of each author are as follows: SdS: study design, study protocol creation, literature search, data collection, data analysis, data interpretation, figure and table creation, manuscript writing. OT: study design, data collection, manuscript revision. IP: study design, data collection, manuscript revision. J-LF: study design, manuscript revision. PM: study design, manuscript revision. CT: study design, study protocol creation, data analysis, data interpretation, figure and table creation, manuscript correction.

Competing interests

The authors declare that they have no competing interests.

Author details

[1]Division of Abdominal Surgery, Geneva University Hospitals, Faculty of Medicine, Rue Gabrielle-Perret-Gentil 4, 1205, Geneva, Switzerland. [2]Division of Gastro-intestinal Disease and Hepatology, Geneva University Hospitals, Faculty of Medicine, Geneva, Switzerland. [3]Hepato-pancreatico-biliary Center, Geneva University Hospitals, Faculty of Medicine, Geneva, Switzerland.

References

1. Stinton LM, Shaffer EA. Epidemiology of Gallbladder Disease: Cholelithiasis and Cancer. Gut Liver. 2012;6(2):172–87.
2. Everhart JE, Khare M, Hill M, Maurer KR. Prevalence and Ethnic Differences in Gallbladder Disease in the United States. 1999. p. 632–9.
3. Horwood J, Akbar F, Katherine D, Morgan R. Prospective evaluation of a selective approach to cholangiography for suspected common bile duct stones. Ann R Coll Surg Engl. 2010;92(3):206–10. doi:10.1308/003588410X12628812458293.
4. Maple JT, Ben-Menachem T, Anderson MA, et al. The role of endoscopy in the evaluation of suspected choledocholithiasis. Gastrointest Endosc. 2010; 71(1):1–9. doi:10.1016/j.gie.2009.09.041.
5. Iranmanesh P, Frossard J-L, Mugnier-Konrad B, et al. Initial cholecystectomy vs sequential common duct endoscopic assessment and subsequent cholecystectomy for suspected gallstone migration: a randomized clinical trial. JAMA. 2014;312(2):137–44. doi:10.1001/jama.2014.7587.
6. Frossard JL, Hadengue A, Amouyal G, et al. Choledocholithiasis: a prospective study of spontaneous common bile duct stone migration. Gastrointest Endosc. 2000;51(2):175–9. doi:10.1016/S0016-5107(00)70414-7.
7. Takada T, Strasberg SM, Solomkin JS, Pitt HA, Gomi H, Yoshida M. TG13 : Updated Tokyo Guidelines for the management of acute cholangitis and cholecystitis. 2013. p. 1–7. doi:10.1007/s00534-012-0566-y.
8. Agresta F, Campanile FC, Vettoretto N, et al. Laparoscopic cholecystectomy : consensus conference-based guidelines. Langenbecks Arch Surg. 2015;429-453. doi:10.1007/s00423-015-1300-4.
9. Buddingh KT, Bosma BM, Ploeg RJ, et al. Kumar versus Olsen cannulation technique for intraoperative cholangiography : a randomized trial. Surg Endosc. 2013;957-963. doi:10.1007/s00464-012-2540-9.
10. Sato N, Shibao K, Akiyama Y. Routine Intraoperative Cholangiography During Single-Incision Laparoscopic Cholecystectomy : a Review of 196 Consecutive Patients. J Gastrointest Surg. 2013;668-674. doi:10.1007/s11605-012-2123-z.
11. Experience F, Vauthey JN, Dindo D, Schulick RD, Santiban E De. The Clavien-Dindo Classification of Surgical Complications. 2009;250(2):187-196. doi:10.1097/SLA.0b013e3181b13ca2.
12. Yang MH, Chen TH, Wang SE, et al. Biochemical predictors for absence of common bile duct stones in patients undergoing laparoscopic cholecystectomy. Surg Endosc. 2008;22(7):1620–4. doi:10.1007/s00464-007-9665-2.
13. Barkun AN, Barkun JS, Fried GM, et al. Useful predictors of bile duct stones in patients undergoing laparoscopic cholecystectomy. McGill Gallstone Treatment Group. Ann Surg. 1994;220(1):32–9. doi:10.1097/00000658-199407000-00006.
14. Gurusamy KS, Giljaca V, Takwoingi Y, et al. Endoscopic retrograde cholangiopancreatography versus intraoperative cholangiography for diagnosis of common bile duct stones. Cochrane Database Syst Rev. 2015; 2(2):CD010339. doi:10.1002/14651858.CD010339.pub2.
15. Eikermann M, Siegel R, Broeders I, et al. Prevention and treatment of bile duct injuries during laparoscopic cholecystectomy: The clinical practice guidelines of the European Association for Endoscopic Surgery (EAES). Surg Endosc Other Interv Tech. 2012;26(11):3003–39. doi:10.1007/s00464-012-2511-1.
16. Buscarini E, Tansini P, Vallisa D, et al. EUS for suspected choledocholithiasis : Do benefits outweigh costs ? A prospective, controlled study. Gastrointest Endosc. 2003;57(4):510–8. doi: 10.1067/mge.2003.149.
17. Tse F, Liu L, Barkun AN. ORIGINAL ARTICLE : Clinical Endoscopy EUS : a meta-analysis of test performance in suspected choledocholithiasis. Gastrointest Endosc. 2008;67(2):235–44. doi:10.1016/j.gie.2007.09.047.
18. Canto MIF, Chak A, Stellato T, et al. Endoscopic ultrasonography versus cholangiography for the diagnosis of choledocholithiasis. Gastrointest Endosc. 1998;47(6):439–48.
19. Aljebreen A, Azzam N, Eloubeidi MA. Prospective study of endoscopic ultrasound performance in suspected choledocholithiasis. J Gastroenterol Hepatol. 2008;23(5):741–5. doi:10.1111/j.1440-1746.2008.05318.x.
20. Nathanson LK, O'Rourke NA, Martin IJ, et al. Postoperative ERCP versus laparoscopic choledochotomy for clearance of selected bile duct calculi: a randomized trial. Ann Surg. 2005;242(2):188–92. doi:10.1097/01.sla.0000171035.57236.d7.
21. Poh BR, Ho SPS, Sritharan M, et al. Randomized clinical trial of intraoperative endoscopic retrograde cholangiopancreatography *versus* laparoscopic bile duct exploration in patients with choledocholithiasis. Br J Surg. 2016;103(9): 1117–24. doi:10.1002/bjs.10207.
22. Bansal VK, Misra MC, Rajan K, et al. Single-stage laparoscopic common bile duct exploration and cholecystectomy versus two-stage endoscopic stone extraction followed by laparoscopic cholecystectomy for patients with concomitant gallbladder stones and common bile duct stones: A randomized con. Surg Endosc Other Interv Tech. 2014;28(3):875–85. doi:10.1007/s00464-013-3237-4.
23. Tzovaras G, Baloyiannis I, Zachari E, et al. Laparoendoscopic Rendezvous Versus Preoperative ERCP and Laparoscopic Cholecystectomy for the Management of Cholecysto-Choledocholithiasis. Ann Surg. 2012;255(3):435–9. doi:10.1097/SLA.0b013e3182456ec0.

21

Proteinuria can predict prognosis after liver transplantation

Heng-Chih Pan[1], Ying-Jen Chen[2], Jhe-Ping Lin[3], Ming-Jung Tsai[3], Chang-Chyi Jenq[3,4], Wei-Chen Lee[3,5*], Ming-Hung Tsai[3,6], Pei-Chun Fan[4], Chih-Hsiang Chang[4], Ming-Yang Chang[3,4], Ya-Chung Tian[3,4], Cheng-Chieh Hung[3,4], Ji-Tseng Fang[3,4], Chih-Wei Yang[3,4] and Yung-Chang Chen[3,4*]

Abstract

Background: Proteinuria is a manifestation of renal dysfunction and it has been demonstrated to be a significant prognostic factor in various clinical situations. The study was designed to analyze prognosis of patients receiving liver transplantation as well as to determine predictive performance of perioperative proteinuria.

Methods: We retrospectively reviewed data of patients who had received a liver transplant in a medical center between 2002 and 2010. Demographic information and clinical characteristic parameters were recorded on the day of intensive care unit admission before operation and on postoperative days 1, 7, and 14.

Results: Among a total of 323 patients, in-hospital mortality and 90-day mortality rates were 13.0 % (42/323) and 14.2 % (46/323), respectively. Patients with proteinuria on admission had higher rates of acute kidney injury (26.8 % vs. 8.8 %, $p < 0.001$), severe infection episodes (48.8 % vs. 30.7 %, $p = 0.023$), hospital death (31.1 % vs. 10.1 %, $p < 0.001$), and 90-day mortality (37.7 % vs. 10.9 %, $p < 0.001$). Multivariate analysis showed that proteinuria on admission and Sequential Organ Failure Assessment (SOFA) score were independent predictors of in-hospital mortality. The discriminatory ability of proteinuria plus SOFA was even better than that of SOFA alone, especially on postoperative day 1.

Conclusions: The presence of proteinuria before liver transplantation is supposed to be recognized as a negative predictor for in-hospital survival. Moreover, the presence of proteinuria after liver transplantation can assist in the early prediction of poor short-term prognosis for patients receiving liver transplantation.

Keywords: Liver transplantation, Proteinuria, SOFA, Prognosis, Mortality

Background

Proteinuria has been suggested to be a predictive factor and an important tool for differentiating the etiology of renal dysfunction in various clinical scenarios [1, 2]. The good predictive performance of preoperative proteinuria utilized for the development of renal failure after operation has been reported [3]. Lin et al. also demonstrated that the presence of proteinuria in patients with end-stage liver disease is associated with increased risk of intensive care unit (ICU) mortality and poor short-term outcome [4].

In the literature, prognostic significance of several scoring systems for end-stage liver disease has been validated [5–7]. Wong and colleagues further compared the predictive accuracy of the commonly used scores in 149 end-stage liver disease patients undergone liver transplantation. The Sequential Organ Failure Assessment (SOFA) system was found to be superior to Child-Pugh points (CP points) and Model for End-Stage Liver Disease (MELD) score, and postoperative day 7 SOFA had the best discriminative power for predicting 3-month and 1-year mortality after liver transplantation [8].

Renal dysfunction is one of the most significant adverse events in patients awaiting or undergoing a liver transplant, and its occurrence generally indicates a high rate of poor prognosis [9, 10]. Prediction of acute kidney

* Correspondence: weichen@cgmh.org.tw; cyc2356@gmail.com
[3]Chang Gung University College of Medicine, Taoyuan, Taiwan
Full list of author information is available at the end of the article

injury (AKI) is important for clinical decision making. Numerous researches have demonstrated that the presence of proteinuria provides a clue to the structural impairment of the kidney and reflects increased risk of developing AKI in general population [11, 12]. In spite of the fact that proteinuria has been increasingly considered as a significant manifestation of acute or chronic renal disease [13], no study clarify the association between presence of proteinuria and prognosis of patients undergoing liver transplant. This study aims to assess proteinuria as an early marker of renal dysfunction for liver transplant as well as to compare the outcome prediction efficacy of proteinuria with that of the main scores in the setting of liver transplant.

Methods

Patient information and data collection

This research was performed from October 2002 to December 2010 in a 2000-bed medical center in Taiwan. A total of 323 patients with end-stage liver disease and acute liver failure received liver transplant were included. Patients less than 18 years of age, patients who had previously received liver transplant, and patients with end-stage renal disease were excluded.

We retrospectively reviewed following data: demographic information, aetiologies of primary liver disease, clinical parameters, donor type, anesthesia time, operation time, duration of hospitalization and ICU stay, and outcome. Illness severity was evaluated on the day of ICU admission before operation and on postoperative day 1, 7, and 14. The primary outcome of this research was in-hospital mortality rate. Follow-up at 90-day after transplantation was performed by chart records review or telephone interview [8].

Definitions

Urine dipstick analysis was used to detect proteinuria. The results were graded as negative (less than 15 mg/dL), trace (15 to 30 mg/dL), 1+ (30 to 100 mg/dL), 2+ (100 to 300 mg/dL), 3+ (300 to 1000 mg/dL) or 4+ (more than 1000 mg/dL). In this study, proteinuria was defined as presence (urine dipstick reading trace, or $\geq$ 1+) or absence (negative urine dipstick reading). The urinary analysis was performed on ICU admission and postoperative days 1, 7, and 14 [4].

Severity of liver disease was assessed by CP points and MELD score [14, 15]. Severity of illness was also graded by SOFA score according to the six organ systems. AKI was diagnosed according to definition of the RIFLE criteria (Table 1). The RIFLE classification was also used to classify patients into risk (RIFLE-R), injury (RIFLE-I), and failure (RIFLE-F) groups [16]. No patient met the criteria for classification of loss of kidney function (RIFLE-L) or end-stage renal disease (RIFLE-E). The following simple model for mortality was constructed: non–acute kidney injury (0 points), RIFLE-R (1 point), RIFLE-I (2 points), and RIFLE-F (3 points) [15]. The worst values measured on the day of ICU admission and postoperative days 1, 7, and 14 were recorded.

Statistical analysis

Data analyses were performed using the statistical package SPSS 19.0 (SPSS, Inc., Chicago, IL, USA). All statistical tests are 2-tailed. A *p*- value of <0.05 is considered to represent statistical significance. Continuous variables were presented as means and standard derivations, and categorical data were summarized as frequency and percentage unless otherwise stated. Hospital survivors were compared with nonsurvivors in the primary analysis. Kolmogorov–Smirnov test was employed for testing normal distribution. Normally distributed continuous variables were compared by Student's *t*-test and non-normally distributed ones were compared by Mann–Whitney *U* test. Categorical data were tested by the chi-square test. The risk factors for in-hospital mortality were assessed by univariate analysis, and statistically significant variables were included in the multivariate analysis. For analyzing these variables, backward multiple logistic regression model was employed.

Hosmer–Lemeshow goodness-of-fit test was used to examined calibration and compare the number of predicted and observed mortality. Discrimination in predicting 90-day mortality was assessed by area under the receiver operating characteristic (AUROC) curve. Nonparametric approach was used to compare the AUROC values. Analyses of the ROC curves were applied for calculating sensitivity, specificity, and overall correctness. The cutoff value was decided according to the ability to offer the highest Youden index [17]. Cumulative survival curves were plotted using the Kaplan-Meier method and compared by the log rank test. Correlation of proteinuria and serum creatinine (SCr) measured on ICU admission was measured by Pearson analysis and linear regression. The prevalence of proteinuria before operation, and on postoperative day 1, 7, and 14 were compared between 90-day survivors and nonsurvivors by repeated-measures analysis of variance using the general linear model procedure.

Results

Patient characteristics

Three hundred and twenty-three patients who received liver transplant from October 2002 to December 2010 were enrolled. Overall in-hospital mortality rate was 13.0 % (42/323). Table 2 listed patient data and

Table 1 The criteria of SOFA score and RIFLE classification

SOFA Score	0	1	2	3	4
Respiration					
PaO2/FiO2	>400	>300–≤ 400	>200–≤ 300	>100–≤ 200 with ventilator	≤100 with ventilator
Coagulation					
Platelets, $\times 10^3/mm^3$	>150	>100–≤ 150	>50–≤ 100	>20–≤ 50	≤20
Liver					
Bilirubin, mg/dL (μmol/L)	<1.2 (<20)	≥1.2–< 2.0 (20–32)	≥2.0–< 6.0 (33–101)	≥6.0–< 12.0 (102–204)	≥12.0 (>204)
Cardiovascular					
Hypotension	MAP ≥ 70 mm Hg	MAP <70 mm Hg	Dopamine ≤5 or dobutamine (any dose)[a]	Dopamine >5 or epi ≤0.1 or norepi ≤0.1[a]	Dopamine >15 or epi >0.1 or norepi >0.1[a]
CNS					
Glasgow Coma Score	15	13–14	10–12	6–9	<6
Renal					
Creatinine, mg/dL (μmol/L) or urine output	<1.2 (<110)	≥1.2–< 2.0 (110–170)	≥2.0–< 3.5 (171–299)	≥3.5–< 5.0 (300–440) or <500 mL/day	≥5.0 (>440) or <200 mL/day

RIFLE Classification	SCr criteria	UO Criteria
Definition	SCr changes over 1–7 days, sustained for more than 24 h	UO < 0.5 ml/kg/h × 6 h
Risk	Increase in SCr ≥ 1.5 × baseline or decrease in GFR ≥ 25 %	UO < 0.5 ml/kg/h × 6 h
Injury	Increase in SCr ≥ 2.0 × baseline or decrease in GFR ≥ 50 %	UO < 0.5 ml/kg/h × 12 h
Failure	Increase in SCr ≥ 3.0 × baseline or an absolute serum creatinine ≥ 4.0 mg/dl with an acute rise of at least 0.5 mg/dl or decrease in GFR ≥ 75 %	UO < 0.5 ml/kg/h × 24 h or anuria × 12 h
Loss	Complete loss of kidney function > 4 weeks	
ESRD	End-stage renal disease (>3 months)	

[a]Abbreviations: *SOFA* the sequential organ failure assessment, *RIFLE* risk of renal failure, injury to kidney, failure of kidney function, loss of kidney function, and end-stage renal failure, *SCr* serum creatinine, *UO* urine output, *hrs* hours, *ESRD* end-stage renal disease, *RRT* renal replacement therapy

clinical characteristics of both survivors and non-survivors. Mean patient age was 51 years; 231 were male (71 %) and 92 were female (29 %). Ninety-one patients (28.2 %) received deceased-donor grafts. Mean length of ICU stay was 21 days. There was no significant difference in age or gender between survivors and non-survivors. Table 3 listed primary liver diseases and presumptive causes of AKI on the first day after transplantation. In this research, hepatitis B virus infection (34 %) was the leading cause of liver diseases, followed by hepatitis B virus infection with hepatoma (15 %). Patient who developed AKI tended to attribute to multiple reasons (23 %), followed by infection (13 %).

Risk factors for adverse outcomes

Table 4 listed the correlation of operation time and newly onset proteinuria after transplantation. Among patients who received deceased-donor grafts,

Table 2 Patient demographic data and clinical characteristics according to in-hospital mortality

	All patients ($n = 323$)	Survivors ($n = 281$)	Non-survivors ($n = 42$)	P-value
Age (years)	50.8 ± 10.4	50.9 ± 9.8	50.3 ± 13.8	NS (0.753)
Gender (M/F)	231/92	199/82	32/10	NS (0.583)
BMI on admission (kg/m^2)	24.3 ± 4.0	24.7 ± 4.0	21.1 ± 2.4	**<0.001**
History of diabetes mellitus (yes/no)	55/268	46/235	9/33	NS (0.387)
History of chronic kidney disease (yes/no)	31/292	22/259	9/33	**0.005**
Proteinuria on admission (yes/no)	45/278	31/250	14/28	**<0.001**
Hemoglobin on admission (g/dL)	10.6 ± 2.2	10.7 ± 2.2	9.8 ± 2.1	**0.008**
Leukocytes on admission (× 10^9/L)	2.9 ± 3.7	2.8 ± 3.5	3.3 ± 4.9	NS (0.569)
Platelets on admission (× 10^9/L) [median]	72.7 [60]	72.9 ± [60]	71.1 [59]	NS (0.809)
Prothrombin time INR on admission	1.8 ± 0.7	1.8 ± 0.7	1.9 ± 0.7	NS (0.050)
Serum sodium on admission (mmol/L)	137.8 ± 5.7	137.9 ± 5.4	137.0 ± 8.0	NS (0.471)
AST on admission (U/L) [median]	88.8 [62]	87.5 [64]	98.3 [51]	NS (0.498)
ALT on admission (U/L) [median]	67.2 [39]	67.4 [40]	65.8 [34]	NS (0.938)
Total bilirubin on admission (μmol/L) [median]	145.4 [51]	130.0 [50]	244.5 [96]	**0.003**
A-a gradient on admission (mmHg) [median]	25.1 [17]	22.8 [17]	43.3 [18]	**0.039**
Serum creatinine on admission (μmol/L) [median]	97.2 [77]	92.2 [75]	114.9 [84]	NS (0.064)
Hepatorenal syndrome, n (%)	29 (9)	22 (8)	7 (17)	NS (0.079)
MAP on admission (mmHg)	86.1 ± 12.4	86.3 ± 12.7	84.7 ± 10.3	NS (0.427)
Child-Pugh points on admission	10.1 ± 2.6	9.9 ± 2.7	11.1 ± 2.0	**0.010**
MELD score on admission	17.6 ± 9.0	17.1 ± 8.9	21.4 ± 9.7	**0.025**
RIFLE on admission (No AKI/Risk/Injury/Failure)	286/16/9/12	250/13/9/9	36/3/0/3	NS (0.449)
SOFA score on admission	5.1 ± 2.7	4.8 ± 2.5	6.7 ± 3.3	**0.001**
Anesthesia time during operation (hours)	12.1 ± 1.8	12.1 ± 1.9	12.4 ± 1.5	NS (0.362)
Donor type (DDLT /LDLT)	91/232	74/207	17/25	**0.018**
Total operative time (mins) [median]	687.1 [683]	685.6 [683]	697.2 [682]	NS (0.589)
Cold ischemia time (mins) [median]	85.0 [15]	74.8 [15]	166.4 [17]	NS (0.125)
Warm ischemia time (mins) [median]	128.2 [122]	126.3 [121]	141.1 [129]	NS (0.115)
Graft-to-recipient weight ratio (%)	1.0 ± 0.3	1.0 ± 0.3	1.1 ± 0.5	NS (0.125)
Blood loss volume during operation (ml) [median]	3034 [2000]	2672 [1840]	4430 [2000]	**0.014**
Length of ICU stay (days) [median]	21.0 [14]	19.2 [14]	33.6 [24]	**0.002**
Length of hospital stay (days) [median]	47.8 [38]	46.7 [38]	54.7 [44]	NS (0.215)

Values in bold are statistically significant (P-value < 0.05)

There were significant differences in BMI on admission, history of chronic kidney disease, presence of proteinuria on admission, hemoglobin on admission, total bilirubin on admission, A-a gradient on admission, Child-Pugh points on admission, MELD score on admission, SOFA score on admission, blood loss volume during operation, and length of ICU stay

Abbreviation: *M* male, *F* female, *ICU* intensive care unit, *MAP* mean arterial pressure, *INR* international normalized ratio, *AST* aspartate aminotransferase, *ALT* alanine aminotransferase, *DM* diabetes mellitus, *MELD* model for end-stage liver disease, *SOFA* sequential organ failure assessment, *AKI* acute kidney injury, *DDLT* deceased donor liver transplantation, *LDLT* living donor liver transplantation

Table 3 Primary liver diseases and presumptive causes of AKI after operation according to in-hospital mortality

	All patients $n = 323$	Survivors $n = 281$	Non-survivors $n = 42$	*P*-value
Primary liver disease	323 (100)	281 (100)	42 (100)	
Alcoholic, n (%)	16 (5)	12 (4)	4 (10)	NS (0.254)
Hepatitis B, n (%)	111 (34)	100 (36)	11 (26)	NS (0.848)
Hepatitis C, n (%)	31 (10)	23 (8)	8 (19)	**0.003**
Hepatoma, n (%)	3 (1)	3 (1)	0 (0)	NS (1.000)
Alcoholic + hepatitis B, n (%)	21 (6)	15 (7)	2 (5)	NS (1.000)
Alcoholic + hepatitis C, n (%)	5 (2)	5 (2)	0 (0)	NS (1.000)
Alcoholic + hepatoma, n (%)	3 (1)	3 (1)	0 (0)	NS (1.000)
Hepatitis B + hepatitis C, n (%)	17 (5)	14 (5)	3 (7)	NS (0.723)
Hepatitis B + hepatoma, n (%)	49 (15)	43 (15)	6 (14)	NS (0.172)
Hepatitis C + hepatoma, n (%)	31 (10)	29 (10)	2 (5)	NS (0.134)
Alcoholic + hepatitis B + hepatoma, n (%)	2 (1)	1 (1)	1 (2)	NS (0.429)
Other causes, n (%)[a]	34 (10)	29 (10)	5 (12)	NS (0.787)
Presence of AKI after transplantation (Post-OP day1)	125 (39)	101 (36)	24 (57)	**0.011**
Prerenal type of AKI, n (%)	2 (1)	2 (1)	0 (0)	NS (1.000)
Infection related AKI, n (%)	42 (13)	31 (11)	11 (26)	**0.006**
Nephrotoxic agent exposure related AKI, n (%)	6 (2)	6 (2)	0 (0)	NS (0.601)
Mixed type and other causes of AKI, n (%)[b]	75 (23)	62 (22)	13 (31)	NS (0.236)

Values in bold are statistically significant (*P*-value < 0.05)
Hepatitis C virus infection was independently associated with in-hospital mortality
Presence of infection related AKI on the first day after transplantation was independently associated with in-hospital mortality
[a]Biliary cirrhosis, biliary sclerosis, autoimmune hepatitis, Wilson's disease, polycystic liver disease, drugs, and unknown causes
[b]Multifactor related, ischemia/reperfusion injury, or unknown cause

those with newly onset proteinuria tended to have longer cold ischemia time. While in patients who received living-donor grafts, those with newly onset proteinuria tended to have longer warm ischemia time.

The univariate analysis showed that 9 (Table 5) out of the 31 variables (Table 2) were good prognostic indicators for in-hospital mortality. On performing the multivariate analysis, we recognized presence of proteinuria and SOFA determined on the first day of ICU admission as having independent prognostic significance (Table 5). Regression coefficients of these variables were used to calculate the odds of death in each patient as follows:

Logarithm of odds of death = $-2.471 + 1.320 \times$ Proteinuria + $0.157 \times$ SOFA score.

Table 4 Operation time according to newly onset proteinuria after transplantation

	Patients with no proteinuria on admission	Patients with newly onset proteinuria on post-OP day 1	Patients with no newly onset proteinuria on post-OP day 1	*P*-value
LDLT	$n = 208$	$n = 65$ (31.2 %)	$n = 143$ (68.8 %)	
Total operative time (mins) [median]	703.9 [695]	789.3 [811]	707.6 [691]	NS (0.087)
Cold ischemia time (mins) [median]	85.4 [14]	27.9 [15]	21.9 [13]	NS (0.659)
Warm ischemia time (mins) [median]	128.2 [130]	194.0 [182]	127.6 [133]	**0.004**
DDLT	$n = 70$	$n = 47$ (67.1 %)	$n = 23$ (32.9 %)	
Total operative time (mins) [median]	640.0 [633]	646.2 [653]	625.8 [632]	NS (0.876)
Cold ischemia time (mins) [median]	651.3 [583]	756.5 [634]	552.0 [541]	**0.039**
Warm ischemia time (mins) [median]	113.5 [91]	114.0 [90]	101.4 [90]	NS (0.737)

Values in bold are statistically significant (*P*-value < 0.05)
In the LDLT group, patients with newly onset proteinuria had significantly longer warm ischemia time
In the DDLT group, patients with newly onset proteinuria had significantly longer cold ischemia time
Abbreviation: *DDLT* deceased donor liver transplantation, *LDLT* living donor liver transplantation

Table 5 Variables showing prognostic significance for in-hospital mortality

Parameters	Beta Coefficient	Standard error	Odds ratios (95 % CI)	*P*-value
Univariate logistic regression				
BMI on admission (kg/m^2)	−0.247	0.050	0.781 (0.708–0.861)	**<0.001**
History of chronic kidney disease	1.167	0.437	3.211 (1.364–7.557)	**0.008**
Proteinuria on admission	1.480	0.398	4.391 (2.011–9.587)	**<0.001**
Hemoglobin on admission (g/dL)	−0.218	0.083	0.804 (0.683–0.947)	**0.009**
Total bilirubin on admission (mg/dL)	0.037	0.011	1.038 (1.015–1.061)	**0.001**
Donor type (DDLT /LDLT)	−0.41	0.169	0.664 (0.477–0.925)	**0.015**
A-a gradient on admission	0.009	0.003	1.009 (1.002–1.016)	**0.007**
Child-Pugh points on admission	0.176	0.070	1.193 (1.040–1.368)	**0.012**
MELD score on admission	0.046	0.056	1.047 (0.999–1.098)	NS (0.056)
SOFA score on admission	0.219	0.057	1.245 (1.114–1.391)	**<0.001**
Blood loss volume during operation (ml)	<0.001	<0.001	1.000 (1.000–1.000)	**0.003**
Length of ICU stay (days)	0.018	0.006	1.018 (1.007–1.029)	**0.002**
Multivariate logistic regression				
Proteinuria on admission	1.320	0.478	3.745 (1.468–9.554)	**0.006**
SOFA on admission	0.157	0.067	1.170 (1.027–1.333)	**0.019**
Constant	−2.471	0.245	0.085	**<0.001**

On performing multivariate logistic regression, the presence of proteinuria on admission and SOFA score on admission had independent prognostic significance for assessing in-hospital mortality
Abbreviation: *MELD* model for end-stage liver disease, *SOFA* sequential organ failure assessment

Calibration and discrimination of the scoring systems

Table 6 showed values of calibration and discrimination of proteinuria, CP points, MELD, RIFLE, and SOFA in predicting 90-day mortality. For assessing calibration, the number of observed and predicted mortality was compared by Hosmer-Lemeshow goodness-of-fit. Discriminatory power was assessed by AUROC. On basis of the ROC analysis, discriminatory ability of SOFA and MELD determined on preoperative, postoperative days 1, 7, and 14 were better than that of CP points and proteinuria.

The proteinuria plus SOFA score [following variables were applied for the calculation: presence of proteinuria (1 point) and SOFA] was defined as the addition of the two variables, with sum ranging from 0 to 25 [4]. The discriminatory ability of this score seemed to be superior to that of other evaluating systems, including proteinuria, CP points, MELD, RIFLE, SOFA, and proteinuria plus nonrenal SOFA scores. AUROC curves were highest for proteinuria plus SOFA on postoperative day 7 to predict 90-day mortality (0.907 ± 0.041). AUROC value for proteinuria plus SOFA determined on postoperative day 1 was significantly higher than that for proteinuria, RIFLE, CP points, and MELD. AUROC for proteinuria plus SOFA determined on postoperative day 7 and 14 were significantly higher than that for proteinuria, RIFLE, and CP points.

Indices for predicting short-term prognosis

For evaluation and validation of the scoring systems, we compared the sensitivity, specificity, and overall correctness of prediction at cut-off values which could offer the highest Youden index (Table 7). At preoperative, postoperative days 1, 7, and 14, The proteinuria plus SOFA had the best Youden index and overall correctness in predicting 90-day mortality

In this study population, 45 patients had proteinuria while 278 patients had no proteinuria on ICU admission. Patients with proteinuria on admission had higher incidence of AKI (26.8 % vs. 8.8 %, $p < 0.001$), severe infection episodes requiring prolonged courses of antibiotics or inotropic agents (48.8 % vs. 30.7 %, $p = 0.023$), hospital death (31.1 % vs. 10.1 %, $p < 0.001$), and 90-day mortality (37.7 % vs. 10.9 %, $p < 0.001$) than those without proteinuria.

Figure 1 illuminates the significantly different cumulative survival rates between patients with and without proteinuria as well as the similar cumulative survival rates between patients with and without SCr level elevation (Increase in SCr ≥ 1.5 × baseline) on ICU admission (before transplantation). Fig. 2 shows the weak correlation of proteinuria and SCr measured on ICU admission ($P = 0.143$). Fig. 3 illustrates significant increases in the prevalence of proteinuria during the time (starting before transplantation to 14 days postoperatively) among hospital and 90-day mortality groups but not survival groups.

Table 6 Calibration and discrimination for the scoring methods used in predicting 90-day mortality

	Calibration			Discrimination		
	Goodness-of-fit (x^2)	df	*p*	AUROC ± SE	95 % CI	*P*
On admission						
Proteinuria	-	-	-	0.582 ± 0.053	0.479–0.685	NS (0.100)
Child-Pugh points	10.157	7	0.180	0.580 ± 0.041	0.499–0.662	NS (0.087)
MELD score	5.845	8	0.665	0.609 ± 0.067	0.418–0.680	NS (0.067)
RIFLE	—	—	—	0.577 ± 0.067	0.355–0.618	NS (0.845)
SOFA	1.618	5	0.899	0.648 ± 0.049	0.552–0.745	**0.002**
Proteinuria plus SOFA	1.047	5	0.959	0.659 ± 0.052	0.557–0.761	**0.002**
Proteinuria plus nonrenal SOFA	6.347	6	0.385	0.658 ± 0.055	0.550–0.765	**0.002**
Postoperative day 1						
Proteinuria	-	-	-	0.609 ± 0.090	0.432–0.786	NS (0.240)
Child-Pugh points	2.438	5	0.786	0.639 ± 0.062	0.479–0.721	NS (0.142)
MELD score	5.947	8	0.653	0.705 ± 0.044	0.620–0.791	**<0.001**
RIFLE	2.684	2	0.261	0.626 ± 0.048	0.531–0.720	**0.007**
SOFA	3.063	8	0.930	0.761 ± 0.043	0.676–0.845	**<0.001**
Proteinuria plus SOFA	7.406	6	0.285	0.828 ± 0.062	0.707–0.949	**<0.001**
Proteinuria plus nonrenal SOFA	11.595	5	0.041	0.823 ± 0.078	0.670–0.977	**0.001**
Postoperative day 7						
Proteinuria	-	-	-	0.757 ± 0.056	0.647–0.866	**<0.001**
Child-Pugh points	6.365	4	0.173	0.750 ± 0.065	0.593–0.847	**0.001**
MELD score	26.161	8	0.001	0.856 ± 0.038	0.782–0.930	**<0.001**
RIFLE	9.602	2	0.008	0.825 ± 0.042	0.742–0.908	**<0.001**
SOFA	6.073	6	0.415	0.899 ± 0.031	0.838–0.961	**<0.001**
Proteinuria plus SOFA	8.625	6	0.196	0.907 ± 0.041	0.825–0.988	**<0.001**
Proteinuria plus nonrenal SOFA	7.856	6	0.249	0.903 ± 0.038	0.828–0.978	**<0.001**
Postoperative day 14						
Proteinuria	-	-	-	0.773 ± 0.067	0.642–0.904	**0.005**
Child-Pugh points	3.469	3	0.325	0.783 ± 0.052	0.682–0.885	**<0.001**
MELD score	134.84	8	<0.001	0.850 ± 0.056	0.740–0.960	**<0.001**
RIFLE	1.658	2	0.436	0.780 ± 0.050	0.681–0.879	**<0.001**
SOFA	24.495	7	0.001	0.892 ± 0.044	0.806–0.978	**<0.001**
Proteinuria plus SOFA	3.987	7	0.781	0.900 ± 0.042	0.819–0.982	**<0.001**
Proteinuria plus nonrenal SOFA	5.009	7	0.659	0.894 ± 0.038	0.819–0.969	**<0.001**

Values in bold are statistically significant (*P*-value < 0.05)

On ICU admission day (before transplantation): The prediction accuracy of the SOFA score was better than those of the Child-Pugh points, MELD score and RIFLE. The proteinuria plus SOFA score has an even better discriminatory power than the SOFA score

On post-transplant day 1, 7, 14: The prediction accuracy of the SOFA and MELD score was better than that of the Child-Pugh points. The proteinuria plus SOFA score has an even better discriminatory power than the SOFA score

Abbreviation: MELD, model for end-stage liver disease; SOFA, sequential organ failure assessment; df, degree of freedom; AUROC, areas under the receiver operating characteristic curve; SE, standard error; CI, confidence intervals; NS, not significant

Discussion

In the current research, overall hospital survival rate was 87.0 % (281/323), which is in agreement with what had been presented in the literature [8, 18, 19]. Our investigation found that both presence of proteinuria and SOFA score determined on the first day of admission to the ICU were significantly correlated to in-hospital mortality (Tables 2 and 5). Analytical results also proved that discriminatory ability of SOFA was better than those of CP points, RIFLE, and MELD. One notable finding of this study was that presence of proteinuria in combination with SOFA has an even more superior discriminatory

Table 7 Prediction of subsequent 90-day mortality

Predictive factors	Cutoff point	Youden index	Sensitivity (%)	Specificity (%)	Overall correctness (%)
Proteinuria					
On admission	positive	0.16	28	88	58
Postoperative day 1	positive	0.22	64	58	61
Postoperative day 7	positive	0.51	85	66	76
Postoperative day 14	positive	0.55	90	65	77
Child-Pugh points					
On admission	12	0.17	95	22	59
Postoperative day 1	10	0.26	90	37	64
Postoperative day 7	9	0.42	60	82	71
Postoperative day 14	8	0.42	50	92	71
MELD score					
On admission	15	0.19	65	56	61
Postoperative day 1	22	0.27	60	71	66
Postoperative day 7	20	0.58	69	87	78
Postoperative day 14	23	0.62	75	87	81
RIFLE					
On admission	I category	0.04	7	97	52
Postoperative day 1	I category	0.20	57	64	61
Postoperative day 7	I category	0.56	72	82	77
Postoperative day 14	R category	0.60	74	82	78
SOFA					
On admission	5	0.23	52	71	62
Postoperative day 1	11	0.41	77	64	71
Postoperative day 7	7	0.70	83	87	84
Postoperative day 14	7	0.69	85	84	84
Proteinuria plus SOFA					
On admission	5	0.26	57	70	63
Postoperative day 1	12	0.54	79	75	77
Postoperative day 7	8	0.72	85	85	85
Postoperative day 14	8	0.72	89	83	86
Proteinuria plus nonrenal SOFA					
On admission	5	0.26	54	76	63
Postoperative day 1	12	0.54	54	100	77
Postoperative day 7	8	0.68	86	82	84
Postoperative day 14	7	0.67	100	67	84

Optimal cutoff points for predicting 3-month mortality were derived from receiver operator characteristic analysis. On admission (pre-transplant), post-transplant day 1, 7, and 14, the Youden index and overall correctness for predicting 3-month mortality were higher for the proteinuria plus SOFA score than those for the proteinuria, Child-Pugh points, MELD score, RIFLE criteria, SOFA, and proteinuria plus nonrenal SOFA scores
Abbreviation: *MELD* model for end-stage liver disease, *SOFA* sequential organ failure assessment

power than SOFA alone (Table 6). Moreover, proteinuria plus SOFA also had the highest Youden index and the best overall correctness of prediction (Table 7).

AKI is a common complication in patients with decompensated liver disease, and its occurrence is correlated to poor prognosis [20]. Recently, several promising urinary protein biomarkers have been proved to be remarkably helpful for detecting AKI, such as Calprotectin, neutrophil gelatinase-associated lipocalin (NGAL), cystatin C, interleukin-18 (IL-18), kidney injury molecule-1 (KIM-1), and L-type or liver-type fatty acid-bind protein (LFABP) [2, 21–24]. The presence of protein in urine might reflect structural or functional defects of the glomerular capillary barrier or the reabsorption receptors in the

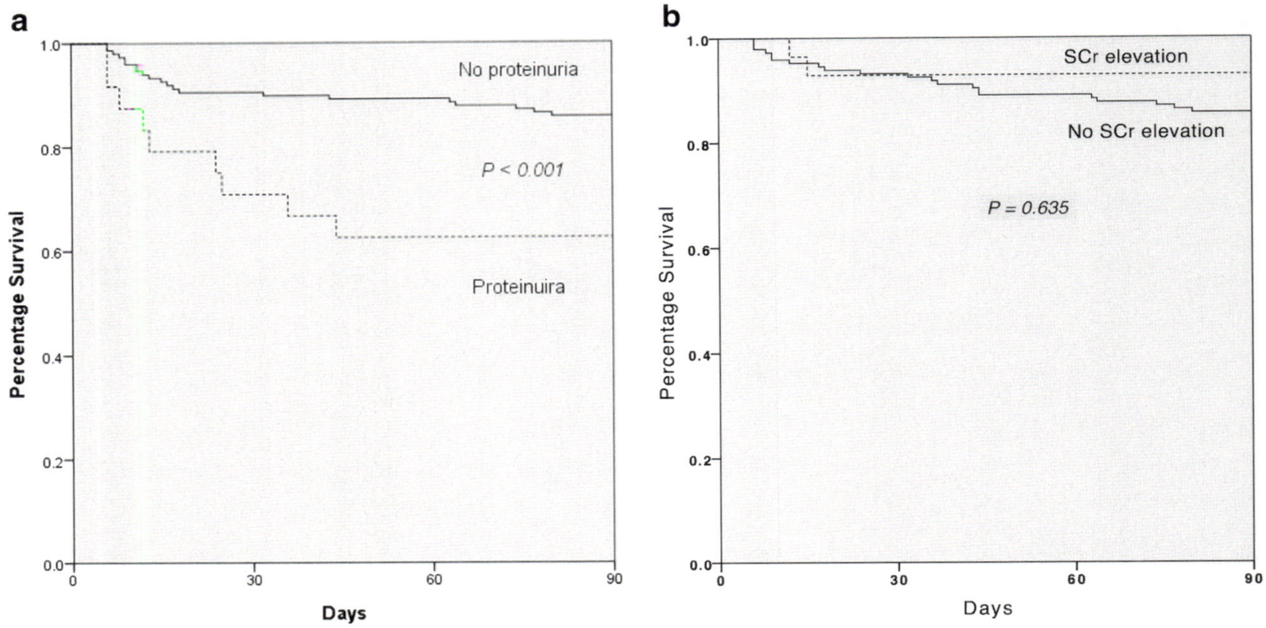

Fig. 1 Survival Functions Kaplan-Meier survival analysis in 323 patients according to the data measured before receiving liver transplantation. **a** Cumulative survival rates differed significantly for patients with proteinuria ($n = 45$) and those without proteinuria ($n = 278$) on the first day of ICU admission. **b** Cumulative survival rates did not differ significantly for patients with SCr level elevation (Increase in SCr ≥ 1.5 × baseline) ($n = 28$) and those without SCr elevation ($n = 295$) on the first day of ICU admission. *Abbreviation: SCr, serum creatinine

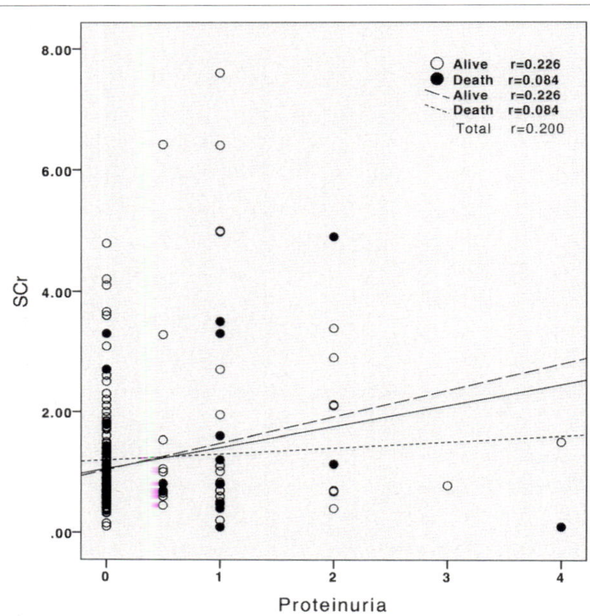

Fig. 2 Correlations of proteinuria and SCr measured on the first day of ICU admission for in-hospital mortality. The proteinuria is not correlated significantly ($p = 0.143$) with SCr. *Abbreviation: SCr, serum creatinine

renal proximal tubules. Proteinuria is not only a sensitive indicator but also a risk factor for acute kidney injury [25]. Increasing evidence has indicated that proteinuria itself may activate intrarenal complement cascade, upregulate proximal tubular inflammatory and fibrogenic gene, trigger apoptotic response, and further lead to spreading of renal tubulointerstitial damage and adverse outcomes [26–31]. In the literature, urine albumin to creatinine ratio (UACR) is a precise method for measurement of albuminuria and identification of renal dysfunction [32, 33]. Nevertheless, previous study had documented that preoperative proteinuria could accurately predict the development of AKI in patients undergoing operation, irrespective of it is determined by UACR or urine dipstick analysis [34]. Previous reports also demonstrated that calculating urinary calprotectin/creatinine or NGAL/creatinine ratio does not lead to higher prediction accuracy than using urinary calprotectin or NGAL alone [2, 24]. In this study, proteinuria was detected with the dipstick analysis, the advantages of this examination are inexpensive and easily performed and interpreted. Analyzed data showed presence of proteinuria on ICU admission (before transplantation) was correlated to increased risks of AKI, severe infection episodes, in-hospital mortality, and 90-day mortality (Fig. 1). The occurrence of AKI after transplantation,

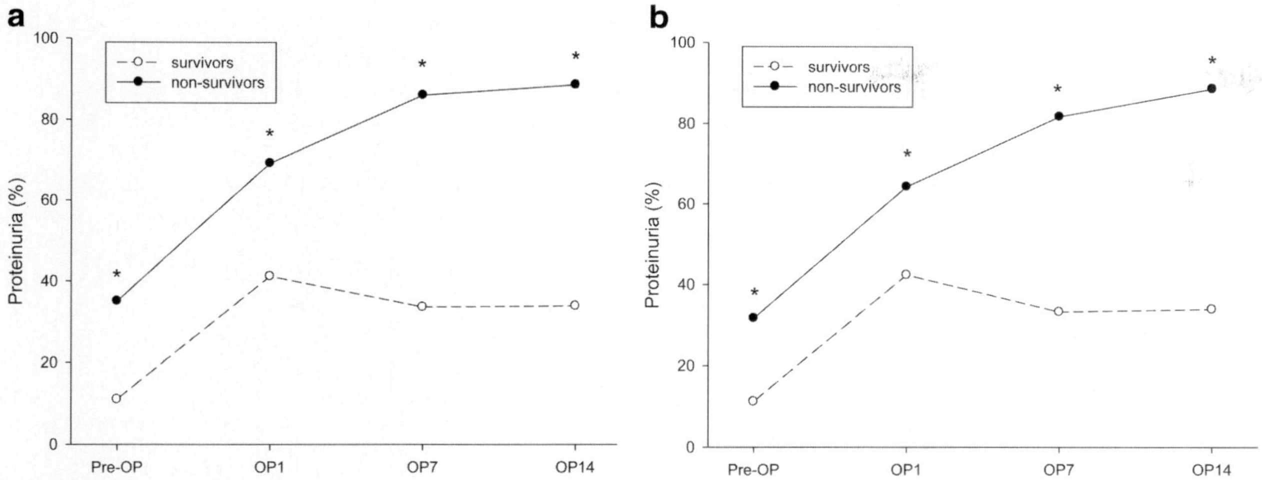

Fig. 3 The prevalence of proteinuria for the (**a**) in-hospital survival group (living, $n = 281$) and mortality group (dead, $n = 42$) and (**b**) 90-day survival group (living, $n = 277$) and mortality group (dead, $n = 46$) during the ICU admission day and postoperative days 1, 7, and 14. The prevalence of proteinuria significantly increased during this period among the in-hospital and 90-day mortality groups but not in the survivor groups (* $P < 0.05$)

especially infection related AKI, was correlated to a markedly lower chance of survival (Table 3). Measurement of preoperative proteinuria might be useful to preemptively identify patients who have increased risk of AKI and severe infection episodes. Based on the observed results, it seems that avoiding nephrotoxic agents and choosing therapy carefully are crucial ways of renoprotection for patients present with proteinuria before transplant. More intensive postoperative care and infection prevention strategies, such as more aggressive prophylactic antimicrobial regimens and strict practice for infection prophylaxis, might also help to prevent further adverse outcomes for these patients. Further well-powered research is needed to study this issue.

Among patients undergoing liver transplant, development of renal dysfunction may be attributed to intraoperative caval cross-clamping with vascular outflow obstruction, reperfusion injury, significant infectious event, bleeding, perioperative hypotension with high vasopressor requirement, large-volume transfusions, exposure to nephrotoxic agents or use of calcineurin inhibitors [35–37]. As part of the acute phase response, general vascular permeability increases and the urinary excretion of protein and albumin occur within several hours after operation [38]. In our study, the decreased-donor graft recipients who had prolonged cold ischemia time and the living-donor graft recipients who had longer warm ischemia time, were found to have significantly higher incidences of newly onset proteinuria on the first day after operation. These findings are consistent with previous studies [39–43]. Moreover, the prevalence of proteinuria decreased significantly within 7 days after operation in the in-hospital and 90-day survival groups but not in the mortality groups (Fig. 3). It implies that patients with poor physiologic adaptability are much more intolerable to the transient hemodynamic change of kidney. In addition, the persistence of proteinuria in serial assessment after liver transplantation might represent delayed recovery from the major operation and signify poor short-term prognosis.

Early detection of AKI after liver transplant could potentially retard the progression of renal dysfunction and prevent further adverse outcomes by prompt intervention [36, 44]. Many researches have shown that SOFA can completely present courses of major organ dysfunction and dynamic changes of illness severity after acute insults [45]. We have proposed that SOFA determined on postoperative day 7 has good predictive performance in short-term outcome of patients receiving liver transplant [8]. However, the renal parameter of the SOFA score, SCr concentration, does not seem to elevate until decline of renal function over than 50 %. This means that early detecting AKI by SOFA is hardly possible [36]. Our data revealed that absolute concentration and relative change of SCr levels are not significantly correlated to the presences of proteinuria and patient outcomes (Table 2, Figs. 1, 2), which highlights that SCr concentration is inaccurate for discovering kidney injury among patients with decompensated liver disease [46]. On the contrary, the occurrence of proteinuria might represent subtle renal function changes, and it also signifies generalized inflammatory environment and poor prognosis (correlation between proteinuria and CRP, before operation: *$P < 0.001$*; postoperative day 1: $P = 0.005$). In this study, the combination of proteinuria improves the flaws of SCr and the prediction ability of SOFA during perioperative time, particularly on postoperative day 1 (an increase in the AUROC from 0.761 to 0.828) (Tables 6). These exciting findings seem to demonstrate that presence of proteinuria could provide outstanding early prognostic prediction for patients undergoing liver transplantation.

Despite the promising results obtained in this research, there are some possible limitation should be acknowledged. Firstly, this research was performed in just one tertiary medical center, so our results might not be exactly generalized to dissimilar patient population. Secondly, owing to the retrospective nature of our study, not every clinical factor was available. Thirdly, the patient population contained a high proportion of hepatitis B viral infection (34 %) and may present as a special subgroup in the cirrhotic patients. Fourthly, predictive precision of logistic regression models is not perfect and flawless. Finally, the prognostic tools were applied on patients already admitted to the ICU, and were not used as a preadmission screening test, this might skew the analyses.

Conclusions

To conclude, this study showed that preoperative proteinuria is a significant risk factor of hospital mortality in patients undergoing liver transplantation. For patients exhibiting proteinuria before transplant, we suggest watch out for infection episodes, carefully choose therapy and do prompt intervention to prevent further adverse outcomes. Avoiding prolonged cold or warm ischemia time of transplantation could also reduce organ injury from reperfusion. The presence of proteinuria in serial assessment after liver transplantation has been proven to have early prognostic predictive effect and to assist the SOFA score with better discriminatory power in predicting short-term outcome. For these reasons, we recommend surveying the presence of proteinuria in preoperative and postoperative serial assessment. Proteinuria is supposed to be recognized as an important negative predictor for short-term survival of liver transplant patients.

Abbreviations

AKI: Acute kidney injury; AUROC: Area under the receiver operating characteristic curve; CP points: Child-pugh points; ICU: Intensive care units; MELD: Model for end-stage liver disease; OP: Operation; RIFLE: The risk of renal failure, injury to the kidney, failure of kidney function, loss of kidney function, and end-stage renal failure; SCr: Serum creatinine; SOFA: Sequential organ failure assessment; TIPS: Transjugular intrahepatic portosystemic shunt; UACR: Urine albumin-creatinine ratio

Acknowledgements

The authors thank the staff of the Core Lab and Liver Transplantation Team of the Chang Gung Memorial Hospital for technical assistance. We also express our sincere gratitude to all participants of the CGMH Critical Care Team.

Funding

None.

Authors' contributions

YCC and HCP contributed to the conception and design of this research. HCP contributed to collection and interpretation of data. HCP, JPL, and MJT contributed to manuscript drafting. WCL provided patient information and participated in the design and coordination. YJC, JPL, MJT, CCJ, MHT, PCF, CHC, MYC, YCT, CHC, CCH, JTF, and CWY contributed to offering intellectual content of the work and were involved in editing and revising the manuscript. All authors discussed and contributed to the final manuscript version.

Competing interests

The authors declare that they have no competing interests.

Author details

[1]Department of Nephrology, Chang Gung Memorial Hospital, Keelung, Taiwan. [2]Division of General Internal Medicine and Geriatrics Medicine, Chang Gung Memorial Hospital, Taipei, Taiwan. [3]Chang Gung University College of Medicine, Taoyuan, Taiwan. [4]Kidney Research Center, Department of Nephrology, Chang Gung Memorial Hospital, Taipei, Taiwan. [5]Laboratory of Immunology, Department of General Surgery, Chang Gung Memorial Hospital, Taipei, Taiwan. [6]Division of Gastroenterology, Chang Gung Memorial Hospital, Taipei, Taiwan.

References

1. Glassock RJ. Is the presence of microalbuminuria a relevant marker of kidney disease? Curr hypertens rep. 2010;12:364–8.
2. Heller F, Frischmann S, Grunbaum M, Zidek W, Westhoff TH. Urinary calprotectin and the distinction between prerenal and intrinsic acute kidney injury. Clin J Am Soc Nephrol. 2011;6:2347–55.
3. Huang T-M, Wu V-C, Young G-H, Lin Y-F, Shiao C-C, Wu P-C, et al. Preoperative proteinuria predicts adverse renal outcomes after coronary artery bypass grafting. J Am Soc Nephrol. 2011;22:156–63.
4. Lin LY, Jenq CC, Liu CS, Huang CS, Fan PC, Chang CH, et al. Proteinuria can predict short-term prognosis in critically ill cirrhotic patients. J Clin Gastroenterol. 2014;48:377–82.
5. Wehler M, Kokoska J, Reulbach U, Hahn EG, Strauss R. Short-term prognosis in critically ill patients with cirrhosis assessed by prognostic scoring systems. Hepatology. 2001;34:255–61.
6. Cholongitas E, Senzolo M, Patch D, Shaw S, Hui C, Burroughs AK. Review article: scoring systems for assessing prognosis in critically ill adult cirrhotics. Aliment Pharmacol Ther. 2006;24:453–64.
7. Pan HC, Jenq CC, Tsai MH, Fan PC, Chang CH, Chang MY, et al. Scoring systems for 6-month mortality in critically ill cirrhotic patients: a prospective analysis of chronic liver failure - sequential organ failure assessment score (CLIF-SOFA). Aliment Pharmacol Ther. 2014;11:12953.
8. Wong CS, Lee WC, Jenq CC, Tian YC, Chang MY, Lin CY, et al. Scoring short-term mortality after liver transplantation. Liver transpl: official publication of the American Association for the Study of Liver Diseases and the International Liver Transplantation Society. 2010;16:138–46. doi:10.1002/lt.21969.
9. Fraley DS, Burr R, Bernardini J, Angus D, Kramer DJ, Johnson JP. Impact of acute renal failure on mortality in end-stage liver disease with or without transplantation. Kidney Int. 1998;54:518–24.
10. Barri YM, Sanchez EQ, Jennings LW, Melton LB, Hays S, Levy MF, et al. Acute kidney injury following liver transplantation: definition and outcome. Liver Transpl. 2009;15:475–83.
11. James MT, Hemmelgarn BR, Wiebe N, Pannu N, Manns BJ, Klarenbach SW, et al. Glomerular filtration rate, proteinuria, and the incidence and consequences of acute kidney injury: a cohort study. Lancet. 2010;376:2096–103.
12. Hsu RK, C-y H. Proteinuria and reduced glomerular filtration rate as risk factors for acute kidney injury. Curr Opin Nephrol Hypertens. 2011;20:211–7.
13. Levey A, Atkins R, Coresh J, Cohen E, Collins A, Eckardt K, et al. Chronic kidney disease as a global public health problem: approaches and initiatives–a position statement from Kidney Disease Improving Global Outcomes. Kidney Int. 2007;72:247–59.
14. Wiesner R, Edwards E, Freeman R, Harper A, Kim R, Kamath P, et al. Model for end-stage liver disease (MELD) and allocation of donor livers. Gastroenterology. 2003;124:91–6. doi:10.1053/gast.2003.50016.

15. Pan HC, Jenq CC, Lee WC, Tsai MH, Fan PC, Chang CH, et al. Scoring Systems for Predicting Mortality after Liver Transplantation. PLoS One. 2014;9:e107138.
16. Bellomo R, Ronco C, Kellum JA, Mehta RL, Palevsky P, Workgroup A. Acute renal failure - definition, outcome measures, animal models, fluid therapy and information technology needs: the Second International Consensus Conference of the Acute Dialysis Quality Initiative (ADQI) Group. Crit Care. 2004;8:R204–12. doi:10.1186/cc2872.
17. Youden W. Index for rating diagnostic tests. Cancer. 1950;3:32–5.
18. Akyildiz M, Karasu Z, Arikan C, Kilic M, Zeytunlu M, Gunsar F, et al. Impact of pretransplant MELD score on posttransplant outcome in living donor liver transplantation. Transplant Proc. 2004;36:1442–4. doi:10.1016/j.transproceed.2004.05.004.
19. Leppke S, Leighton T, Zaun D, Chen SC, Skeans M, Israni AK, et al. Scientific Registry of Transplant Recipients: collecting, analyzing, and reporting data on transplantation in the United States. Transplant Rev (Orlando). 2013;27:50–6. doi:10.1016/j.trre.2013.01.002.
20. Pan HC, Jenq CC, Tsai MH, Fan PC, Chang CH, Chang MY, et al. Risk models and scoring systems for predicting the prognosis in critically ill cirrhotic patients with acute kidney injury: a prospective validation study. PLoS One. 2012;7:7.
21. Coca SG, Yalavarthy R, Concato J, Parikh CR. Biomarkers for the diagnosis and risk stratification of acute kidney injury: a systematic review. Kidney Int. 2008;73:1008–16.
22. Chen YCFJ, Yang CW. Acute kidney injury biomarkers. Taiwan Crit Care Med. 2009;10:121–8.
23. Belcher JM, Sanyal AJ, Peixoto AJ, Perazella MA, Lim J, Thiessen-Philbrook H, et al. Kidney biomarkers and differential diagnosis of patients with cirrhosis and acute kidney injury. Hepatology. 2014;60:622–32.
24. Chang CH, Yang CH, Yang HY, Chen TH, Lin CY, Chang SW, et al. Urinary Biomarkers Improve the Diagnosis of Intrinsic Acute Kidney Injury in Coronary Care Units. Medicine. 2015;94:0000000000001703.
25. Abbate M, Zoja C, Remuzzi G. How does proteinuria cause progressive renal damage? J Am Soc Nephrol. 2006;17:2974–84.
26. Nangaku M, Pippin J, Couser WG. Complement membrane attack complex (C5b-9) mediates interstitial disease in experimental nephrotic syndrome. J Am Soc Nephrol. 1999;10:2323–31.
27. Morigi M, Macconi D, Zoja C, Donadelli R, Buelli S, Zanchi C, et al. Protein overload-induced NF-kB activation in proximal tubular cells requires H2O2 through a PKC-dependent pathway. J Am Soc Nephrol. 2002;13:1179–89.
28. Abbate M, Zoja C, Rottoli D, Corna D, Tomasoni S, Remuzzi G. Proximal tubular cells promote fibrogenesis by TGF-&bgr; 1–mediated induction of peritubular myofibroblasts. Kidney Int. 2002;61:2066–77.
29. Nangaku M, Pippin J, Couser WG. C6 mediates chronic progression of tubulointerstitial damage in rats with remnant kidneys. J Am Soc Nephrol. 2002;13:928–36.
30. Tang S, Leung JC, Abe K, Chan KW, Chan LY, Chan TM, et al. Albumin stimulates interleukin-8 expression in proximal tubular epithelial cells in vitro and in vivo. J Clin Investig. 2003;111:515–27.
31. Erkan E, Garcia CD, Patterson LT, Mishra J, Mitsnefes MM, Kaskel FJ, et al. Induction of renal tubular cell apoptosis in focal segmental glomerulosclerosis: roles of proteinuria and Fas-dependent pathways. J Am Soc Nephrol. 2005;16:398–407.
32. Ciavarella A, Silletti A, Forlani G, Morotti L, Borgnino L, D'Apote M, et al. A screening test for microalbuminuria in type 1 (insulin-dependent) diabetes. Diabetes Res Clin Pract. 1989;7:307–12.
33. Eknoyan G, Levin NW. K/DOQI clinical practice guidelines for chronic kidney disease: evaluation, classification, and stratification. Am J Kidney Dis. 2002;39:S1–S266.
34. Coca SG, Jammalamadaka D, Sint K, Thiessen Philbrook H, Shlipak MG, Zappitelli M, et al. Preoperative proteinuria predicts acute kidney injury in patients undergoing cardiac surgery. J Thorac Cardiovasc Surg. 2012;143:495–502.
35. Cabezuelo JB, Ramirez P, Rios A, Acosta F, Torres D, Sansano T, et al. Risk factors of acute renal failure after liver transplantation. Kidney Int. 2006;69:1073–80.
36. Wagener G, Minhaz M, Mattis FA, Kim M, Emond JC, Lee HT. Urinary neutrophil gelatinase-associated lipocalin as a marker of acute kidney injury after orthotopic liver transplantation. Nephrol Dial Transplant. 2011;26:1717–23.
37. Nastos C, Kalimeris K, Papoutsidakis N, Tasoulis M-K, Lykoudis PM, Theodoraki K, et al. Global Consequences of Liver Ischemia/Reperfusion Injury. Oxidative Med Cell Longev. 2014;2014:13. doi:10.1155/2014/906965.
38. Gosling P, Shearman CP, Gwynn BR, Simms MH, Bainbridge ET. Microproteinuria: Response to operation. Br Med J (Clin Res Ed). 1988;296:338.
39. Paugam-Burtz C, Kavafyan J, Merckx P, Dahmani S, Sommacale D, Ramsay M, et al. Postreperfusion syndrome during liver transplantation for cirrhosis: outcome and predictors. Liver Transpl. 2009;15:522–9.
40. Lee HT, Park SW, Kim M, D'Agati VD. Acute kidney injury after hepatic ischemia and reperfusion injury in mice. Lab Invest. 2009;89:196–208.
41. Heidenhain C, Pratschke J, Puhl G, Neumann U, Pascher A, Veltzke-Schlieker W, et al. Incidence of and risk factors for ischemic-type biliary lesions following orthotopic liver transplantation. Transpl Int. 2010;23:14–22.
42. Wang B, Zhang Q, Zhu B, Cui Z, Zhou J. Protective effect of gadolinium chloride on early warm ischemia/reperfusion injury in rat bile duct during liver transplantation. PLoS One. 2013;8:14.
43. Xia Y, Gong JP. Impact of recombinant globular adiponectin on early warm ischemia-reperfusion injury in rat bile duct after liver transplantation. Sci Rep. 2014;4:6426.
44. Yalavarthy R, Edelstein CL, Teitelbaum I. Acute renal failure and chronic kidney disease following liver transplantation. Hemodial Int. 2007;11:S7–S12.
45. Goldhill DR, Sumner A. Outcome of intensive care patients in a group of British intensive care units. Crit Care Med. 1998;26:1337–45.
46. Pan HC, Chien YS, Jenq CC, Tsai MH, Fan PC, Chang CH, et al. Acute Kidney Injury Classification for Critically Ill Cirrhotic Patients: A Comparison of the KDIGO, AKIN, and RIFLE Classifications. Sci Rep. 2016;6:23022. doi:10.1038/srep23022.

Preliminary experience in laparoscopic resection of hepatic hydatidectocyst with the Da Vinci Surgical System (DVSS)

Haibo Zou, Lanyun Luo, Hua Xue, Guan Wang*, Xiankui Wang, Le Luo, Yutong Yao, Guangming Xiang and Xiaolun Huang

Abstract

Background: At present, Da Vinci robotic assisted hepatectomy has been routinely carried out in conditional units. But there is no report concerning the use of Da Vinci robots for hepatic hydatid cystectomy and experience on this aspect is seldom mentioned before. This study was to summarize the preliminary experience in laparoscopic resection of hepatic hydatidectocyst with the Da Vinci Surgical System (DVSS).

Case presentation: A 29-year-old female diagnosed as hepatic hydatid in the right anterior lobe of liver was treated with laparoscopic resection by the DVSS under general anesthesia. Appropriate disposal of tumor cell in vascular system and disinfection of surgical field with hypertonic saline were conducted. The hepatic hydatidectocyst was resected completely with an operation time of 130 min, an intraoperative blood loss of 200 ml and a length of hospital stay for five days. The vital signs of patient were stable and no cyst fluid allergy occurred after operation.

Conclusions: Our result showed that laparoscopic resection of hepatic hydatidectocyst by using the DVSS is safe and feasible on the basis of hospitals have rich experience in treatment of cystic echinococcosisliver, resection with DVSS and laparoscopic excision.

Keywords: Hepatic hydatidectocyst, DVSS, Laparoscopic operation

Background

As a common parasitic disease, cystic echinococcosis (echinococcosisgranulosa) is distributed worldwide [1]. In many developing countries, such as Peru, Argentina and western China, cystic echinococcosis is considered an epidemic [2]. For patients with cystic echinococcosis, surgical resection has been the gold standard for this disease. In recent years, alternative methods have facilitated the treatment of specific patients and now become first-line treatment options. Conservative treatment, percutaneous therapy, surgical resection and chemotherapy are the most common treatment strategies. [3]. With the advancement and improvement of laparoscopic technique, laparoscopic hepatectomy is becoming more and more mature in recent years [4, 5], which provides a technical basis for minimally invasive surgery for hepatic hydatidosis [6]. Minimally invasive surgical treatment of hepatic hydatid disease is considered to be safe [7]. However, for the cases with poor exposure and complex operation, laparoscopic surgery has its inherent shortcomings which limit its application.

Over the last decade, robotic surgery has played an increasingly important role in gynecology [8, 9]. The superiority of robot assisted laparoscopic surgery have been reported in many papers. At present, robotic surgery is widely used in a variety of surgical procedures, such as cholecystectomy, esophagectomy, thymectomy, et al. [10]. The advantages of robotic surgery mainly include three dimensional (3D) vision, reduced operator fatigue, more dexterous and penetration of the surgeon's

* Correspondence: wangguan_99@126.com
Department of Hepatobiliary Surgery, Sichuan Academy of Medical Sciences and Sichuan Provincial People's Hospital, #32, Section 2, West 1st Ring Road, Chengdu 610072, China

natural tremor. [11, 12]. The robot-aided thymectomy was firstly conducted by Yoskino et al. for the treatment of thymoma. Their experience suggested that a surgical robot has a great potential for facilitating precise surgery in a narrow area [13]. During surgery, a doctor operates the DVSS arms inserted through the surgical ports used in conventional Video-assisted Thoracoscopic Surgery. In addition, the endoscope of DVSS could provide a 3D high-resolution binocular view of the surgical field, which is far larger than that of video-assisted thoracoscopic surgery, thus the surgical convenience and safety is improved. [14]. The operability around anatomic structures was improved as the Endo-Wrist system can articulate and rotate 360 degrees [15]. Furthermore, the physiological vibrations of the surgeons' hands can be eliminated via the Endo-Wrist system [14].

Based on the mature technology of laparoscopic resection of hepatic cystic echinococcosis, the world's first Da Vinci robot assisted resection of hepatic cystic echinococcosis was successfully implemented in 11th March, 2016. Now the preliminary treatment experience are reported as follows.

Case presentation

A 29-year-old woman of Han nationality with a history of chronic hepatitis B presented more-than-one-year persistent right epigastric pain. She was a long-term resident of the pastoral area of Aba in Sichuan Province and raised dogs at home. The BMI assessed at admission was 23.9 kg. m^2, the nutritional risk score was 1, the ability of daily living (ADL) grade was I and ECOG score was 0. Physical examination showed normal vital signs; skin and sclera without yellow dye; no abnormal cardiopulmonary function and palpable superficial lymph nodes; liver and spleen were impalpable. Auxiliary examination showed HBsAg(+), HBeAg(+), HBcAb(+), Pre-S1Ag(+);HBV-DNA:5.7E + 04 IU/ml;ALT: 118 U/L, AST: 92 U/L,normal PT, ALB, TBIL, liver function: Child A; ICG R15:5.4% (DDG-3300 K, Nihon Kohden); normal serum AFP (chemiluminescence analysis); liver ultrasound imaging: hepatic cystic echinococcosis; contrast-enhanced CT: no hydatid lesion was found in head and lungs; an about 6 cm cystic mass with a little marginal calcification, which down into the gap of liver and kidney, was found on the anterior lobe of the right liver (Fig 1 and 1b). The cystic fluid was slightly turbid, and the cystic mass was diagnosed as hepatic cystic echinococcosis.

Half an hour before surgery, a dose of antibiotics (ceftazidime, 1.0 g) was used to prevent infection. The patient was treated with 100 mg hydrocortisone and rapid fluid infusion of 2000 ml before operation, the CVP was required to fall below 12 cm H_2O during operation. After general anesthesia and tracheal intubation, the patient was placed in a 15° reverse Trendelenburg position (head-high, feet-low). The pneumoperitoneum pressure was maintained at 15 mmHg.

The distribution of Troca was shown in Fig. 2 and Da Vinci robot assisted resection was performed as follows: The right side of the umbilicus was selected as observation hole and the left side of the umbilicus was selected as auxiliary hole; No. 1 arm located below the left costal margin in the mid-clavicular line; No. 2 arm located 3 cm above the umbilical level on the right anterior axillary line; No. 3 arm located 3 cm above the umbilical level on the left anterior axillary line,. A straight needle with thread was punctured into the round ligament. After crossing the round ligament in the abdominal cavity, the thread was pierced from the opposite side. Lifting the thread to fully expose the surgical site. Then the liver and abdominal cavity was examined after successful puncture.

The adhesion between the cyst and omentummajus, colon and stomach was severed with the ultrasound knife (Fig 3a). Free the lower edge of the cyst with the ultrasound knife. The operation should be careful,

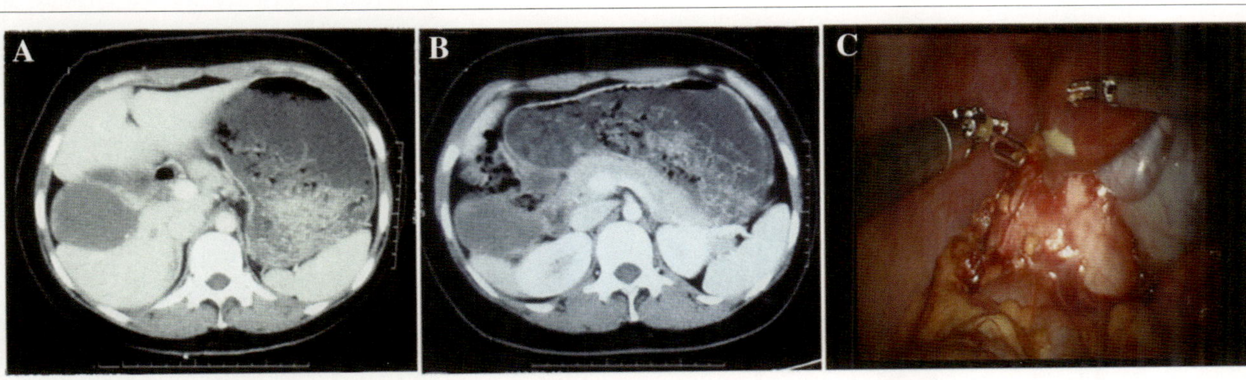

Fig. 1 **a** CT showedabnormal morphology of the right liver, spins to the right; **b** CT showed a hepatic hydatid cyst located in the anterior segment of the right lobe of the liver; **c** Intraoperative visual field showed hydatid cysts adjacent to the gallbladder and liver spins to the right

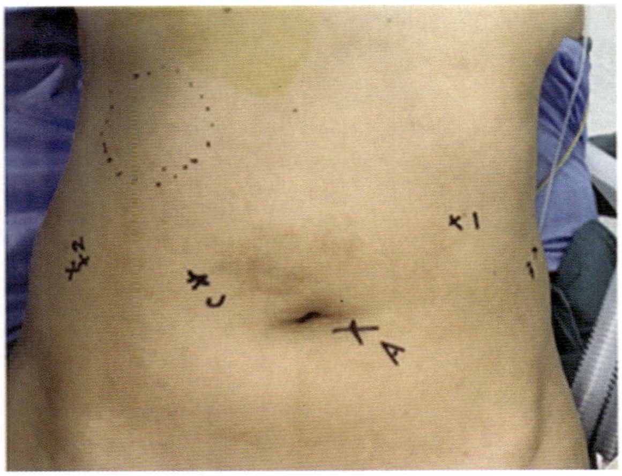

Fig. 2 Abdominal wall incisions

titanium clip was used for clamping (Fig 3b). During the propulsion process, the cyst was pressed from inside to outside with an aspirator by the assistant to maintain a certain tension and good vision of the space. Promote in the same plane from top to bottom, from front to back, until the specimen was completely free. No visible spill of cystic contents was observed during the operation. Then the outer capsule of the hydatid cyst was completely removed. Biliary ducts were seen during the operation, but no major biliary duct was observed. A complete removal of the external capsule was performed during our operation, so there was no residual cystic cavity, and only the interface between the liver and the cyst were left after resection. So omentum was not used to obliterate the cyst cavity.

After resection, the cyst was loaded into the specimen bag and then the contents of the cyst were suck out with a puncture needle. Bleeding points were treated with electrocoagulation and suture (Fig 3c). Electrocoagulation hook (Johnson & Johnson, US) was mainly used for electrocoagulation of wound oozing blood and small bleeding point. No vessel sealing system was used in this study. Larger tubes (such as portal branch, branch of hepatic vein, small bile duct and hepatic artery) were treated with titanium clips and sutures. Before the end of the operation, the dissection plane of the liver parenchyma and surgical field were immersed with hypertonic saline for 10 min to kill potential echinococcus (Fig 3d) and an abdominal drainage tube was placed in the liver

especially to prevent the rupture of colon. To find the space between fibrous capsule and hepatic tissue, the liver capsule and part of the liver parenchyma was dissected with an ultrasound knife along the junction of hydatid cyst and normal liver tissue. Then the space was deepened gradually via a series of measures such as pushing, squeezing, sub and hook. The blood oozing and crushing tissues were scraped and sucked out by aspirator to make the operation field clearer. When encountered a pipe structure larger than 3 mm, the

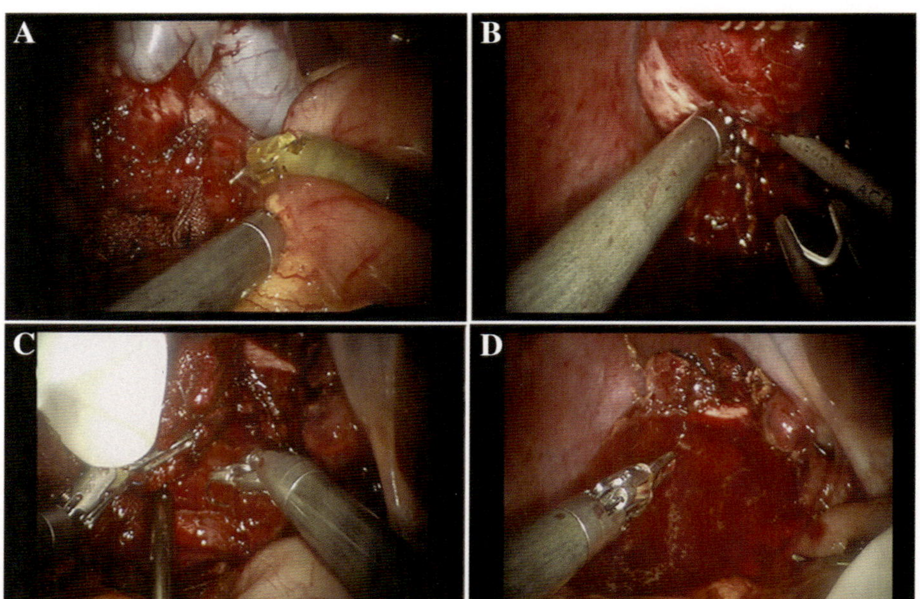

Fig. 3 **a** The separation of the omentum and the colon wrapped cyst; **b** Clamping large vessels and bile ducts; **c** Suture the bleeding point; **d** The operative field was soakedwith hypertonic saline

sections postoperatively. The drainage fluid was a pale bloody liquid (mainly from small amount of blood oozing from the wound surface). No bile or other liquid was observed. To prevent recurrence and reinfection, oral albendazole (15 mg/kg/d) therapy against parasites was initiated half a month after surgery and lasted for one year.

After operation, the patient was educated with diet, hand hygiene, and proper knowledge for keeping dogs. The volume of blood loss was about 200 ml during operation. The main cause of bleeding was the small nutrient vessels and the hepatic parenchymal hemorrhage when the hydatid cyst was separated. In addition, since the sixth branch of the middle hepatic vein was close to the cyst, a small break may occur during the process of cyst separation, which also lead to small amount of bleeding. Reliable hemostasis was achieved after suture. The surgery time was 130 min. The patient's vital signs were stable, no cystic allergies appeared. Subhepatic drainage was left for 24 h. On the first day after surgery, only liquid peroral diet was allowed. No complications such as postoperative bile leakage and bleeding were observed. The patient was discharged 5 days later. Cystic echinococcosis was confirmed by postoperative pathology. Excellent result was obtained in the laparoscopic resection of hepatic hydatidectocyst by the Da Vinci Surgical System (DVSS) in our study.

Discussion and conclusions

At present, Da Vinci robotic assisted hepatectomy has been routinely carried out in conditional units. But there is no report concerning the use of DaVinci robots for hepatic hydatid cystectomy and experience on this aspect was seldom mentioned before. Through this surgical treatment, we summarized that liver hydatid cyst grows slowly and is prone to produce vascular and bile duct pushing, oppression and infringement. For lesions located on the edge of the liver, the dense pipe system outside the capsule fiber layer should be clamped and sutured to reduce the incidence of postoperative bleeding and bile leakage. Due to the technical advantages of 3D magnification vision and multi DOF manipulator of the Da Vinci robot, the operation is more simple, flexible and precise compared with laparoscopic surgery. For the separation, suture, knotting and other complex operations, the advantages of Da Vinci robot surgery is particularly evident. It can reduce the probability of fluid leakage due to cyst rupture, reduce the operation time, improve the operation precision, and reduce the postoperative complications such as bleeding and bile leakage.

Compared with the traditional operation, the advantages of laparoscopic resection of hepatic hydatid cyst of the external capsule are: 1. compared with liver laparotomy for more than 20 cm of incision, it can greatly reduce the length of the incision and minish the abdominal trauma and scar; 2. It can reduce abdominal adhesions [16], and provide better conditions for the reoperation of possible recurrence; 3. In the operation, the magnified view of laparoscopy can be used to deal with finer bile ducts and blood vessels, and reduce the complications such as bleeding and bile leakage. It can not only achieve the effect of radical resection, but also maximize the retention of normal liver tissue; 4. After surgery, the patient can get out of bed earlier and resume the diet earlier, which shorten the hospitalization time [17]. Da Vinci robotic surgery retains the advantages of laparoscopic surgery, and at the same time, more complex surgery can be implemented because of its excellent operation advantages.

With the improvement of laparoscopic technique, there are almost no restricted areas of hepatic lobectomy[18]. Due to the inherent limitations of laparoscopy and the characteristics of hydatid cysts, more stringent surgical indications are often needed for the implementation of laparoscopic liver hydatid cysts. Poor exposure can greatly increase the risk of rupture and bleeding [19]. Because of its technical advantages, the indications of Da Vinci robot assisted surgery can be more extensive than laparoscopic surgery. Robotic surgery has shown a greater advantage over laparoscopic and open surgery during liver surgery in terms of 3D imaging, increased range of motion within the abdominal cavity and fine control of dissection. Therefore, DVSS may play a vital role in the treatment of posterior cysts close to the vena cava and cysts with thickened and calcified walls.

Preoperative imaging was obtained to assess the relationship between the cyst and the major vessels and bile ducts. The difficulty of surgery will be greatly increased if there is large blood vessel or bile duct invasion. For patients with multiple lesions and the lesions cannot be removed by one-time surgery, the merits of Da Vinci surgery may be extremely limited. Therefore, if there are S7, S8 and other poor exposure lesions, open surgery is still the best choice. For lesions that are well exposed but located at different sites, the distance between the operating arms of the Da Vinci robot should be considered. The interference and collision between the operating arms should be avoided, and the position of Troca should be re-selected if necessary. There are four stages in the surgical methods of hepatic hydatid cyst: internal capsule excision, cyst wall resection, subtotal resection and complete removal of external capsule. Because of high recurrence rate and complications, internal capsule excision and cyst wall resection has been eliminated gradually. At present, the removal of the external capsule and the resection of the liver are considered as radical resection method. Removal of external capsule has increasingly widespread due to its advantage of retention of more normal liver tissue on the premise of radical resection.

Hepatococcal cysts have a gap between the fibrous layer and the liver tissue, which is quite important to identify. It should be noted that this gap is often flat staggered, if the surgery is not timely adjusted, increased bleeding or cyst rupture may occur. Hydatid cyst fluid contains allergens that can cause severe allergic reactions [20]. To prevent the occurrence of allergic reactions, patients were treated routinely with hydrocortisone 200 mg before surgery. Attention should be paid to observe the vital signs of patient during surgery and corresponding preparations for rescue should be made in advance. Once the cyst ruptures, timely and appropriate decompression is needed, and then wet dressing or soaking of hypertonic saline should be performed. The treatment of operative field with hypertonic saline is of great significance for the prevention of cyst recurrence and planting metastasis [21].

Most of the patients with hepatic hydatididae come from pastoral areas, the living environment of which is likely to cause re-infection, thus postoperative antiparasitic drugs and health education are needed. Minimally invasive surgery is the main theme of surgery in 21 century [22]. Through the above operation, we concluded that the indications of Da Vinci robot assisted surgery may be more extensive than laparoscopic surgery. For patients with hydatid cysts extrusion and multiple piping systems, which need to carry out suture and ligation and other complex operations, the advantages of Da Vinci robot assisted surgery are particularly evident. In theory, it can also reduce the risk of allergy, implant and metastasis caused by the rupture of cyst. However, further study and results are still needed.

This case report suggested that laparoscopicresection of hepatic hydatidectocyst with the DVSS is safe and feasible on the basis of hospitals have rich experience in treatment of cystic echinococcosisliver, resection with DVSS and laparoscopic excision.

Acknowledgments
Not applicable.

Funding
This work was supported by Health and Family Planning Commission of Sichuan Province research item 16PJ448.

Authors' contributions
Conception and design, HZ and GW; Data collection, LY L, HX and XW; Data analysis and Manuscript preparation, HZ, LL, YY, GX and XH. All Authors approved the current version of the article.

Competing interests
The authors declare that they have no competing interests.

References

1. Budke CM, Deplazes P, Torgerson PR. Global socioeconomic impact of cystic echinococcosis. Emerg Infect Dis. 2006;12:296–303.
2. Craig PS, McManus DP, Lightowlers MW, Chabalgoity JA, Garcia HH, Gavidia CM, Gilman RH, Gonzalez AE, Lorca M, Naquira C, et al. Prevention and control of cystic echinococcosis. Lancet Infect Dis. 2007;7:385–94.
3. Agudelo Higuita NI, Brunetti E, McCloskey C. Cystic Echinococcosis. J Clin Microbiol. 2016;54:518–23.
4. Mathoulin-Pelissier S, Chevreau C, Bellera C, Bauvin E, Saves M, Grosclaude P, Albert S, Goddard J, Le Guellec S, Delannes M, et al. Adherence to consensus-based diagnosis and treatment guidelines in adult soft-tissue sarcoma patients: a French prospective population-based study. Ann Oncol. 2014;25:225–31.
5. Thomas M, Thepot S, Galic N, Jouanne-Pin S, Remoue C, Goldringer I. Diversifying mechanisms in the on-farm evolution of crop mixtures. Mol Ecol. 2015;24:2937–54.
6. Powell HA, Baldwin DR. Multidisciplinary team management in thoracic oncology: more than just a concept? Eur Respir J. 2014;43:1776–86.
7. Lai CL, Yuen MF. Prevention of hepatitis B virus-related hepatocellular carcinoma with antiviral therapy. Hepatology. 2013;57:399–408.
8. Iavazzo C, Gkegkes ID. The role of uterine manipulators in endometrial cancer recurrence after laparoscopic or robotic procedures. Arch Gynecol Obstet. 2013;288:1003–9.
9. Iavazzo C, Gkegkes ID. Robotic retroperitoneal lymph node dissection in gynaecological neoplasms: comparison of extraperitoneal and transperitoneal lymphadenectomy. Arch Gynecol Obstet. 2016;293:11–28.
10. Tomulescu V, Stanciulea O, Balescu I, Vasile S, Tudor S, Gheorghe C, Vasilescu C, Popescu I. First year experience of robotic-assisted laparoscopic surgery with 153 cases in a general surgery department: indications, technique and results. Chirurgia (Bucur). 2009;104:141–50.
11. Krill LS, Bristow RE. Robotic surgery: gynecologic oncology. Cancer J. 2013;19:167–76.
12. Ohuchida K, Hashizume M. Robotic surgery for cancer. Cancer J. 2013;19:130–2.
13. Yoshino I, Hashizume M, Shimada M, Tomikawa M, Tomiyasu M, Suemitsu R, Sugimachi K. Thoracoscopic thymomectomy with the da Vinci computer-enhanced surgical system. J Thorac Cardiovasc Surg. 2001;122:783–5.
14. Kajiwara N, Kakihana M, Kawate N, Ikeda N. Appropriate set-up of the da Vinci Surgical System in relation to the location of anterior and middle mediastinal tumors. Interact Cardiovasc Thorac Surg. 2011;12:112–6.
15. Hashizume M, Konishi K, Tsutsumi N, Yamaguchi S, Shimabukuro R. A new era of robotic surgery assisted by a computer-enhanced surgical system. Surgery. 2002;131:S330–3.
16. Huang G, Lau WY, Shen F, Pan ZY, Fu SY, Yang Y, Zhou WP, Wu MC. Preoperative hepatitis B virus DNA level is a risk factor for postoperative liver failure in patients who underwent partial hepatectomy for hepatitis B-related hepatocellular carcinoma. World J Surg. 2014;38:2370–6.
17. Branch Association of Hepatology. Chinese Medical Association, Guide to prevention and treatment of chronic hepatitis (The 2010 edition). Chinese Journal of Internal Medicine. 2011;14:1–12.
18. Lau WY, Lai EC. Hepatocellular carcinoma: current management and recent advances. Hepatobiliary Pancreat Dis Int. 2008;7:237–57.
19. Lau WY, Leung TW, Lai BS, Liew CT, Ho SK, Yu SC, Tang AM. Preoperative systemic chemoimmunotherapy and sequential resection for unresectable hepatocellular carcinoma. Ann Surg. 2001;233:236–41.
20. Lau WY, Lai EC. Salvage surgery following downstaging of unresectable hepatocellular carcinoma–a strategy to increase resectability. Ann Surg Oncol. 2007;14:3301–9.
21. Choi JW, Park JY, Ahn SH, Yoon KT, Ko HK, Lee DY, Lee JT, Kim KS, Choi JS, Han KH, et al. Efficacy and safety of transarterial chemoembolization in recurrent hepatocellular carcinoma after curative surgical resection. Am J Clin Oncol. 2009;32:564–9.
22. Morimoto M, Numata K, Kondou M, Nozaki A, Morita S, Tanaka K. Midterm outcomes in patients with intermediate-sized hepatocellular carcinoma: a randomized controlled trial for determining the efficacy of radiofrequency ablation combined with transcatheter arterial chemoembolization. Cancer. 2010;116:5452–60.

Selective versus routine lymphadenectomy in the treatment of liver metastasis from colorectal cancer: a retrospective cohort study

Daniel Pindak[1,2*], Jana Pavlendova[1,2], Miroslav Tomas[1,2], Jozef Dolnik[2], Robert Duchon[2] and Juraj Pechan[1,2]

Abstract

Background: Limited data are available on the importance of routine lymphadenectomy of the hepatoduodenal ligament in the treatment of liver metastasis from colorectal cancer in the literature.

Methods: A single center retrospective cohort study was conducted to evaluate morbidity and long-term survival in patients who had undergone selective versus routine lymphadenectomy during surgery for colorectal liver metastasis. From January 2006 to December 2009, eighty-one patients undergoing radical resection due to liver metastasis from colorectal cancer were included. The combination of two surgical teams with different approaches to hepatoduodenal ligament lymphadenectomy at our institution allowed us to select two cohorts of patients undergoing selective or routine lymphadenectomy.

Results: No significant differences between the cohorts were found in age, American Society of Anesthesiology score or Fong's prognostic criteria. Patients with pN+ disease had significantly inferior survival compared to patients with pN0 disease (hazard ratio [HR] = 6.33, 95% CI 2.16–18.57, $p = 0.0001$). No significant difference in postoperative morbidity was observed in the group undergoing routine opposed to selective lymphadenectomy (13.63% vs. 8.69%, $p = 0.36$). There was no difference in long-term survival between the groups (HR = 0.90, 95% CI 0.52–1.58, $p = 0.70$). There were also no significant differences in the subgroup of patients with pN0 stage (HR = 1.17, 95% CI 0.6–2.11, $p = 0.60$).

Conclusions: These data suggest that there is no survival benefit from the use of routine lymphadenectomy during surgery for colorectal liver metastasis, but these data should be confirmed in a prospective randomized study.

Keywords: Colorectal, Liver, Metastasis, Lymphadenectomy, Survival

Background

The liver is the most common site of metastatic spread after curative treatment of colorectal cancer (CRC), and approximately 50% of all patients with CRC will develop liver metastases [1]. Liver resection represents the best treatment option, with a long-term survival rate of 30%. Resectability is recommended only in approximately 20% of patients, mainly due to the presence of extrahepatic disease [2]. The infiltration of lymph nodes (LN) in the hepatic pedicle and the coeliac region is considered an extrahepatic disease, and many authors still consider its involvement to be a contraindication for liver resection, especially if they are in the coeliac region. Limited data are available on the importance of routine lymphadenectomy of the hepatoduodenal ligament in the literature. Moreover, its survival benefit for both prophylactic and therapeutic indications is not clear [2]. To date, there have been no prospective randomized studies published on this topic. The combination of two different surgical teams with different approaches to lymphadenectomy during liver resection in CRC, at the National Cancer Institute Bratislava Slovakia (NCI), gave us the

* Correspondence: pindakd@zoznam.sk; daniel.pindak@nou.sk
[1]Department of Surgical Oncology, Slovak Medical University, Bratislava, Slovakia
[2]National Cancer Institute, Klenova 1, 833 10 Bratislava 3, Slovakia

opportunity to conduct a study with the aim of evaluating the role of routine lymphadenectomy during liver resection in patients with CRC.

Methods

This retrospective cohort study was conducted to determine the influence of routine lymphadenectomy of the hepatoduodenal ligament on postoperative morbidity and long-term survival in patients with clinically negative nodal status in the hepatoduodenal ligament according to preoperative computed tomography (CT) scans.

Patient selection

From January 2006 to December 2009, eighty-one patients underwent liver resection due to CRC metastases at the National Cancer Institute Bratislava. Patients were divided into two cohorts: patients with or without a routine lymphadenectomy (Fig. 1). This was possible due to the existence of two different hepatobiliary surgical teams working during that time period in the NCI with different approaches to lymphadenectomy. At that time, the presence of nodal involvement in the hepatic pedicle and coeliac region was considered a contraindication for hepatic resection, so all patients who underwent liver resection had clinically negative nodes. At that time, no patient received neoadjuvant or "conversion" chemotherapy before hepatic resection; thus, its influence is of no concern for survival analysis. Administration of adjuvant chemotherapy was considered individually, on the basis of an overall assessment of the below-mentioned prognostic factors. The most commonly used regimen was fluoropyrimidine plus oxaliplatin. Unfortunately different institutions in Slovakia delivered subsequent oncological treatment, so we did not have data about adjuvant chemotherapy available in all patients.

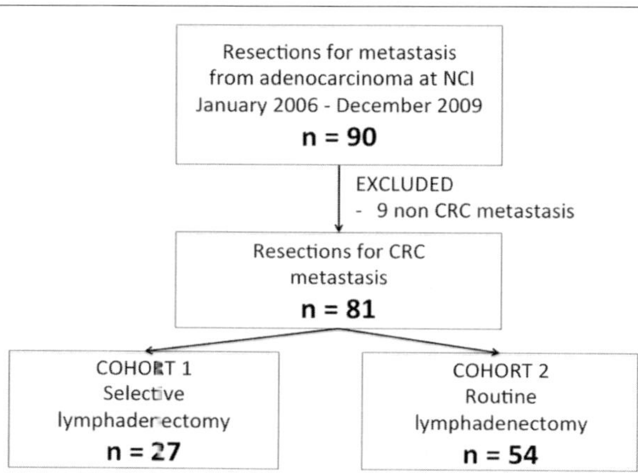

Fig. 1 Patients' selection

Data collection

From the patient's medical records and the National Center of Medical Information and Population Register, we constructed specific case report forms with clinical features and survival information. These features included age, gender, American Society of Anesthesiologists (ASA) score, number and size of liver metastases, disease-free interval (from the treatment of the CRC primary tumor), level of preoperative carcinoembryonic antigen (CEA), positivity of pathological nodal staging (pN+) of the primary tumor, definitive histology finding (only hematoxylin and eosin staining was used for the evaluation of nodal status), presence of postoperative complications and their classification according to the Clavien Dindo system [3], 30-day postoperative mortality and overall survival.

Surgical technic

In cohort 1, no standard lymphadenectomy was performed; nodal sampling (selective lymphadenectomy) was performed only if there was a suspicion for nodal involvement according to macroscopic assessment or intraoperative palpation. In cohort 2, routine lymphadenectomy that included nodes in hepatoduodenal ligament and along the common hepatic artery, coeliac trunk and retropancreatic region was performed.

Statistical analysis

Statistical relationships were evaluated by different tests depending on the data characteristics (Kolmogorov-Smirnov, *t* test, Fisher-Freeman-Halton test), and Kaplan-Meier's method and Log-rank test were used to evaluate differences between the groups in terms of survival analysis. All of the statistical hypotheses were tested with a significance level of alpha = 0.05, and the data cut-off for survival analysis was 31 May 2016. The study was approved by the institutional review board of the NCI Bratislava, Slovakia, and a waiver of consent was granted.

Results

Cohort characteristics

There were 55 men (66.7%) and 26 women (33.3%) included in the study. The median age was similar in both cohorts: 57 (42–88) versus 61 (38–82) years old, respectively ($p = 0.63$). The ASA score was also not different between the groups ($p = 0.42$). The most important and well-accepted prognostic criteria (metastasis size, number of metastases, preoperative CEA level, disease free interval from the treatment of the primary CRC and the nodal status of primary CRC), as counted both separately and by Fong's clinical score [4], were equal and exhibited no significant differences ($p = 0.08$). All of the data are shown in Table 1. The cohorts were well

Table 1 Cohort comparisons with no significant differences in any prognostic factors

	Cohort 1 Selective lymphadenectomy $n = 27$	Cohort 2 Routine lymphadenectomy $n = 54$	p value
Age median (min/max)	57 (42–88)	61 (38–82)	0.63[a]
ASA score (1/2/3/4) %	5/68/27/0	18/68/14/0	0.42[a]
Fong's score (0–2)/(3–5) %	96.97/3.03	83.33/16.67	0.08[b]
MTS size (mm) median (min/max)	21 (10–40)	20 (8–130)	0.12[a]
MTS number median (min/max)	1 (1–8)	2 (1–7)	0.25[a]
CEA level μg/l median (min/max)	5.7 (0.3–850)	6.62 (0.4–850)	0.97[a]
pN+ primary %	41.67	29.09	0.29[a]
disease free < 12 month %	70.37	74.07	0.14[a]

[a]t test
[b]Fisher-Freeman-Halton test

balanced regarding known prognostic factors. The mean number of lymph nodes harvested in patients with routine lymphadenectomy was 4.6 (2–13) per patient. Overall, only one lymph node was sampled in 5 patients in the cohort with selective lymphadenectomy.

Postoperative morbidity

We found a higher rate of postoperative complications in the group of patients undergoing routine lymphadenectomy (13.63%) compared to the group of patients with selective lymphadenectomy (8.69%), but this difference did not reach statistical significance ($p = 0.36$).

The severity of complications evaluated by Clavien Dindo classification system also showed no significant differences ($p = 0.61$).

Survival

The median length of follow up was 61.67 (0.33–122.93) months.

There were 6 patients with positive nodes in cohort 2 (routine lymphadenectomy) and 1 patient with positive nodes in cohort 1 (selective lymphadenectomy), for a prevalence of 11.11% and 3.7% of histological nodal positivity, respectively. Using the Kaplan-Meier method and Log-rank test, we found a significant difference in survival between the patients with positive and negative nodes (median overall survival (mOS) 29.6 vs. 66.97 months, respectively, hazard ratio (HR) 6.33 95% CI 2.16–18.57, $p = 0.0001$) (Fig. 2).

There were no significant differences in long-term survival between cohorts 1 and 2 (median survival 61.62 vs. 60.16 months, respectively, HR 0.90 95% CI 0.52–1.58, $p = 0.7$) (Fig. 3). The 3- and 5-year survival rates were 59.25 and 51.85% vs. 66.67 and 48.15% in cohorts 1 and 2, respectively.

To evaluate the prophylactic potential of lymphadenectomy, we selected patients with pN0 nodal status

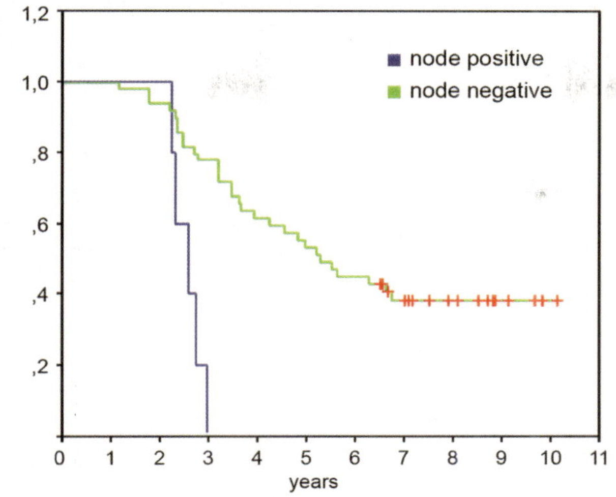

Fig. 2 Survival according to histological nodal status. Kaplan-Meier curves showing the difference in overall survival in patients with positive lymph nodes in hepatic pedicle ($n = 7$) compared to patients with negative nodes ($n = 74$). The *green line* indicates patients with negative nodes, the *blue line* patients with positive nodes. The vertical lines on the curve mark censored data. The difference is statistically significant HR 6.33 95% CI 2.16–18.57, $p = 0.0001$

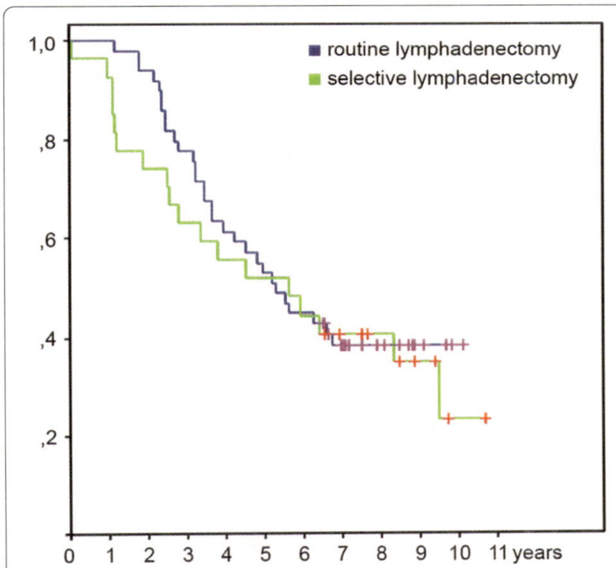

Fig. 3 Survival for selective vs. routine lymphadenectomy in all patients. Kaplan-Meier curves showing the difference in overall survival between patients' cohorts with selective ($n = 27$) and routine ($n = 54$) lymphadenectomy. The *green line* indicates cohort with selective and the *blue line* indicates cohort with routine lymphadenectomy. The vertical lines on the curve mark censored data. Using Log-rank test we found no statistical difference between cohorts HR 0.90 95% CI 0.52–1.58, $p = 0.7$

after definitive histology and found no significant difference in survival (HR 1.17 95% CI 0.6–2.11, $p = 0.6$) (Fig. 4).

Discussion

The indication for lymphadenectomy of the hepatoduodenal ligament during liver resection for CRC metastasis remains controversial. It is still unclear whether the lymph node dissection imparts a survival advantage or merely allows a more complete staging of the disease [2]. The metastatic involvement of nodes is considered one of the worst prognostic factors [5, 6] and was once a contraindication for liver resection because the 5 year survival ranged between 0 and 4.3% [7, 8]. The location of the involved nodes also played an important role, as stated by Adam et al: for those who had metastases in the hepatic pedicle and underwent hepatectomy, the 5 year survival was better (25%) than that observed in patients with positive nodes in the coeliac and paraaortic regions (0%) [9]. In our study, we performed en bloc lymphadenectomy, so the subclassification of nodes to different stations was not possible, but none of our node-positive patients survived for 3 years, despite the use of adjuvant chemotherapy. We can therefore confirm that nodal positivity is a negative prognostic factor: node-positive patients exhibited a median survival of 29.6 months vs. 66.97 for node-negative patients.

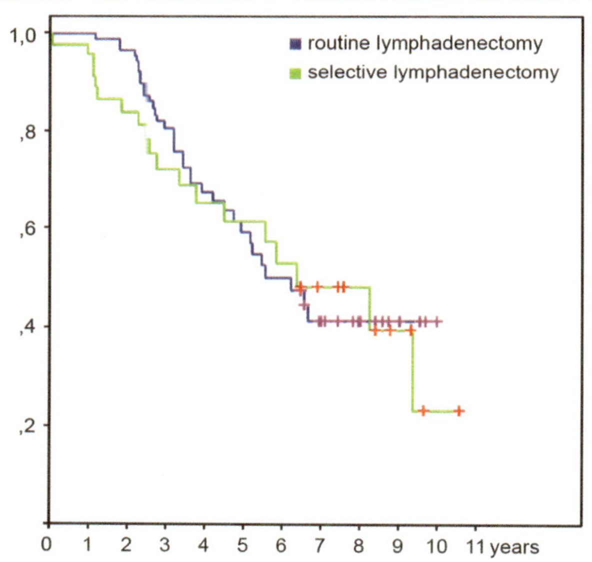

Fig. 4 Survival for selective vs. routine lymphadenectomy in pN0 patients. Kaplan-Meier curves showing the difference in overall survival in the subgroup of patients with confirmed pN0 stage. The *green line* indicates cohort with selective and the *blue line* indicates cohort with routine lymphadenectomy. The vertical lines on the curve mark censored data. Using Log-rank test we found no significant difference in survival HR 1.17 95% CI 0.6–2.11, $p = 0.6$ between patients' cohorts with selective ($n = 26$) and routine ($n = 48$) lymphadenectomy

The overall prevalence of positive lymph nodes was reported to be 8.4%, ranging between 5.4 and 27.9% after routine lymphadenectomy and between 4.0 and 22.5% after selective lymphadenectomy. Koti et al. reported that the prevalence was not correlated to the extent or approach (routine/selective) of lymphadenectomy [10]. In our study, the prevalence was higher in the group of patients undergoing routine lymphadenectomy compared to selective lymphadenectomy (11.11% vs. 3.7%), which can be explained by patient selection for those with cN0 stage. During the study period, the clinical positivity of extrahepatic nodes was considered a contraindication for liver resection.

Regardless of the extent of lymphadenectomy that was performed, we found equal survival in patients with and without routine lymphadenectomy (median survival 61.62 vs. 60.16 months, respectively, HR 0.90 95% CI 0.52–1.58, $p = 0.7$).

To evaluate the "prophylactic" potential of lymphadenectomy, we excluded all patients with proven positive nodes. We assumed, that routine lymphadenectomy in patients with pN0 nodal status could improve survival through the eliminating potential site of future recurrence, as in the cohort with selective lymphadenectomy, patients were expected to have residual nodal disease. We also found no survival advantage of routine lymphadenectomy over no lymphadenectomy (HR 1.17 95% CI 0.6–2.11).

Although the routine lymphadenectomy of the hepatoduodenal ligament in the treatment of liver metastasis from CRC is, according to our results, a safe procedure with acceptable morbidity that is not higher than after liver resection only ($p = 0.36$), we found no survival benefit from its use. Therefore, we suggest considering routine lymphadenectomy during liver resection individually until evidence from high-quality studies supports its use.

Our results do not support the use of routine lymphadenectomy; therefore, we suggest to not perform it as a standard procedure, although its morbidity is the same as after liver resection only ($p = 0.36$). The quality of data in the literature is unclear, and the conclusions are controversial; thus, we suggest that patients be enrolled in prospective clinical studies, which we are currently performing.

Conclusion

Although the routine lymphadenectomy of the hepatoduodenal ligament in the treatment of liver metastasis from CRC is, according to our results, a safe procedure with acceptable morbidity, we found no survival benefit from its use. Therefore, we suggest considering routine lymphadenectomy during liver resection individually until evidence from high-quality studies supports its use. We confirmed the presence of nodal metastasis as a negative prognostic marker with zero percent 3-year survival.

Abbreviations

ASA: American Society of Anesthesiologists; CEA: Carcinoembryonic antigen; CRC: Colorectal cancer; CT: Computed tomography; HR: Hazard ratio; LN: Lymph nodes; NCI: National Cancer Institute Bratislava Slovakia; pN+: positivity of pathological nodal staging; vs.: versus

Acknowledgements

Special thanks to Dr. Michal Mego from NCI for reviewing important intellectual content and language corrections.

Funding

Not applicable.

Authors' contributions

Authors contributed to the conception and design (DP, JP), to the writing of the manuscript (DP), and the acquisition of data, statistical analysis and interpretation of data (JP, DP, MT). All authors read and approved the final manuscript.

Competing interests

The authors declare that they have no competing interests.

References

1. Gurusamy KS, Imber C, Davidson BR. Management of the hepatic lymph nodes during resection of liver metastases from colorectal cancer: a systematic review. HPB Surg. 2008; doi:10.1155/2008/684150
2. Bradatsch A, Kornprat P, Bacher H, Cerwenka H, Haybaeck J, Mischinger HJ. The Value of Lymph Node Dissection in the Surgery of Colorectal Cancer Liver Metastases. Anticancer Res. 2016;36:2993–7.
3. Dindo D, Demartines N, Clavien PA. Classification of surgical complications: a new proposal with evaluation in a cohort of 6336 patients and results of a survey. Ann Surg. 2004;240(2):205–13.
4. Fong Y, Fortner J, Sun RL, Brennan MF, Blumgart LH. Clinical score for predicting recurrence after hepatic resection for metastatic colorectal cancer: analysis of 1001 consecutive cases. Ann Surg. 1999;230(3):309–18.
5. Rodgers MS, McCall JL. Surgery for colorectal liver metastases with lymph node involvement: a systematic review. Br J Surg. 2000; doi:10.1046/j.1365-2168.2000.01580.x
6. Poston GJ, Adam R, Alberts S, Curley S, Figueras J, Haller D, et al. OncoSurge: a strategy for improving resectability with curative intent in metastatic colorectal cancer. J Clin Oncol. 2005; doi:10.1200/JCO.2005.08.722
7. Jaeck D, Nakano H, Bachellier P, Inoue K, Weber JC, Oussoultzoglou E, et al. Significance of hepatic pedicle lymph node involvement in patients with colorectal liver metastases: a prospective study. Ann Surg Oncol. 2002;9(5):430–8.
8. Laurent C, Cunha AS, Rullier E, Smith D, Rullier A, Saric J. Impact of microscopic hepatic lymph node involvement on survival after resection of colorectal liver metastasis. J Am Coll Surg. 2004; doi: 10.1016/j.jamcollsurg.2004.01.017
9. Adam R, de Haas RJ, Wicherts DA, Aloia TA, Delvart V, Azoulay D, et al. Is hepatic resection justified after chemotherapy in patients with colorectal liver metastases and lymph node involvement? J clin Oncol. 2008; doi:10.1200/JCO.2007.15.7297
10. Koti RS, Simillis C, Gurusamy KS. Jacovides M, Davidson BR. Management of the Hepatic Lymph Nodes During Resection of Liver Metastases from Colorectal Cancer: A Systematic Review. Curr Colorectal Cancer Rep. 2013; doi: 10.1007/s11888-013-0165-6

Extended left hepatectomy for intrahepatic cholangiocarcinoma: hepatic vein reconstruction with in-situ hypothermic perfusion and extracorporeal membrane oxygenation

Deniz Balci[1*], Menekse Ozcelik[2], Elvan Onur Kirimker[1], Arda Cetinkaya[1], Evren Ustuner[3], Mehmet Cakici[4], Bahadir Inan[4], Zekeriyya Alanoglu[2], Sadik Bilgic[3] and Ahmet Ruchan Akar[4]

Abstract

Background: Liver resection for intrahepatic cholangiocarcinoma (ICC) with invasion of the inferior vena cava (IVC) and hepatic veins (HV) is a challenging procedure.

Case presentation: We report a case of a 63-year-old woman with a 6-cm, centrally located liver mass. Her biochemistry results were normal except for a Ca19–9 level of 1199 U/ml. The liver biopsy was consistent with ICC and 60% macrosteatosis. Abdominal CT scans revealed a large central mass invading the left HV, middle HV and right HV, infringing on their junction with the vena cava. An operation was planned using a 3-dimensional (3D) computer simulation model using dedicated software. We also describe a novel veno-portal-venous extracorporeal membrane oxygenation (VPV-ECMO) support with in-situ hypothermic perfusion (IHP) during this procedure. We aimed to perform an extended left hepatectomy and reconstruct 3 right HV orifices with an interposition jump graft to the IVC with total vascular exclusion (TVE) and IHP A supplemental video describing the preoperative planning, the operative procedure with the postoperative follow-up in detail is presented. After the patient was discharged, she developed a hepatic venous outflow obstruction 3 months postoperatively, which was effectively managed with hepatic venous stenting by interventional radiology. She is currently symptom free and without tumour recurrence at the 1-year follow-up.

Conclusions: This report demonstrates that extended left hepatectomy for IHC with IHP and VPV-ECMO is safe and feasible under the supervision of a highly experienced team.

Keywords: Intrahepatic cholangiocarcinoma, ECMO, Total vascular exclusion, In-situ hypothermic perfusion

Background

Liver resection offers curative treatment for intrahepatic cholangiocarcinoma (ICC), with 5-year survival reported between 30 and 50% after curative resection in both western and eastern populations [1]. Depending on tumour location and size, hepatic resection could be challenging, requiring thorough preoperative evaluation and planning. For complex liver resections, computer-assisted surgical planning using software for 3-dimensional (3D) reconstruction of the liver anatomy with better interpretation of a tumour's relationship with critical vascular structures was reported to facilitate intraoperative decision-making with increased safety during resection [2]. In cases with invasion of the inferior vena cava (IVC) and hepatic veins where resection of these structures is required, additional safety measures, such as total vascular exclusion (TVE) to minimize bleeding, veno-venous bypass (VVB) for venous

* Correspondence: denizbalci1@yahoo.com
This study was presented as an oral video abstract at the European-African Hepatobiliary Surgery Association Meeting on May 2017; Mainz, Germany.
[1]Department of General Surgery, Ankara University School of Medicine, K4 06590 Sihhiye, Ankara, Turkey
Full list of author information is available at the end of the article

return and to prevent splanchnic congestion, and in-situ hypothermic perfusion (IHP) for liver preservation and complex reconstructions, may be required [3]. However, all these measures can potentially complicate the operation and the postoperative outcome. Normothermic liver ischaemia, especially for more than 60 min, and subsequent ischaemia-reperfusion injury elicit a risk of postoperative complications such as bleeding and liver failure (PLF) [4]. To decrease these risks, IHP with TVE is required so that the future liver remnant (FLR) can tolerate the ischaemia-reperfusion injury, which is critical for safe patient recovery [5]. Recently, the use of veno-venous extracorporeal membrane oxygenation (VV-ECMO) in the liver transplant setting was reported to be beneficial in facilitating operations in critical patients with complex comorbidities where prolonged cardiopulmonary support is required [6].

Here, we report a case of ICC with involvement of the IVC and hepatic veins. Using a 3D computer simulation model, we performed an extended left hepatectomy and reconstruction of 3 right hepatic veins under IHP and veno-portal-venous extracorporeal membrane oxygenation (VPV-ECMO) support.

Case presentation

A 63-year-old obese, diabetic woman with a history of previous cholecystectomy was admitted to our institution with right upper quadrant pain. Her body mass index was 36. She was positive for Factor 5 Leiden heterozygous mutation. Abdominal Ultrasonography (USG) revealed a centrally located 6-cm mass with grade 3 hepatosteatosis. Fine needle biopsy was consistent with adenocarcinoma of biliary origin, which was interpreted as intrahepatic cholangiocarcinoma (ICC). Abdominal computed tomography (CT) scans revealed a large central mass invading the left (LHV), middle (MHV) and right hepatic veins (RHV) infringing upon their junction with the vena cava. An additional movie file shows this in more detail (see Additional file 1: Video S1). Her biochemistry results were normal other than a Ca19–9 level of 1199 U/ml. Positron Emission Tomography confirmed liver-only disease and a single liver mass with SUV Max: 7.5.

Operation plan

The operation was planned using computer assisted 3-dimensional (3D) modelling software for 3D reconstruction of the liver scan images (Myrian, Intrasense France). The IVC and the RHV, MHV and LHV junction were affected by the tumour. Therefore, resection and reconstruction of these structures were planned. The resection plane was modified to obtain the maximum volume of the FLR, including segments 5–6-7 of the right lobe (61% of total liver volume), because of the patient's age and the degree of hepatosteatosis. It was estimated that the critical part of the parenchymal transection would be providing a safety margin while following an initially anatomical and then non-anatomical resection plane to find the junction where the RHV separated into 3 branches before invasion by the tumour. We planned to resect and reconstruct the IVC followed by a jump graft reconstruction of the 3-orifice junction to the IVC. We intended to perform the critical transection and reconstruction steps using TVE and VPV-ECMO with IHP for FLR protection. The submitted multimedia (see Additional file 1: Video S1) shows the operative plan with 3D reconstruction.

The patient was taken to the OR, but during the initial phase of anaesthesia induction, she experienced an anaphylactic reaction in the form of severe bronchoconstriction associated with increased airway pressure, profound hypoxaemia and hypercarbia. Despite all efforts with conventional medical treatment for severe bronchoconstriction and lung protective ventilation strategies, the patient did not recover until reversal of the neuromuscular blocker rocuronium with sugammadex, a reversal agent for rocuronium. The operation was cancelled to allow the patient to recover and detailed allergy tests were conducted. After comprehensive studies with the objective of determining safe anaesthetic agents, including neuromuscular blockers, the operation was performed 2 weeks later. Anaesthetic induction was maintained with thiopental, vecuronium, fentanyl and midazolam without any adverse events. The right femoral artery was cannulated with a 5 Fr central venous cannula for advanced haemodynamic monitoring of continuous cardiac output with pulse contour analysis (FloTrac system, software version 1.01; Edwards Lifesciences, Irvine, CA, USA). To derive more detailed haemodynamic data, including tissue oxygenation, an 8 Fr pulmonary artery catheter (CCombo, Edwards Lifesciences, Irvine, CA, USA) was inserted into the left internal jugular vein.

We planned to use VPV-ECMO rather than standard VV-Bypass to provide not only perfusion but also support for oxygenation and respiratory function and to avoid splanchnic congestion during the course of the procedure.

The VPV-ECMO setup

The ECMO circuit used in this case was a continuous flow centrifugal pump (JostraRotaflow®; Maquet Cardiopulmonary, Rastatt, Germany), oxygenator (JostraQuadrox®; Maquet Cardiopulmonary, Rastatt, Germany), and heat exchanger. After heparin administration (5000 IU), USG-guided right common femoral vein (RCFV) puncture was performed. A flexible J-tip guide-wire was advanced through the RCFV. Using the Seldinger technique, a 21 Fr multi-perforated venous cannula (HLS®Cannulae, Maquet®, Rastatt, Germany) was inserted over the guide-wire up to the infra-hepatic IVC. The position was confirmed with manual palpation of the catheter tip within the IVC, located just below the level of the left renal vein. Another 17 Fr cannula (Arterial ®Cannulae, Maquet®, Rastatt, Germany) was inserted over a guide-wire through the right internal jugular vein (RIJV) down to the right atrium under transesophageal echocardiography guidance. Furthermore, a 16 Fr venous cannula (Edwards Lifescience, TF016L, LLC, Irvine, CA, USA) was inserted to the portal vein (PV). The RCFV and PV cannulas served as drainage cannulas and the RIJV cannula served as a supplying cannula for the VPV-ECMO set-up. Using flow sensors, we monitored flow ratios in the draining cannulas during the procedure; maximum VPV-ECMO flow was 3.2 L/min and maximum PV flow was 0.5 L/min. PO_2, PCO_2, SO_2, pH and lactate levels were monitored via right radial arterial blood samples. Maximum serum lactate was 2.75 mmol/Lt during the procedure.

The operation

A median laparotomy was performed. The operation started with TVE of the liver for inflow and outflow control (see Additional file 1: Video S1). An intraoperative USG examination was performed by an experienced radiologist (EU) to confirm the tumour's relationship with vascular structures and the anticipated tumour-free FLR. The hepatoduodenal ligament was dissected, isolating the main (MPV), right (RPV) and left portal (LPV) veins, followed by left (LHA) and right hepatic artery (RHA) dissection.

Hepatoduodenal ligament dissection was completed after a 16 Fr IHP cannula was inserted from the LPV. Selective control of the left hilar pedicle by tying both the LHA and LPV revealed a demarcation line on the liver and parenchymal transection proceeded using an ultrasonic surgical aspirator (Sonastar, Misonix USA) following the MHV until the point of preoperatively planned deviation using the 3D model from the anatomical line (MHV) was reached. At this point, although we had planned to resect the IVC with the tumour, we were able to dissect and preserve it using the ultrasonic surgical aspirator. In this step, we obtained three frozen biopsies from the tissue showing a desmoplastic reaction between the IVC and liver capsula, demonstrating an invasion-free IVC.

IHP was initiated before the LHV, MHV and RHV were cut and the liver was elevated through the incision for the final critical step of parenchymal transection. The 3 right hepatic vein branches were exposed (see Additional file 1: Video S1). After the hepatectomy was completed, an 8-cm interposition cadaveric IVC graft was used for reconstruction of the three hepatic vein orifices, joining them with the patient's preserved IVC. We first anastomosed the right hepatic vein junction with the IVC graft that matched the total diameter of the 3 RHV orifices using 4.0 prolene in an end-to-end fashion. Then, we anastomosed the graft to the RHV orifice on the IVC that was enlarged in both inferior and medial directions, finally matching the diameter of the graft. After the reconstruction was complete, we terminated IHP and removed the ECMO cannula in the MPV. During and immediately after reperfusion, we kept the femoral vein cannula in place and the ECMO system running. The RCFV and RIJV cannulae were removed after haemostasis and confirmation of haemodynamic and respiratory stability.

The total duration of the operation was 12 h. Four units of erythrocytes and 3 l of HTK solution were required for IHP, which was performed for a total of 82 min.

The patient was discharged from the ICU 48 h after the operation with gradual improvement of liver function. Pathology confirmed a 6-cm, grade 2 adenocarcinoma of biliary origin. The tumour showed lymphovascular invasion. Three hepatoduodenal lymph nodes were negative and the operation was considered an R0 resection with a less than 1-mm surgical margin in the parenchymal transection line close to the hepatic veins.

On postoperative day 5, despite anticoagulation prophylaxis, the patient experienced pulmonary embolism, which caused haemodynamic instability and required intubation, mechanical ventilation, and inotropic support. She was readmitted to the ICU. However, there was no evidence of myocardial injury as indicated by a negative cardiac troponin test. Unfractionated heparin was administered as an intravenous bolus followed by a therapeutic dose of low-molecular weight heparin. After a gradual recovery, she was ambulated and discharged after 32 days of hospitalization.

At 3 months, she experienced abdominal pain, ascites and jaundice. A triphasic CT scan showed outflow obstruction with kinking of the venous graft due to extensive liver regeneration. The patient's condition deteriorated, with an increase in total bilirubin to 9 mg/dl and massive ascites and hydrothorax. The patient was taken to an angiography suite where a metallic stent was inserted, resulting in rapid recovery of liver function and the patient's condition (see Additional file 1: Video S1).

At the 1-year follow up, she is symptom-free. Her Ca19–9 level is 35 U/ml. Her follow-up CT scan shows no tumour recurrence and normal liver function tests.

Discussion and conclusions

Over the last 2 decades, advances in surgical techniques, perioperative care and interdisciplinary teamwork represent a paradigm shift for patients undergoing complex liver reconstruction with vascular resection. In recent years, technological advances have been established for preoperative planning and perioperative support, which may affect operative mortality, morbidity, and long-term outcomes of these patients in experienced centres [5, 7].

In complex liver resections requiring HV-IVC reconstruction, TVE becomes an important safety measure when bleeding is anticipated, but haemodynamic instability with splanchnic venous congestion causes ischaemia and eventually reperfusion injury (IRI) after declamping. Hepatic IRI, an inflammatory response that follows hepatic ischaemia and is characterized by overproduction of reactive oxygen species (ROS), has detrimental effects on FLR recovery after extended liver resections. To avoid this, IHP has been reported to be a protective manoeuvre that may potentially increase the liver's tolerance to ischaemia and may be helpful in the recovery of hepatic function and regeneration in the normal liver, but it has not been thoroughly studied in the context of damaged liver parenchyma [8]. The patient in the case reported here was relatively older with a significant degree of parenchymal steatosis (60% macrovesicular), which are both reported significant risk factors for severe morbidity and mortality after major liver resection [9]. To optimize FLR recovery, parenchymal preservation with IHP and the use of TVE with VPV-ECMO provide additional safety measures for patients with significant comorbidities. To our best knowledge, this is the first report of VPV-ECMO support in extended left hepatectomy, which was designed and configured by our multidisciplinary team (ARA, DB, MO). Recently, we reported the effective use of VPV-ECMO support in critically ill liver transplant recipients during IVC resection and reconstruction in the LDLT setting [10]. There are several advantages of VPV-ECMO support during hepatectomy over conventional techniques. In brief, VPV-ECMO 1) drains portal circulation and mitigates splanchnic congestion and edema, 2) provides partial or complete support for oxygenation and respiratory function, 3) allows ventilation with lower tidal volumes and lower pressures, and 4) provides better myocardial oxygenation and 5) pulmonary vasodilation. Furthermore, VV-ECMO support can be continued after surgery if required. However, the technique requires expertise and has several disadvantages, including an increased risk of bleeding during surgery because of moderate anticoagulation during support, a potential inflammatory response to extracorporeal circulation, and a risk of vascular complications.

For preoperative planning of complex liver resections, 3D reconstructions with computer simulation models are showing broader clinical application for volumetric calculations and parenchymal transection plane determination [11]. We used a similar approach to choose the FLR and determine the parenchymal transection plane and for planning the outflow reconstruction with 3 RHV junctions to the IVC. Although outflow reconstruction using a native IVC graft enabled successful recovery of the patient in the early period, after 3 months, graft regeneration in the anterior-posterior and lateral to medial directions resulted in graft tension and kinking, with symptoms of outflow obstruction requiring endovascular intervention. Outflow reconstruction problems have been studied in detail in the living-donor liver transplantation (LDLT) setting and the general solution is to create larger openings with consideration of graft regeneration patterns [12]. However, in LDLT, the distance between the graft RHV and the recipient IVC is much shorter than an atypical resection as presented here that created a longer gap. Alternatively, a ringed Gore-tex or a dacron graft could be a better choice than a native graft due to better patency, but timely diagnosis and endovascular hepatic venous stenting is helpful in this clinical scenario [13].

This report demonstrates that complex liver resection with vascular reconstruction is safe and feasible with preoperative planning using 3D computer simulation, intraoperative VPV-ECMO for cardiorespiratory support and a close postoperative follow-up using a multidisciplinary team approach. Using a combination of techniques described could potentially increase the number of patients with centrally located liver tumors of either metastatic or primary disease (ie. cholangiocellular carcinoma) with various degree of liver parenchymal quality and function who could safely undergo complex liver surgeries that is otherwise unresectable.

Abbreviations

3D: 3-dimensional; CT: Computed tomography; FLR: Future liver remnant; ICC: Intrahepatic cholangiocarcinoma; IHP: In-situ hypothermic perfusion; IVC: Inferior vena cava; PV: Portal vein; RCFV: Right common femoral vein; RIJV: Right internal jugular vein; TVE: Total vascular exclusion; VPV-ECMO: Veno-portal-venous extracorporeal membrane oxygenation; VVB: Veno-venous bypass

Acknowledgements

We sincerely thank Neslihan Alkis, MD for her support as the co-chair of Anesthesiology and the ICU. We also thank our perfusionists Altan Ada and Emre Özsoylu for VPV-ECMO set-up and management. Finally, we would like thank Cumhur Çeken for the 3D-computer simulation model and Celal Bayar for editing and preparing the supplemental video.

Funding

Not applicable.

Authors' contributions

DB, MO, EOK, AC, EU, MC, BI, ZA and ARA participated in the surgery of this case. DB, MO, EOK drafted the manuscript. MC, AC, BI collected the data. ARA, SB, EU, ZA revised the manuscript. All authors read and approved the final manuscript.

Competing interests

The authors declare that they have no competing interests.

Author details

[1]Department of General Surgery, Ankara University School of Medicine, K4 06590 Sihhiye, Ankara, Turkey. [2]Department of Anesthesiology, Ankara University School of Medicine, Ankara, Turkey. [3]Department of Radiology, Ankara University School of Medicine, Ankara, Turkey. [4]Department of Cardiovascular Surgery, Ankara University School of Medicine, Ankara, Turkey.

References

1. Doussot A, Gonen M, Wiggers JK, Groot-Koerkamp B, RP DM, Fuks D, et al. Recurrence patterns and disease-free survival after resection of intrahepatic cholangiocarcinoma: preoperative and postoperative prognostic models. J Am Coll Surg. 2016;223:493–505.e2.

2. Soon DSC, Chae MP, Pilgrim CHC, Rozen WM, Spychal RT, Hunter-Smith DJ. 3D haptic modelling for preoperative planning of hepatic resection: a systematic review. Ann Med Surg. 2016;10:1–7.
3. Azoulay D, Eshkenazy R, Andreani P, Castaing D, Adam R, Ichai P, et al. *In situ* hypothermic perfusion of the liver versus standard total vascular exclusion for complex liver resection. Ann Surg. 2005;241:277–85.
4. Emond JC, Kelley SD, Heffron TG, Nakagawa T, Roberts JP, Lim RC Jr. Surgical and anesthetic management of patients undergoing major hepatectomy using total vascular exclusion. Liver Transpl Surg. 1996;2:91–8.
5. Azoulay D, Lim C, Salloum C, Andreani P, Maggi U, Bartelmaos T, et al. Complex liver resection using standard total vascular exclusion, venovenous bypass, and *in situ* hypothermic portal perfusion: an audit of 77 consecutive cases. Ann Surg. 2015;262:93–104.
6. Nandhabalan P, Loveridge R, Patel S, Willars C, Best T, Vercueil A, et al. Extracorporeal membrane oxygenation and pediatric liver transplantation, "a step too far?": results of a single-center experience. Liver Transpl. 2016;22:1727–33.
7. Hemming AW, Reed AI, Langham MR, Fujita S, Howard RJ. Combined resection of the liver and inferior vena cava for hepatic malignancy. Ann Surg. 2004;239:712–21.
8. Reiniers MJ, Olthof PB, van Golen RF, Heger M, van Beek AA, Meijer B, et al. Hypothermic perfusion with retrograde outflow during right hepatectomy is safe and feasible. Surgery. 2017;162:48–58.
9. Belghiti J, Hiramatsu K, Benoist S, Massault P, Sauvanet A, Farges O. Seven hundred forty-seven hepatectomies in the 1990s: an update to evaluate the actual risk of liver resection. J Am Coll Surg. 2000;191:38–46.
10. Balci D, Kirimker EO, Akar AR. A new technique for living donor liver transplantation: backtable outflow reconstruction and bicaval anastomosis with veno-venous bypass: back to basics. In: Video presented at international liver transplantation society annual congress: 24th May 2017; Prague, Czech Republic; 2017.
11. Oshiro Y, Ohkohchi N. Three-dimensional liver surgery simulation: computer-assisted surgical planning with three-dimensional simulation software and three-dimensional printing. Tissue Eng Part A. 2017;23:474–80.
12. Hwang S, Ha TY, Ahn CS, Moon DB, Song GW, Kim KH, et al. Hemodynamics-compliant reconstruction of the right hepatic vein for adult living donor liver transplantation with a right liver graft. Liver Transpl. 2012;18:858–66.
13. Lee JM, Ko GY, Sung KB, Gwon DI, Yoon HK, Lee SG. Long-term efficacy of stent placement for treating inferior vena cava stenosis following liver transplantation. Liver Transpl. 2010;16:513–9.

Hepatectomy for liver metastases from gastric cancer

Ying-Yang Liao[1†], Ning-Fu Peng[2†], Di Long[3], Peng-Cheng Yu[3], Sen Zhang[3], Jian-Hong Zhong[2*] and Le-Qun Li[2]

Abstract

Background: Official guidelines recommend palliative treatments for patients with liver metastases from gastric cancer. However, many case series reported that hepatectomy for such cases is safe and effective. This systematic review compares the overall survival between hepatectomy and palliative therapy in patients with liver metastases from gastric cancer.

Methods: Two independent reviewers performed a systematic search of literature in EMBASE and PubMed, updated until 26 October 2016. The Newcastle-Ottawa score for cohort studies was used for quality assessment of included studies.

Results: A total of eight cohort studies involving 196 patients in the hepatectomy arm and 481 in the palliative arm were included. Median overall survival of patients in the two arms was 23.7 (range, 13.0 to 48.0) and 7.6 (range, 5.5 to 15.2), respectively. Median rates of overall survival of the two arms were 69, 40, 33 and 27, 8, 4% at 1, 2, and 3 years, respectively. Comparing with palliative therapy, hepatectomy was associated with significantly lower mortality at 1 year (odds ratio 0.17, $P < 0.001$) and 2 years (odds ratio 0.15, $P < 0.001$). Among the patients who underwent hepatectomy, Asian cohorts showed higher median rates of overall survival than Western cohorts at 1 year (76 vs. 60%), 2 years (47 vs. 30%) and 3 years (39 vs. 23%).

Conclusions: Hepatectomy in the management of liver metastases from gastric cancer can be considered effective. In the elective setting, hepatectomy provides a potential alternative to palliative therapy.

Keywords: Gastric cancer, Hepatectomy, Liver metastases, Systematic review

Background

As the sixth highest incidence and the second leading cause of cancer deaths worldwide, gastric cancer is the most common form of cancer, with more than 951,000 new cases worldwide diagnosed in 2012 [1]. Due to late onset and nonspecific symptoms, the majority of gastric cancer cases present in advanced stage, with less than 30% of patients eligible for curative resection [2]. In recent decade, treatment of gastric cancer has been significantly improved, and the 5-year overall survival of patients with T1 tumors is up to 95% [3]. However, the prognoses of patients represented by peritoneal or liver metastases is extremely poor, with a 3-year overall survival lower than 10% after chemotherapy [4, 5].

Gastrectomy is more used in Eastern centers than Western centers. And Eastern patients' prognoses after gastrectomy are better than those in Western [6]. According to the guideline of the Japanese Classification of Gastric Carcinoma [7], liver metastases from gastric cancer is categorized as stage IV disease. This guideline [7] and the National Comprehensive Cancer Network guideline [8, 9] do not recommend surgery for stage IV gastric cancer, which lead to most patients with liver metastases of gastric cancer receive palliative treatment (such as chemotherapy). Though the necessity of hepatectomy for liver metastases of gastric cancer is still controversial, the Guidelines Committee of the Japan Gastric Cancer Association reconsidered the treatment of potentially resectable M1 disease [10].

* Correspondence: zhongjianhong66@163.com; zhongjianhong@gxmu.edu.cn
†Equal contributors
[2]Hepatobiliary Surgery Department, Affiliated Tumor Hospital of Guangxi Medical University, Nanning 530021, Guangxi Province, China
Full list of author information is available at the end of the article

Recently, many case-control or case series studies of liver metastases from gastric cancer have been reported. However, most of these studies are presented from a single center, have a small sample size, and/or include old cases from the 1960s and 1980s [11–20]. Therefore, it is important to thoroughly analyze the significance of hepatectomy for liver metastases from gastric cancer, and compare the efficacy of hepatectomy with palliative therapy for such patients in recent two decades (1990–2016) with a systematic review.

Methods

Two independent authors performed a systematic review (Y.-Y.L, D.L) according to the Preferred Reporting Items for Systematic Reviews and Meta-Analyses (PRISMA) statement [21]. A study protocol was followed which defined the study objectives, eligibility criteria, outcome measures, search strategy and methodology of analysis. The quality of included studies was assessed using the Newcastle-Ottawa score for cohort studies [22]. This tool was chosen because of the unavailability of randomized controlled trials and large heterogeneity between studies.

Search strategy

A systematic search of literature, updated until 26 October 2016, was performed by two independent reviewers (Y.-Y.L, D.L). The EMBASE and PubMed databases were searched using MeSH and free text words. MeSH and free text words concerning gastric cancer and metastasis were used. No language or time period restrictions were applied. Titles and abstracts retrieved from the search were screened for relevance and selected studies. Disagreements during the search and selection process were resolved by discussion and, if needed, a third reviewer (N.-F.P) was consulted to reach consensus. Reference lists of all included articles were screened for additional eligible papers.

The following search strategy was used in PubMed (Medline):

((“cancer” [Mesh] AND “gastric Neoplasms” [Mesh]) OR “neoplasm, stomach” [Mesh] OR stomach neoplasm*[tw] OR gastric neoplasm*[tw] OR cancer of stomach*[tw] OR stomach cancer*[tw] OR gastric cancer*[tw]) AND (“Metastases, Neoplasm” [Mesh] OR metastasis*[tw] OR metastases*[tw]) AND (surgery*[tw] OR resection*[tw] OR hepatectomy*[tw]) AND (hepatic*[tw] OR liver*[tw]).

Eligibility criteria and data extraction

Criteria for final study inclusion were: (1) study population formed by patients with liver metastases from gastric cancer in the absence of peritoneal metastasis or extractable from studies in which hepatectomy was performed; (2) sufficient description of the study population; (3) description of patient survival rates for at least 1 year after hepatectomy; (4) the study had a randomized control, cohort, or case-control design. In order to reduce the bias of diagnosis, original treatments, neoadjuvant and adjvuant treatments, only cases after 1990 may be included. In cases in which a study was followed by a more complete study or studies that included the original data set, the most recent and complete report was chosen. Such linked studies were identified on the grounds of authorship, institutions, design, length of follow-up, and study populations. If additional data or results were needed, the corresponding author of each report was contacted by e-mail.

Data were extracted by two authors (Y.-Y.L, D.L) using standardized forms. The following data were collected: author details, country, recruitment period, study design, median follow-up, sample size, gender, positive and negative findings, and methodological quality. A third author (N.-F.P) checked the extracted data against the original studies. Survival data were taken directly from tables or the text whenever possible; if such data were presented only in graphs, they were extracted by manual interpolation. *P* values associated with inter-group differences in mortality were extracted directly from survival curves, text, or tables wherever possible.

Statistical analysis

Meta-analysis was performed on an intention-to-treat basis. To assess attrition bias, we calculated mortality using a ‘worst-case’ approach in which patients with missing data were counted as treatment failures (death). For patients with missing data, we ’carried forward’ data from the most recent measurement.

Outcomes are displayed as they were reported in the original article. All statistical tests for this meta-analysis were performed using Stata 11.0 softwares. Due to the high likelihood of mortality, odds ratio (ORs) with corresponding 95% confidence intervals (95% CIs) were calculated for dichotomous outcomes using the Mantel-Haenszel method. Point estimates of RR were considered statistically significant when $P < 0.05$. Statistical heterogeneity was explored by inconsistency (I^2) statistics; in particular, I^2 values of <25% was interpreted as low heterogeneity, between 25 and 50% as medium, between 50 and 75% as substantial and above 75% as considerable [23].

Results

A total of 3629 records were identified. Following screening for duplications, 2108 articles remained. After screening by title and abstract, a further 2057 records were excluded. Of the remaining 52 articles which need full-text assessment, 35 were studies with single arm investigating the role of hepatectomy for liver metastases from gastric cancer [11–20, 24–48]. In the end, only 8 studies compared the efficacy of hepatectomy to that of other palliative treatments met the eligibility criteria and were included in a quantitative synthesis [49–56]. Details are listed in Fig. 1.

Baseline characteristics

Five of the studies based on Eastern population [49, 50, 52, 53, 56] while the other three based on Western population [51, 54, 55]. These eight studies included 196 patients in the hepatectomy arm and 481 in the palliative arm. Most patients in the hepatectomy arm (70%) underwent minor hepatectomy. No study described complications during or after hepatectomy. Patient demographics and characteristics of liver metastases from gastric cancer are summarized in Table 1. The median follow-up was 13.2 months.

Efficacy

Median overall survival of patients in the hepatectomy arm and those in the palliative arm was 23.7 (range, 13.0 to 48.0) and 7.6 (range, 5.5 to 15.2), respectively. Median rates of overall survival of the two arms were 69, 40, 33 and 27, 8, 4% at 1, 2, and 3 years, respectively (Table 2).

Comparing with palliative therapy, hepatectomy was associated with significantly lower mortality at 1 year (OR 0.17, 95% CI 0.11–0.26, $P < 0.001$; Fig. 2) and 2 years (OR 0.15, 95% CI 0.09–0.25, $P < 0.001$; Fig. 3).

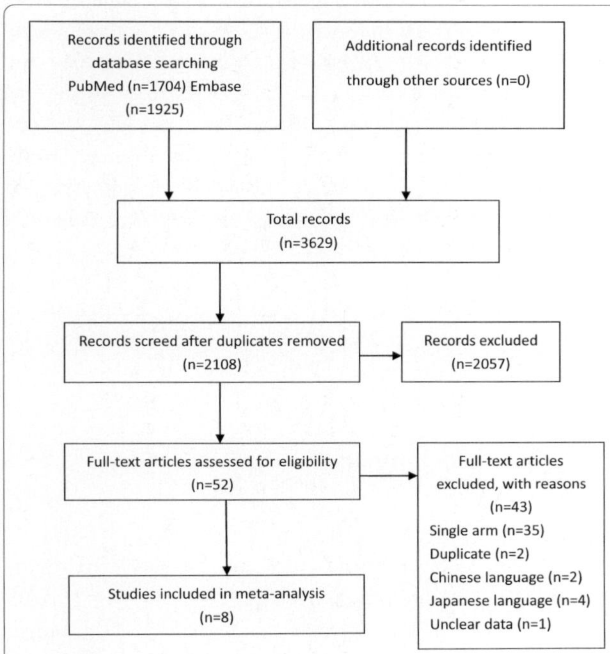

Fig. 1 Flow chart of study selection

Among the patients who underwent hepatectomy, comparison of studies performed in Asian countries (5 studies, 117 patients) and Western countries (3 studies, 79 patients) indicated that Asian cohorts showed higher median rates of overall survival at 1 year (76 vs. 60%), 2 years (47 vs. 30%) and 3 years (39 vs. 23%).

Quality assessment

Details on individual quality of studies are displayed in Table 3. Among the 8 cohort studies, only one had eight stars [50], one had seven stars [52], and the remaining 6 studies had six stars [49, 51, 53–56].

Discussion

Among all included studies in this systematic review, a total of 196 patients were treated with hepatectomy for liver metastases from gastric cancer. Hepatectomy was associated significantly better overall survival than palliative therapy for such patients. Our results were consistent with previous reviews [57–60].

The liver is a common site of distant metastasis from gastrointestinal tract cancer, including gastric cancer. Hepatectomy is now widely accepted as a potentially curative treatment for hepatocellular carcinoma [61, 62] and colorectal liver metastases [63], with reported 5-year overall survival of 40–50% [61–63]. Moreover, indications of hepatectomy for hepatocellular carcinoma and colorectal liver metastases have been expanded by progress in surgical procedures, perioperative care and/or chemotherapy. Liver metastases from gastric cancer not only show more aggressive oncological behavior and heterogeneous characteristics, but also are with frequently other metastatic extrahepatic lesions, such as peritoneal seeding or extensive lymph node metastases, leading to a dismal prognosis and debatable benefits of hepatectomy. Therefore, chemotherapy is regarded as the first-choice treatment in most guidelines. However, a lot of case reports and case series supported the role of hepatectomy for liver metastases from gastric cancer [11–20, 24–48], which lead to Japanese guideline reconsidered the role of hepatecotmy for such patients [10].

Previous systematic reviews [57–60] were mainly based on some part of the case series [11–20, 24–48]. Many of the quoted and included studies of these systematic reviews are of small studies stretching back in some cases to the 1960's. This leads to many concerns over the diagnosis, original treatments, neoadjuvant and adjuvant treatments in such a big time span. Assessment of metastatic disease in the pre multilevel computer tomography and positron emission tomography era is also doubtful when trying to compare outcomes. In addition, those systematic reviews are not comparing like with like. Those undergoing hepatectomy are a highly selected group with resectable liver disease in the

Table 1 Main characteristics of the retrieved literature regarding hepatectomy for hepatic metastases from gastric cancer

Study	Country	Recruitment period	Sample size (hepatectomy/ palliative therapy)	Hepatectomy arm					
				Median follow-up, mo	Median age, yr	Male/ Female	Single/ Multinodular	Uni/ Bilobar	Synchronous/ Metachronous
Chen 2013	China	2007–2012	20/94	10	57	12/8	8/12	11/9	20/0
Cheon 2008	Korea	1995–2005	41/17	16	60	34/7	28/13	NR	30/11
Dittmar 2012	Germany	1995–2009	15/83	11	57	12/3	8/7	12/3	9/6
Makino 2010	Japan	1992–2007	16/47	NR	NA	13/3	9/7	11/5	9/7
Miki 2012	Japan	1995–2009	25/25	NR	72	23/2	18/7	20/5	16/9
Tiberio 2009	Italy	1990–2004	11/62	19	NR	NR	NR	NR	0/11
Tiberio 2015	Italy	1997–2011	53/142	NR	NR	NR	NR	NR	53/0
Ueda 2009	Japan	1991–2005	15/11	NR	NR	NR	NR	NR	NR

NR not reported

absence of other disease. It is not reasonable to compare this with all comers with widespread metastatic disease. It would be more reasonable to cone in on those studies where comparative outcomes were considered. Therefore, we only focus on cohort studies which comparing hepatectomy and palliative therapy and patients who were included after 1990. Such results may be more reliable than previous.

Our systematic review revealed that median overall survival after hepatectomy was 23.7 (range, 13.0 to 48.0). Median overall survival was ranges from 24 to 40.8 months after hepatectomy among other large scale case series (>60 cases) [40, 46–48]. Hepatectomy for liver metastases from gastric cancer is not performed frequently at present. It is notable that none of the patients who underwent hepatectomy in this systematic review or these case series [40, 46–48] was with peritoneal metastasis. Careful patient selection is likely to be important for ensuring good prognosis after hepatectomy. The number of hepatic tumors (≥3), tumor diameter (≥5), and serosal invasion of the primary tumor were identified as prognostic factors associated with a poor overall survival [19, 37, 40, 46]. Moreover, patients with more risk factors have much poor survival rates at 3 or 5 years after hepatectomy [46]. Therefore, palliative therapy should be considered when any of these factors is recognized at diagnosis. Other indications for hepatectomy included adequate physical condition, preserved liver function, and feasibility of complete tumor resection. In addition, indications for hepatectomy may also need to consider response rate to neoadjuvant chemotherapy in those patients who receive it, since prognosis of non-responders is generally worse than that of responders [64, 65].

The role of neoadjuvant or adjuvant therapy for liver metastases from gastric cancer is still controversial. Of the eight included studies, 16.4% patients received neoadjuvant therapy, while 55.2% received adjuvant therapy. If all case series [11–20, 24–48] and these eight cohort studies [49–56] were included into analysis, the percentage of patients who received neoadjuvant therapy for the primary gastric cancer was 11.3%, and the percentage of patients receiving adjuvant therapy was 55.1%. For patients with gastric cancer with extensive lymph node metastasis, Tsuburaya and coworkers found neoadjuvant chemotherapy with 4-weekly S-1 and cisplatin followed

Table 2 Overall survival of patients with hepatic metastases from gastric cancer after hepatectomy or palliative treatments

Study	Hepatectomy arm				Palliative arm				*P*
	Median survival (moths)	1-year	2-year	3-year	Median survival (moths)	1-year	2-year	3-year	
Chen 2013	22.3	70	30	21	5.5	15	0	0	<0.001
Cheon 2008	18.3	75	38	32	8.1	29	0	0	<0.001
Dittmar 2012	48.0	79	64	55	9.0	42	18	9	<0.001
Makino 2010	38.2	87	68	56	15.2	53	12	4	<0.001
Miki 2012	33.4	74	55	43	8.7	40	18	18	0.045
Tiberio 2009	23.0	80	30	20	6.9	28	6	3	<0.001
Tiberio 2015	13.0	50	21	14	5.5	13	7	2	<0.001
Ueda 2009	-	80	60	60	10.0	36	0	0	<0.001

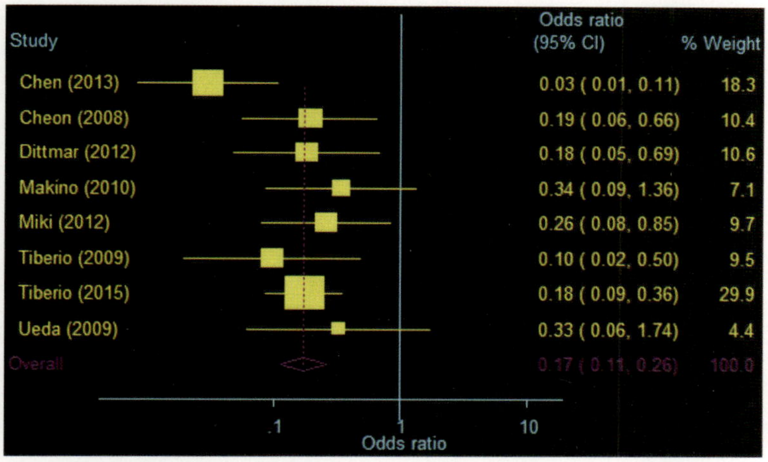

Fig. 2 Meta-analysis of mortality at 1 year after hepatectomy or palliative therapies in patients treated for liver metastases from gastric cancer

by D2 gastrectomy is safe and effective for some patients [66]. Further trials should be performed to investigate the role of neoadjuvant therapy as a biological trial.

We found Asian cohorts showed higher median rates of overall survival than Western cohorts. Western cohorts usually show more advanced stage of disease than Asian cohorts [19, 24, 28, 41, 43, 50, 51, 54, 55]. Such presentation may lead to more Western cases receive chemotherapy while more Asian cases receive curative resection. Even so, there needs to be consideration of the role of chemotherapy versus surgery in the chemotherapy naïve patients. In this systematic review, hepatectomy associated with a median overall survival of 23.7 months. However, median overall survival was only 11.3 to 13.8 months after combination therapy with or without trastuzumb for advanced gastric cancer [4, 67]. Therefore, our results suggest that hepatectomy is associated with substantially longer median overall survival than combination chemotherapy with or without targeted therapy. In selected patients, hepatectomy may be preferable to chemotherapy.

A limitation of our study is the low availability of high level evidence studies in literature. Since all studies were retrospective cohort studies, a potential bias is that the positive effects of hepatectomy are overestimated, as cases of unsuccessful resection are less likely to be reported or published. Moreover, the types and frequency of postoperative complications remain unclear because all of the studies failed to report such data. Most patients underwent minor rather than major hepatectomy. Heterogeneity in surgical technique and skill may also affect patient prognosis.

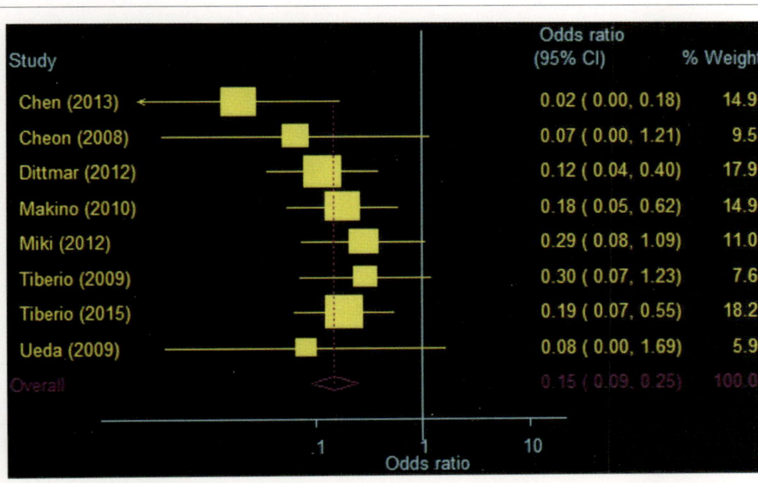

Fig. 3 Meta-analysis of mortality at 2 years after hepatectomy or palliative therapies in patients treated for liver metastases from gastric cancer

Table 3 Newcastle-Ottawa score quality assessment scale for cohort studies

Study	Selection				Comparability		Outcome			Total star
	1	2	3	4	1a	1b	1	2	3	
Chen 2013	a*	a*	a*	a*	a*	b*	d	b	d	6
Cheon 2008	a*	a*	a*	a*	a*	b*	d	a*	a*	8
Dittmar 2012	a*	a*	a*	a*	-	-	d	a*	a*	6
Makino 2010	a*	a*	a*	a*	a*	b*	d	a*	d	7
Miki 2012	a*	a*	a*	a*	a*	-	d	a*	d	6
Tiberio 2009	a*	a*	a*	a*	-	-	d	a*	a*	6
Tiberio 2015	a*	a*	a*	a*	-	-	d	a*	a*	6
Ueda 2009	a*	a*	a*	a*	-	-	d	a*	a*	6

-, no description on comparability

Conclusions

This systematic review provides comprehensive evidence that hepatectomy is associated with longer median overall survival than palliative treatments for selected patients with liver metastases from gastric cancer. If our findings can be verified and extended in a completion of a randomized controlled trial on hepatectomy versus chemotherapy or a high-quality prospective study with long-term follow-up, they make a strong argument for changing current clinical practices and official guidelines to bring them into line with the evidence base.

Abbreviations

CI: Confidence interval; OR: Odds ratio

Acknowledgements

None.

Funding

This work was supported by the Guangxi University of Science and Technology Research Projects (KY2015LX056), the Self-Raised Scientific Research Fund of the Ministry of Health of Guangxi Province (Z2015621, GZZC15-34, Z20165 2), the Innovation Project of Guangxi Graduate Education (YCBZ2015030), and the National Natural Science Foundation of China (81560460/H1602, 81260088/H0322).

Authors' contributions

J-HZ conceived and designed the study. Y-YL, DL, P-CY, and SZ searched the literature and extracted data. NFP and L-QL performed statistical analyses. All authors wrote and reviewed the manuscript. All authors read and approved the final manuscript.

Competing interests

The authors who have taken part in this study declare that they do not have anything to disclose regarding funding or conflicts of interest with respect to this manuscript.

Author details

[1]Nutrition Department, Affiliated Tumor Hospital of Guangxi Medical University, Nanning, China. [2]Hepatobiliary Surgery Department, Affiliated Tumor Hospital of Guangxi Medical University, Nanning 530021, Guangxi Province, China. [3]Colorectal Anal Surgery Department, The First Affiliated Hospital of Guangxi Medical University, Nanning 530021, China.

References

1. http://www.who.int/mediacentre/factsheets/fs297/en/[Internet]. Accessed 19 Sept 2016.
2. National Oesophago-gastric Cancer Audit—2013, Annual report [Internet]. 2013. http://www.hscic.gov.uk/catalogue/PUB11093. Accessed 19 Sept 2016.
3. Yoshikawa T, Sasako M. Gastrointestinal cancer: adjuvant chemotherapy after D2 gastrectomy for gastric cancer. Nat Rev Clin Oncol. 2012;9(4):192–4.
4. Waddell T, Chau I, Cunningham D, et al. Epirubicin, oxaliplatin, and capecitabine with or without panitumumab for patients with previously untreated advanced oesophagogastric cancer (REAL3): a randomised, open-label phase 3 trial. Lancet Oncol. 2013;14(6):481–9.
5. Koizumi W, Narahara H, Hara T, et al. S-1 plus cisplatin versus S-1 alone for first-line treatment of advanced gastric cancer (SPIRITS trial): a phase III trial. Lancet Oncol. 2008;9(3):215–21.
6. Markar SR, Karthikesalingam A, Jackson D, Hanna GB. Long-term survival after gastrectomy for cancer in randomized, controlled oncological trials: comparison between West and East. Ann Surg Oncol. 2013;20(7):2328–38.
7. Japanese Gastric Cancer Association. Japanese classification of gastric carcinoma: 3rd english edition. Gastric Cancer. 2011;14(2):101–12.
8. Strong VE, D'Amico TA, Kleinberg L, Ajani J. Impact of the 7th edition AJCC staging classification on the NCCN clinical practice guidelines in oncology for gastric and esophageal cancers. J Natl Compr Canc Netw. 2013;11(1):60–6.
9. Ajani JA, Bentrem DJ, Besh S, et al. Gastric cancer, version 2.2013: featured updates to the NCCN Guidelines. J Natl Compr Canc Netw. 2013;11(5):531–46.
10. Kodera Y, Fujitani K, Fukushima N, et al. Surgical resection of hepatic metastasis from gastric cancer: a review and new recommendation in the Japanese gastric cancer treatment guidelines. Gastric Cancer. 2014;17(2):206–12.
11. Ambiru S, Miyazaki M, Ito H, et al. Benefits and limits of hepatic resection for gastric metastases. Am J Surg. 2001;181(3):279–83.
12. Fujii K, Fujioka S, Kato K, et al. Resection of liver metastasis from gastric adenocarcinoma. Hepato-Gastroenterology. 2001;48(38):368–71.
13. Miyazaki M, Itoh H, Nakagawa K, et al. Hepatic resection of liver metastases from gastric carcinoma. Am J Gastroenterol. 1997;92(3):490–3.
14. Ochiai T, Sasako M, Mizuno S, et al. Hepatic resection for metastatic tumours from gastric cancer: analysis of prognostic factors. Br J Surg. 1994;81(8):1175–8.
15. Okano K, Maeba T, Ishimura K, et al. Hepatic resection for metastatic tumors from gastric cancer. Ann Surg. 2002;235(1):86–91.
16. Saito A, Korenaga D, Sakaguchi Y, Ohno S, Ichiyoshi Y, Sugimachi K. Surgical treatment for gastric carcinomas with concomitant hepatic metastasis. Hepato-Gastroenterology. 1996;43(9):560–4.
17. Saiura A, Umekita N, Inoue S, et al. Clinicopathological features and outcome of hepatic resection for liver metastasis from gastric cancer. Hepato-Gastroenterology. 2002;49(46):1062–5.
18. Sakamoto Y, Ohyama S, Yamamoto J, et al. Surgical resection of liver metastases of gastric cancer: an analysis of a 17-year experience with 22 patients. Surgery. 2003;133(5):507–11.
19. Schildberg CW, Croner R, Merkel S, et al. Outcome of operative therapy of hepatic metastatic stomach carcinoma: a retrospective analysis. World J Surg. 2012;36(4):872–8.
20. Zacherl J, Zacherl M, Scheuba C, et al. Analysis of hepatic resection of metastasis originating from gastric adenocarcinoma. J Gastrointest Surg. 2002;6(5):682–9.
21. Hutton B, Salanti G, Caldwell DM, et al. The PRISMA extension statement for reporting of systematic reviews incorporating network meta-analyses of health care interventions: checklist and explanations. Ann Intern Med. 2015; 162(11):777–84.
22. Stang A. Critical evaluation of the Newcastle-Ottawa scale for the assessment of the quality of nonrandomized studies in meta-analyses. Eur J Epidemiol. 2010;25(9):603–5.
23. Huedo-Medina TB, Sanchez-Meca J, Marin-Martinez F, Botella J. Assessing heterogeneity in meta-analysis: Q statistic or I2 index? Psychol Methods. 2006;11(2):193–206.

24. Adam R, Chiche L, Aloia T, et al. Hepatic resection for noncolorectal nonendocrine liver metastases: analysis of 1,452 patients and development of a prognostic model. Ann Surg. 2006;244(4):524–35.
25. Aizawa M, Nashimoto A, Yabusaki H, Nakagawa S, Matsuki A. Clinical benefit of surgical management for gastric cancer with synchronous liver metastasis. Hepato-Gastroenterology. 2014;61(133):1439–45.
26. Baek HU, Kim SB, Cho EH, et al. Hepatic resection for hepatic metastases from gastric adenocarcinoma. J Gastric Cancer. 2013;13(2):86–92.
27. Choi SB, Song J, Kang CM, et al. Surgical outcome of metachronous hepatic metastases secondary to gastric cancer. Hepato-Gastroenterology. 2010; 57(97):29–34.
28. Garancini M, Uggeri F, Degrate L, et al. Surgical treatment of liver metastases of gastric cancer: is local treatment in a systemic disease worthwhile? HPB. 2012;14(3):209–15.
29. Hirai I, Kimura W, Fuse A, et al. Surgical management for metastatic liver tumors. Hepato-Gastroenterology. 2006;53(71):757–63.
30. Imamura H, Matsuyama Y, Shimada R, et al. A study of factors influencing prognosis after resection of hepatic metastases from colorectal and gastric carcinoma. Am J Gastroenterol. 2001;96(11):3178–84.
31. Komeda K, Hayashi M, Kubo S, et al. High survival in patients operated for small isolated liver metastases from gastric cancer: a multi-institutional study. World J Surg. 2014;38(10):2692–7.
32. Liu J, Li JH, Zhai RJ, Wei B, Shao MZ, Chen L. Predictive factors improving survival after gastric and hepatic surgical treatment in gastric cancer patients with synchronous liver metastases. Chin Med J. 2012;125(2):165–71.
33. Morise Z, Sugioka A, Hoshimoto S, et al. The role of hepatectomy for patients with liver metastases of gastric cancer. Hepato-Gastroenterology. 2008;55(85):1238–41.
34. Nomura T, Kamio Y, Takasu N, et al. Intrahepatic micrometastases around liver metastases from gastric cancer. J Hepato-Biliary-Pancreat Surg. 2009; 16(4):493–501.
35. Qiu JL, Deng MG, Li W, et al. Hepatic resection for synchronous hepatic metastasis from gastric cancer. Eur J Surg Oncol. 2013;39(7):694–700.
36. Roh HR, Suh KS, Lee HJ, Yang HK, Choe KJ, Lee KU. Outcome of hepatic resection for metastatic gastric cancer. Am Surg. 2005;71(2):95–9.
37. Sakamoto Y, Sano T, Shimada K, et al. Favorable indications for hepatectomy in patients with liver metastasis from gastric cancer. J Surg Oncol. 2007;95(7):534–9.
38. Schmidt B, Look-Hong N, Maduekwe UN, et al. Noncurative gastrectomy for gastric adenocarcinoma should only be performed in highly selected patients. Ann Surg Oncol. 2013;20(11):3512–8.
39. Shirabe K, Shimada M, Matsumata T, et al. Analysis of the prognostic factors for liver metastasis of gastric cancer after hepatic resection: a multi-institutional study of the indications for resection. Hepato-Gastroenterology. 2003;50(53):1560–3.
40. Takemura N, Saiura A, Koga R, et al. Long-term outcomes after surgical resection for gastric cancer liver metastasis: an analysis of 64 macroscopically complete resections. Langenbecks Arch Surg. 2012;397(6):951–7.
41. Thelen A, Jonas S, Benckert C, et al. Liver resection for metastatic gastric cancer. Eur J Surg Oncol. 2008;34(12):1328–34.
42. Tsujimoto H, Ichikura T, Ono S, et al. Outcomes for patients following hepatic resection of metastatic tumors from gastric cancer. Hepatol Int. 2010;4(1):406–13.
43. Vigano L, Vellone M, Ferrero A, Giuliante F, Nuzzo G, Capussotti L. Liver resection for gastric cancer metastases. Hepato-Gastroenterology. 2013; 60(123):557–62.
44. Wang W, Liang H, Zhang H, Wang X, Xue Q, Zhang R. Prognostic significance of radical surgical treatment for gastric cancer patients with synchronous liver metastases. Medical oncology (Northwood, London, England). 2014;31(11).
45. Wang YN, Shen KT, Ling JQ, et al. Prognostic analysis of combined curative resection of the stomach and liver lesions in 30 gastric cancer patients with synchronous liver metastases. BMC Surg. 2012;12:20.
46. Kinoshita T, Saiura A, Esaki M, Sakamoto H, Yamanaka T. Multicentre analysis of long-term outcome after surgical resection for gastric cancer liver metastases. Br J Surg. 2015;102(1):102–7.
47. Markar SR, Mackenzie H, Mikhail S, et al. Surgical resection of hepatic metastases from gastric cancer: outcomes from national series in England. Gastric cancer. 2016. doi:10.1007/s10120-016-0604-6. [Epub ahead of print].
48. Oki E, Tokunaga S, Emi Y, et al. Surgical treatment of liver metastasis of gastric cancer: a retrospective multicenter cohort study (KSCC1302). Gastric Cancer. 2016;19(3):968–76.
49. Chen L, Song MQ, Lin HZ, et al. Chemotherapy and resection for gastric cancer with synchronous liver metastases. World J Gastroenterol. 2013; 19(13):2097–103.
50. Cheon SH, Rha SY, Jeung HC, et al. Survival benefit of combined curative resection of the stomach (D2 resection) and liver in gastric cancer patients with liver metastases. Ann Oncol. 2008;19(6):1146–53.
51. Dittmar Y, Altendorf-Hofmann A, Rauchfuss F, et al. Resection of liver metastases is beneficial in patients with gastric cancer: report on 15 cases and review of literature. Gastric Cancer. 2012;15(2):131–6.
52. Makino H, Kunisaki C, Izumisawa Y, et al. Indication for hepatic resection in the treatment of liver metastasis from gastric cancer. Anticancer Res. 2010; 30(6):2367–76.
53. Miki Y, Fujitani K, Hirao M, et al. Significance of surgical treatment of liver metastases from gastric cancer. Anticancer Res. 2012;32(2):665–70.
54. Tiberio GA, Coniglio A, Marchet A, et al. Metachronous hepatic metastases from gastric carcinoma: a multicentric survey. Eur J Surg Oncol. 2009;35(5):486–91.
55. Tiberio GA, Baiocchi GL, Morgagni P, et al. Gastric cancer and synchronous hepatic metastases: is it possible to recognize candidates to R0 resection? Ann Surg Oncol. 2015;22(2):589–96.
56. Ueda K, Iwahashi M, Nakamori M, et al. Analysis of the prognostic factors and evaluation of surgical treatment for synchronous liver metastases from gastric cancer. Langenbecks Arch Surg. 2009;394(4):647–53.
57. Petrelli F, Coinu A, Cabiddu M, et al. Hepatic resection for gastric cancer liver metastases: a systematic review and meta-analysis. J Surg Oncol. 2015; 111(8):1021–7.
58. Grimes N, Devlin J, Dunne DF, Poston G, Fenwick S, Malik H. The role of hepatectomy in the management of metastatic gastric adenocarcinoma: a systematic review. Surg Oncol. 2014;23(4):177–85.
59. Martella L, Bertozzi S, Londero AP, Steffan A, De Paoli P, Bertola G. Surgery for liver metastases from gastric cancer: a meta-analysis of observational studies. Medicine (Baltimore). 2015;94(31):e1113.
60. Markar SR, Mikhail S, Malietzis G, et al. Influence of surgical resection of hepatic metastases from gastric adenocarcinoma on long-term survival: systematic review and pooled analysis. Ann Surg. 2016;263(6):1092–101.
61. Zhong JH, You XM, Lu SD, et al. Historical comparison of overall survival after hepatic resection for patients with large and/or multinodular hepatocellular carcinoma. Medicine (Baltimore). 2015;94(35):e1426.
62. Zhong JH, Rodriguez AC, Ke Y, Wang YY, Wang L, Li LQ. Hepatic resection as a safe and effective treatment for hepatocellular carcinoma involving a single large tumor, multiple tumors, or macrovascular invasion. Medicine (Baltimore). 2015;94(3):e396.
63. de Jong MC, Pulitano C, Ribero D, et al. Rates and patterns of recurrence following curative intent surgery for colorectal liver metastasis: an international multi-institutional analysis of 1669 patients. Ann Surg. 2009; 250(3):440–8.
64. Cunningham D, Allum WH, Stenning SP, et al. Perioperative chemotherapy versus surgery alone for resectable gastroesophageal cancer. N Engl J Med. 2006;355(1):11–20.
65. Kurokawa Y, Shibata T, Sasako M, et al. Validity of response assessment criteria in neoadjuvant chemotherapy for gastric cancer (JCOG0507-A). Gastric Cancer. 2014;17(3):514–21.
66. Tsuburaya A, Mizusawa J, Tanaka Y, Fukushima N, Nashimoto A, Sasako M. Neoadjuvant chemotherapy with S-1 and cisplatin followed by D2 gastrectomy with para-aortic lymph node dissection for gastric cancer with extensive lymph node metastasis. Br J Surg. 2014;101(6):653–60.
67. Bang YJ, Van Cutsem E, Feyereislova A, et al. Trastuzumab in combination with chemotherapy versus chemotherapy alone for treatment of HER2-positive advanced gastric or gastro-oesophageal junction cancer (ToGA): a phase 3, open-label, randomised controlled trial. Lancet (London, England). 2010;376(9742):687–97.

The value of hepatic resection in metastasic renal cancer in the Era of Tyrosinkinase Inhibitor Therapy

Hans Michael Hau[1*†], Florian Thalmann[1†], Christoph Lübbert[4], Mehmet Haluk Morgul[1], Moritz Schmelzle[2], Georgi Atanasov[2], Christian Benzing[2], Undine Lange[1], Rudolf Ascherl[1], Roman Ganzer[3], Dirk Uhlmann[1], Hans-Michael Tautenhahn[1], Georg Wiltberger[1†] and Michael Bartels[1†]

Abstract

Background: The value of liver-directed therapy (LDT) in patients with metastasic renal cell carcinoma (MRCC) is still an active field of research, particularly in the era of tyrosinkinase inhibitor (TKI) therapy.

Methods: The records of 35 patients with MRCC undergoing LDT of metastasic liver lesions between 1992 and 2015 were retrospectively analyzed. Immediate postoperative TKI was given in a subgroup of patients after LDT for metastasic lesions. Uni- and multivariate models were applied to assess overall survival (OS), progression-free survival (PFS) and disease-free survival (DFS).

Results: Following primary tumor (renal cell cancer) resection and LDT, respectively, median OS was better for a total of 16 patients (41 %) receiving immediate postoperative TKI with 151 and 98 months, when compared to patients without TKI therapy with 61 ($p = 0.003$) and 40 months ($p = 0.032$). Immediate postoperative TKI was associated with better median PFS (47 months versus 19 months; $p = 0.023$), whereas in DFS only a trend was observed (51 months versus 19 months; $p = 0.110$).

Conclusions: LDT should be considered as a suitable additive tool in the era of TKI therapy of MRCC to the liver. In this context, postoperative TKI therapy seems to be associated with better OS and PFS, but not DFS.

Keywords: Liver resection, Metastasic renal cancer, Tyrosinkinase inhibitor agents

Background

Renal cell carcinoma (RCC) is one of the most common tumors with an increasing incidence of approximately 85 new cases and 35 deaths per 100 000 reported in 2012 in Europe [1–3]. The majority of patients with RCC present with an early stage of their disease, 20–30 % have synchronous metastases and 20–50 % of the patients develop metastasic disease after primary tumor resection [4–7].

Most data exist for lung metastases which represent the common sites of distant metastases [5, 8]. Although it is less common, liver metastases were observed in 30–40 % of the patients with metastasic disease [5, 9]. Unfortunately, development of liver metastasis was generally considered as a poor prognostic factor and was frequently associated with more widespread disease [10, 11]. That's the reason why liver resections in these patients are often single decisions and consequently, there is little available literature on this topic. Although larger series were published with a focus on non-colorectal/non-neuroendocrine metastases, patients with RCC represent only a small subgroup and were not the focus of these studies [10, 12].

Unfortunately, the prognosis is poor in MRCC with 5-year survival ranging from 5 to 15 %, because chemotherapy, radiotherapy or immunotherapy have almost no

* Correspondence: HansMichael.Hau@medizin.uni-leipzig.de
Hans Michael Hau and Florian Thalmann are contributed equally to this work and share first authorship. Georg Wiltberger and Michael Bartels are contributed equally to this work and share senior authorship.
†Equal contributors
[1]Department of Visceral, Transplantation, Vascular and Thoracic Surgery, University Hospital of Leipzig, Liebigstrasse 20, 04103 Leipzig, Germany
Full list of author information is available at the end of the article

influence or showed limited response [6, 8, 9, 11, 13–16]. Since several years, antiangiogenic targeted therapies (TT), particularly tyrosinkinse inhibitor (TKI) agents, have become available and showed improved clinical outcomes in large multicenter trials [17–21]. However, a majority of patients treated with TT develop resistance to this drugs and complete response remains extremely rare. Surgical treatment if feasible is the only potentially curative treatment option for patients with MRCC [7, 8, 22]. Complete resection of metastatic lesions is consistently associated with survival benefits as previous studies has noted [23–25]. Thus, some authors reported 25–52 % five-year survival rates in cases of MRCC with complete resection and decreased risk of death from RCC [7, 8, 25–27].

However, little information has been available on the utility and benefit of systemic treatment after complete resection of metastatic lesions. There are only a few reports with small patient numbers reporting low long-term progression-free survival rates after metastasectomy [8, 23, 26, 27]. Most of the studies had a focus on the adjuvant treatment with immunotherapeutic or chemotherapeutic agents [6, 24, 28]. Therefore, understanding the role of surgery in the era of TKI therapy - especially in the neoadjuvant and/or adjuvant multimodal treatment setting - is of increasing importance and interest.

In the present study, we examined besides the efficacy of surgical therapy for MRCC - with a focus to the liver - the different treatment regimens that were received by patients with hepatic metastasized RCC after surgical resections of metastases. In addition, we assessed the effect of immediate postoperative TT on short- and long-term outcome like survival, tumor recurrence and morbidity in patients with MRCC following primary tumor resection and liver-directed therapy, respectively.

Methods

Patient selection and study population

Medical records of patients undergoing liver-directed therapy (liver-directed therapy - LDT) for histologically proven RCC liver metastases (RCCLM) at the Department of Surgery, University Hospital of Leipzig, between 1992 and 2015 were analyzed retrospectively. The study was approved by the local ethical commission board from the University of Leipzig (AZ EK: 243-14-14072014). Due to the retrospective design of the study and accordingly national guidelines, the local ethic committee confirmed, that informed consent was not necessary from participants.

Inclusion criteria consist of patients with metastasic RCC to the liver who underwent LDT. Only patients with complete available follow-up data were included in the study. Patients with extended and unresectable liver tumors, peripheral diffuse metastasic disease, or diffuse hepatic involvements of all liver lobes were excluded from study. Resectable synchronous extra-hepatic site metastases were no contraindications for study inclusion provided that the overall surgical strategy aimed to be curative. All patients underwent staging examinations to determine suitability and eligibility for surgery including physical examination, serum laboratory tests, abdominal ultrasound, computed tomography (CT) (abdomen/chest) or magnetic resonance tomography. In some cases the diagnosis of liver metastasis was confirmed by fine-needle cytology or biopsy. The Karnofsky Performance Scale (KPS) of our study population were not less than 80.

All cases of patients with RCCLM were discussed by a multidisciplinary team to assess the indication and suitability for surgery. The decision for use of neoadjuvant and/or immediate adjuvant targeted therapy following liver metastasectomy was made on an individual basis in oncological tumor board and was not prospectively specified. With regards to survival analysis, patients who are withdrawn from a study as well as patients who are lost to follow-up or alive without the event occurrence at latest follow-up were censored in the survival chart.

The primary aim of the present study was to assess the effect of immediate postoperative TT/TKI therapy on progression-free survival (PFS)/disease-free survival (DFS) of patients with hepatic metastasized renal cell cancer who received metastasectomy of primary metastasic lesions or liver-directed therapy of metastatic hepatic lesions, respectively. The secondary endpoint was to assess the overall survival in the different treatment regimes.

Variables/data collection

Standard clinicopathological and demographic parameters of the study population were collected including: Patient age (years); gender (male versus female); body mass index (kg/m^2); oncological parameters (Eastern Cooperative Oncology Group (ECOG) performance Status (0–5)); primary tumor characteristics (tumor location (right versus left kidney), T-stage (T1-T4), lymph node stage (N0-N2), Fuhrman grading (low (1–2); high (3–4)), histological subtype (clear cell, chromophobe, papillary/other)); treatment of the primary tumor (type of surgery (complete or partial nephrectomy). Variables were also collected on the number (n), location (unilobular versus multilobular); size (cm), weight (g) of hepatic lesions as well as occurrence of liver metastases (synchronous versus metachronous) as well as presence of extrahepatic metastases (yes versus no). A particular interest applied with details of adjuvant TT/TKI therapy (yes versus no) after occurrence of metastasic lesions and liver resection. Additionally, the different TKI treatment regimes, the onset and duration of TKI therapy following liver-directed therapy as well as the efficacy of TKI therapy were examined.

Operative information including type of liver-directed therapy (surgery, interventional procedure (ablation, electroporation), operating time (minutes), intraoperative transfusion (yes vs. no), red blood cell concentrate (RBCC), fresh frozen plasma (FFP), application of vascular inflow occlusion (Pringles manoeuvre: yes vs. no) and extent of resection. Hepatectomy was classified as minor (less than three segments) and major (three or more segments). Margin status (microscopically complete- R0, microscopic (R1) and macroscopic involvement (R2)) was determined based on final pathological assessment. Peri- and postoperative collected data including length of intensive care unit (ICU) stay (days), length of hospital stay (days), tumor recurrence, survival such as morbidity and mortality rate. Postoperative complications are presented according to the Clavien-Dindo-Classification (grade I to V). Therefore, grades I and II were taken together as minor complications and grade III-V as major complications. The perioperative mortality was defined as 30-day mortality.

Overall survival (OS) was either calculated as the time interval between primary tumor operation (renal cell cancer resection) until latest follow-up/or death or secondary tumor operation (liver tumor therapy) until latest follow-up/or death.

Disease-free interval (DFI) was calculated as the time interval from liver-directed therapy until first recurrence at any site. Progression-free survival (PFS) was calculated from time of resection of first metastases/start of TKI therapy until time of progression/recurrence or last follow-up/death. Disease-free survival (DFS) was calculated from date of liver-directed therapy to first recurrence, distant metastases, last follow-up or death.

Statistical analysis

All data are presented as either percentage, mean value with range or median value with interquartal range (IQR). Data were analyzed using Student's *t*-test and Wilcoxon rank sum test for continuous variables, and the chi-squared test or Fisher's exact test for discrete variables, where appropriate. Disease-free survival, progression-free survival and overall survival were examined using the Kaplan-Meier Method and potential prognostic factors were evaluated in univariate analysis by a two-sided log-rank test. A multivariable Cox proportional hazard regression model was used to identify independent prognostic factors for disease recurrence and survival/mortality. Included tested variables in Cox proportional hazard regression analysis were chosen according to the literature and the primary/secondary aims of the study: immediate postoperative targeted Therapy, ECOG performance status >1, synchronous liver metastases and multiple liver metastases. P-values < 0.05 were considered statistically significant. All data were analyzed by using SPSS software (SPSS Inc., Chicago, Illinois, USA, version 19.0).

Results

General and oncological characteristics

The outcome of 35 patients (female = 11, male = 24) with a median age of 65 years (IQR: 59–71) at time of LDT was investigated.

The primary tumor location was nearly equally distributed between the patient collective (right kidney; 21 (60 %)/left kidney; 14 (40 %). Each patient underwent curative surgery for the primary tumor: radical nephrectomy in 31 patients (86 %) and partial nephrectomy in 4 patients (14 %). The majority of patients (60 %) had lymph node metastases associated with the primary tumor (N1; 40 %, N2; 20 %) and most primary tumors were pathologic T2 or T3 lesions (T1: 20 %; T2: 25.8 %; T3, 42.8 %; T4, 11.4 %). The primary tumor could be removed completely in all patients. Fuhrman Grading was low in most patients (grade 1: 2 patients (5.7 %); grade 2: 22 patients (62.9 %); grade 3: 9 patients (25.7 %); grade 4: 2 patients (5.7 %)). The final histology of the primary tumor showed in all patients RCC, compromising a clear cell subtype in 25 patients (71.4 %), followed by chromophobe carcinoma in 6 (17.1 %) and unclassified/papillary subtype in 3 cases (11.5 %). Prognostic criteria using ECOG performance status were 0 in 29 patients (83 %) and >1 in the remaining 6 patients (17 %). The complete list of patient characteristics is shown in Table 1 without relevant differences regarding general and oncological characteristics between the groups.

Most RCCLM were metachronous (n = 29; 82.9 %); the median time interval between the diagnosis of primary tumor and the occurrence of first metastases was 13 months (IQR: 3–36 months), 15 months (IQR: 3–39 months) between primary tumor operation and occurrence of liver metastases. The median time between last staging and liver surgery was 1 month (IQR: 0–2 months). The mean number of hepatic metastatic lesions was 1.7 (range: 1–5) being localized unilobular in the liver (n = 28, 80 %). The median size of the largest lesion was 4.4 cm (IQR: 2.9 – 6.0 cm).

Details of liver-directed therapy

Among the 35 patients with RCCLM, liver-directed treatment consisted of liver resection in 33 patients (94.3 %) and local ablation in 2 patients (5.7 %) (Table 2). In the resection-group, 16 of 35 patients (48.5 %) underwent major liver resections, in 17 patients (51.5 %) minor liver resections were performed. On final pathologic analysis, local R0 (margin free) resection could be achieved in 30 patients (85.7 %); only 5 patients (14.3 %) had microscopic disease at the margin (R1) and none patient had macroscopic disease (R2).

Median operating time was 238 min (IQR: 161.5–276 min), median ICU and hospital stay were 1.9 days (IQR: 1–6 days) and 18.7 (IQR: 11–28 days), respectively.

Table 1 Basic general and oncological characteristics according to state of postoperative Tyrosinkinase Inhibitor (TKI) therapy

Variables	Overall ($n = 35$)	TKI (+) ($n = 16$)	TKI (-) ($n = 19$)	*p*-value
Median Age (years)	65 (59–71)	64.5 (58–71)	69 (62–71)	0.160[a]
Gender	24:11	12:4	12:7	0.452[d]
Male/female	(68.6/31.4 %)	(34.3:11.4 %)	(34.3:20 %)	
Median Body mass index (kg/m2)	26.5 (24.5–28.0)	26.9 (26.0–28.3)	25.9 (24.2–27.7)	0.349[a]
ECOG performance status (%)				
0	29 (82.9 %)	15 (42.9 %)	14 (40 %)	0.117[d]
1	6 (17.1 %)	1 (2.9 %)	5 (14.3 %)	
Primary tumor characteristics				
Right side/left side; n (%)	21/14 (60 %:40 %)	7/9 (20 %:25.7 %)	14/5 (40 %:14.3)	0.072[d]
Primary tumor histology				
Clear cell	25 (71.4 %)	10 (28.6 %)	15 (42.9 %)	0.283[c]
Non-clear cell	10 (28.6 %)	6 (17.1 %)	4 (11.5 %)	
Primary tumor T-stage				
Stage 1–2	16 (45.8 %)	8 (22.9 %)	8 (22.9 %)	0.640[c]
Stage 3–4	19 (54.2 %)	11 (31.3 %)	8 (22.9 %)	
Primary tumor grading				
Low (Fuhrmann 1–2)	24 (68.6 %)	12 (34.3 %)	12 (34.3 %)	0.452[d]
High (Fuhrmann 3–4)	11 (31.4 %)	4 (11.4 %)	7 (20 %)	
Liver tumor distribution				
Unilobular/Multilobular	28:7 (80 %:20 %)	14:2 (40 %:14.3 %)	14:5 (40 %:5.7 %)	0.309[d]
Median tumor size (cm)	4.4 (2.9–6.0)	3.9 (2.5–4.5)	5.6 (3.0–7.5)	0.094[a]
Mean number of hepatic tumor lesions	1.70 (1–5)	1.64 (1–4)	1.74 (1–5)	0.813[b]
Median weight of resected liver (g)	212.5 (39.2–652.5)	81.4 (15.5–265.0)	290 (70–916.3)	0.138[a]
Timing of liver metastases				
Synchronous/	6 (17.1 %)	4 (11.4 %)	2 (5.7 %)	0.258[d]
metachronous	29 (82.9 %)	12 (34.3)	17 (48.6 %)	
Extrahepatic disease at time of liver-directed therapy				
Yes	7 (20 %)	5 (14.3 %)	2 (5.7 %)	0.127[d]
No	28 (80 %)	11 (31.4 %)	17 (48.6 %)	

Used statistical tests:
[a]Student's *t*-test
[b]Wilcoxon rank sum test
[c]chi-squared test
[d]Fisher's exact test

Postoperative complications were classified according to the Clavien-Dindo Classification, with an overall postoperative morbidity in 10 patients (28.5 %). In this context, minor complications (grade I, n =0; 0 %; grade II, $n = 3$; 8.6 %) were observed in 3 patients (8.6 %), major complications occurred in 7 patients (19.9 %) (grade IIIa, $n = 5$, 14.3 %; grade IIIb, $n = 1$, 2.9 %; grade IV, $n = 1$, 2.9 %; grade V, $n =$ 0; 0 %). The 30-day mortality of the study group was 0 %.

Treatment after resection of metastatic lesions/recurrence analysis

At time of liver-directed therapy, the liver was the first and only metastases in 28 patients ($n = 80$ %). Whereas, there was evidence of extrahepatic disease in 7 patients (20 %). These metastases were surgically treated with curative intention before liver resection, or were synchronously discovered at laparotomy and subsequently resected. The most common sites of metastases were the retroperitoneum/local recurrence ($n = 5$; 14.3 %), the lung ($n = 2$; 5.7 %), the adrenal glands ($n = 2$; 5.7 %) and the bone ($n = 1$; 2.8 %).

A total of 16 patients (41 %) received TKI therapy following liver-directed therapy of their metastatic hepatic lesions after a median duration of 2.4 months (IQR: 1–5 months) (Fig. 1). In 3 patients a preoperative targeted therapy was started with median duration of 2.1 months

Table 2 Operative and perioperative details at time of liver-directed therapy of our study population ($n = 35$ patients) according to state of Tyrosinkinase Inhibitor (TKI) Therapy

Variables	Total ($n = 35$)	TKI+ ($n = 16$)	TKI- ($n = 19$)	*p*-value
Extent of resection				
Minor resection	17 (51.5 %)	11 (33.3 %)	6 (18.2 %)	0.008[d]
Major	16 (48.5 %)	3 (9.1 %)	13 (39.4 %)	
Type of liver resection				
Segmental resection	9 (27.3 %)	6 (18.2 %)	3 (9.1 %)	0.13[d]
Anatomical right/left resection	11 (33.3 %)	9 (27.2 %)	2 (6.1 %)	0.003[d]
Extended resection right/left	5 (15.2 %)	4 (12.1 %)	1 (3.1 %)	0.06[d]
Atypical resection	8 (24.2 %)	4 (12.1 %)	4 (12.1 %)	0.61[d]
Resection Margin				
Complete Resection (R0)	30 (85.7 %)	14 (40 %)	16 (45.7 %)	0.78[d]
Microscopically positive margin (R1)	5 (14.3 %)	2 (5.7 %)	3 (8.6 %)	
Transfusion intraoperative				
Substitution	15 (8 %)	9 (4.8 %)	3 (1.6 %)	0.7[d]
- Transfusion erythrocyte concentrations	0.27 (0–6)	0.23 (0–6)	0.36 (0–4)	0.7[d]
- Transfusion Fresh frozen plasma	0.17 (0–8)	0.2 (0–8)	0.03 (0–1)	0.7[d]
Pringle manoeuvre	19 (54.3 %)	6 (17.1 %)	13 (37.1 %)	0.067[c]
Median Hospital stay (days)	18.7 (11–28)	16.6 (11–18)	20.5 (16–24)	0.360[a]
Median Intensive care unit stay (days)	1.9 (1–6)	2.0 (1–6)	1.8 (1–5)	0.716[a]
Median Operating time (min)	238 (161.5–276)	224.5 (164.5–272.5)	242 (155–281)	0.477[a]
Complications				
Grade I	0 (0 %)	0 (0 %)	0 (0 %)	-
Grade II	3 (8.6 %)	2 (5.7 %)	1 (2.9 %)	0.434[d]
Grade IIIa	5 (14.3 %)	4 (11.4 %)	1 (2.9 %)	0.096[d]
Grade IIIb	1 (2.9 %)	0 (0 %)	1 (2.9 %)	0.352[d]
Grade Iva	1 (2.9 %)	1 (2.9 %)	0 (0 %)	0.269[d]
Grade IVb	0 (0 %)	0 (0 %)	0 (0 %)	-
Grade V	0 (0.5 %)	0 (0 %)	0 (0 %)	-

Used Statistical tests:
[a]Student's *t*-test
[b]Wilcoxon rank sum test
[c]chi-squared test
[d]Fisher's exact test

(IQR: 1–25 months) and continued after liver-directed therapy. The given targeted therapy included sunitinib ($n = 10$ patients; 62.5 %), sorafenib ($n = 2$ patients; 12.5 %), pazopanib ($n = 3$ patients; 18.8 %) and everolimus ($n = 1$ patient; 6.2 %).

Of these 16 patients, 10 patients (28.5 %) had ongoing TT after liver-directed therapy for a median duration of 21 months (IQR: 18–49 months) and 6 patients (17.1 %) discontinued TT therapy at a median duration of 13 months (IQR: 7–35 months) without evidence of recurrence. Of the 10 patients with ongoing TT after liver-directed therapy, 4 patients (40 %) experienced relapse/recurrence. Of the 6 patients discontinued TT, 5 patients (83 %) experienced relapse/recurrence.

Of the 19 patients (59 %), who did not receive immediate postoperative targeted therapy, 14 patients (74 %) experienced recurrence after a median time of 11 months (IQR: 4–31 months). In total, 23 patients (66 %) did develop recurrence following LDT within a median time of 16 months (IQR: 5–34 months). Among these patients, the pattern of recurrence was extrahepatic in 13 patients (57 %), intrahepatic in 7 patients (30 %) and both in 3 patients (13 %). At the end of the observation period, 20 patients (57 %) had died. Of the 15 patients (43 %) alive, 8 patients (54 %) remained free of recurrence after a median follow-up of 2.1 years (range: 1–4.3 years). Of the 7 patients (43 %) developed recurrence, only 2 patients had local metastases in the pre-existing site. Lung metastases were developed most frequently ($n = 4$), followed

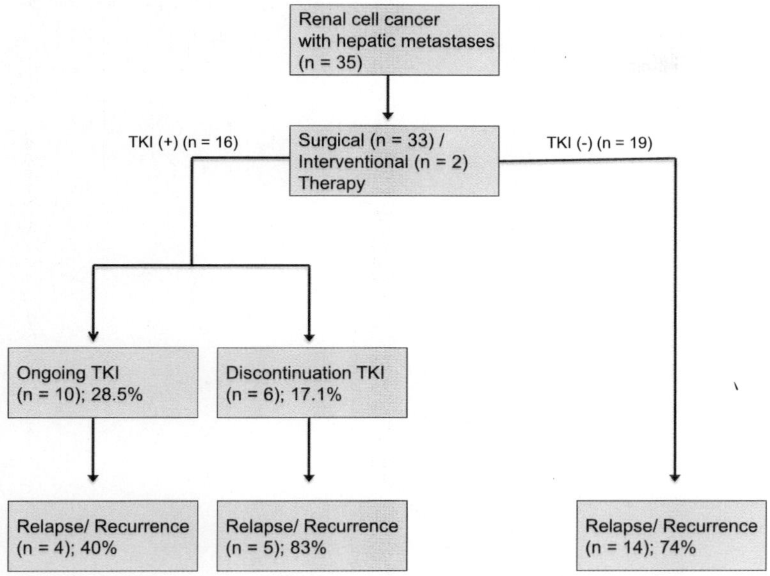

Fig. 1 Treatment algorithm of patients with hepatic metastasized renal cell cancer following liver-directed therapy

by the liver ($n = 2$) and the bone ($n = 1$). Sites of recurrence were not different according to the immediate postoperative TKI therapy.

Median progression-free survival and median disease-free survival was 27 months (IQR: 8–47 months; median follow-up was 3.1 years (IQR: 1.1–4.8 years)) following resection of first metastatic lesions and 19 months (IQR: 7–58 months; median follow-up was 2.1 years (IQR: 1–4.3 years)) following LDT, respectively. One-, 3-, and 5-year progression-free survival following resection of first metastases was 60, 28.6 and 11.4 %, respectively. Following LDT, 1-, 3- and 5-year disease-free survival was 60, 22.9 and 14.3 %, respectively.

In univariate analysis for progression-free survival, immediate postoperative targeted therapy ($p = 0.023$) (Fig. 2), ECOG performance status 0 ($p = 0.015$), metachronous liver metastases ($p = 0.035$), negative resection margins ($p = 0.001$), T-stage 1/2 ($p = 0.027$) and low Fuhrman Grading ($p = 0.002$) were associated with significantely longer progression-free survival rates (Table 3). At multivariable Cox regression analysis, immediate postoperative targeted therapy (HR 0.32, 95 CI: 0.1–0.9, $p = 0.032$) could be identified as a favourable significant independent predictor of good progression-free survival. In contrast, ECOG performance status >1 (HR 3.4, 95 CI 1.2–9.8, $p = 0.023$) could be identified as independent significant predictor associated with disease progression.

Following factors show benefitial effects on disease-free survival in univariate analyses: Negative resection margins ($p = 0.014$) and low Fuhrman grading ($p = 0.001$) (Table 4). Immediate postoperative TKI therapy ($p = 0.1$), ECOG status 0 ($p = 0.1$), metachronous liver metastases ($p = 0.08$) and T-stage 1/2 ($p = 0.07$), however, showed only a trend for a decreased recurrence rate in univariate analysis.

Survival analysis

Median overall survival was 86 months (IQR: 21 – 136 months; median follow-up was 5.1 years (IQR: 1.8 – 8.0 years) following primary tumor resection and 42 months (IQR: 18 – 98 months; median follow-up was 2.2 years (IQR: 1 – 4.8 years) following LDT, respectively. One-, 3-, and 5-year survival following resection of the primary tumor was 88.6, 68.6 and 51.4 %, respectively. Following LDT, 1-, 3- and 5-year survival was 77.1, 45.7 and 20 %, respectively.

In the univariate analysis using the Kaplan-Meier Method, immediate postoperative TKI therapy ($p = 0.032$) (Fig. 3), ECOG performance status 0 ($p < 0.001$), metachronous liver metastases ($p = 0.006$), liver tumor size <45 mm ($p = 0.007$), negative resection margins ($p = 0.013$) and a disease free survival >12 months ($p = 0.002$) were significant predictors of good overall survival following liver-directed therapy (Table 4).

Multivariate survival analysis using a Cox regression model showed that immediate postoperative TKI therapy (HR 0.28, 95CI: 0.1–0.99, $p = 0.046$) was a favourable significant independent predictor of good overall survival. Whereas ECOG performance status >1 (HR 4.6, 95 CI 1.4–14.7, $p < 0.001$) and synchronous liver metastases (HR 5.7 95 CI 1.4–23.8, $p = 0.015$) are significant independent predictors of poor overall survival. Whereas, multiple liver

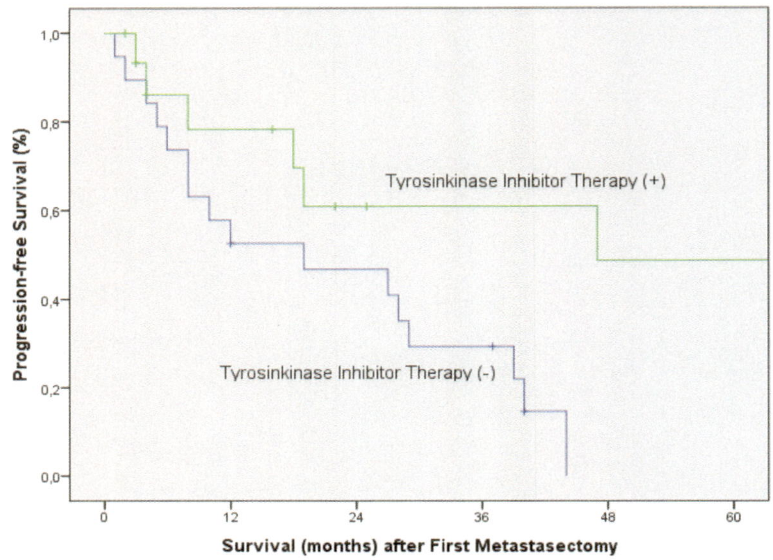

Fig. 2 Kaplan-Meier survival curve representing progression-free survival after first metastasectomy according to immediate postoperative tyrosinkinase inhibitor therapy ($p = 0.023$)

metastases (HR 1.1; 95 CI 0.4–2.9, $p = 0.8$) were no significant independent predictors of overall survival.

Following primary tumor resection, in univariate analysis immediate postoperative TKI therapy ($p = 0.003$), ECOG performance status 0 ($p < 0.001$), metachronous liver metastases ($p = 0.006$), liver tumor size <45 mm ($p = 0.007$) and negative resection margins ($p = 0.041$) were of prognostic impact on good overall survival. Multivariate analysis using a Cox regression model confirmed immediate postoperative TKI therapy (HR 0.14, 95 CI: 0.03–0.6, $p = 0.011$) as a favourable significant independent predictor of good overall survival. In contrast, ECOG performance status >1 (HR 8.3, 95 CI 1.9–18.7, $p < 0.001$) and synchronous liver metastases (HR 5.4 95 CI 1.1–26.8, $p = 0.013$) are significant independent predictors of poor overall survival.

Discussion

To our best knowledge, this is one of the largest studies examining the value of metastasectomy with a special focus on liver resection in patients with MRCC in the era of TKI therapy. We examined whether TKI therapy is associated with MRCC prognosis when it is provided immediately after surgical resection of metastatic hepatic lesions. Uni- and multivariate analyses showed that median overall survival such as progression-free survival were significantly better in patients receiving immediate postoperative TKI therapy following primary tumor resection and LDT, respectively. However, disease recurrence following liver resection showed only a trend to be less common in patients who received immediate postoperative TKI therapy. These results could be a sign that immediate postoperative TKI therapy improves survival and disease control by decreasing tumor recurrence following resection of metastatic hepatic lesions.

Various treatment options have been studied for the therapy of MRCC and the benefits of metastasectomy in these patients could be demonstrated in some retrospective studies [7, 8, 29]. In this context, there is emerging evidence that surgical resection may represent a significant tool in multimodal concepts of MRCC. In accordance with retrospective studies, our study demonstrates liver resection to be safely applicable with comparable survival and recurrence rates for patients with resectable RCCLM [6, 10, 11, 13, 30]. Therefore, selected clinical characteristics and patient-defined variables have been determined to stratify risk for metastasectomy in MRCC patients to help to define groups of patients which benefit most from surgical therapy with a focus on liver metastasectomy. In accordance with previous reports, in our study immediate postoperative TKI therapy, ECOG performance status, timing of liver metastases presence, tumor diameter, primary tumor characteristics (Fuhrman Grading, T-Stage,), negative resection margins and time of disease free interval were of prognostic value for overall survival and recurrence [6, 10, 11, 25, 30–33].

However, the prognostic value of Fuhrman grading in papillary renal cancer is inconsistent and nowdays not considered as the best grading system for non-clear cell renal cancer. In recent studies, nuclear grade seems to be more effective to predict outcome in patients with non-clear cell renal cancer [34]. Other factors like patients' age, number of metastases, presence

Table 3 Univariate analysis of potential prognostic factors for progression-free survival ($n = 35$ patients) and disease-free survival ($n = 35$ patients) following metastasectomy of primary and hepatic metastasic lesions, respectively

		Progression-free Survival after first Metastasectomy		Disease-free Survival after Liver-directed therapy (LDT)	
Variables	n	Median Time (months) with IQR	*p-value*	Median Time (months) with IQR	*p-value*
Gender					
Male	24	8 (5–44)	0.324	15 (5–44)	0.346
Female	11	27 (10–47)		20 (9–58)	
Targeted therapy					
TKI+	16	47 (18–79)	**0.023**	58 (18–79)	0.110
TKI–	19	19 (6–39)		19 (4–46)	
ECOG					
0	29	29 (10–47)	**0.015**	20 (8–71)	0.132
> 1	6	6 (2–28)		15 (1–28)	
Age					
< 65 years	18	19 (8–40)	0.518	19 (5–71)	0.960
> 65 years	17	39 (8–71)		20 (9–58)	
Tumor distribution					
unilobular	28	28 (8–44)	0.772	28 (8–58)	0.981
multilobular	7	19 (3–77)		19 (3–79)	
Extrahepatic Disease					
Yes	28	27 (7–45)	0.412	19 (8–59)	0.962
No	7	29 (4–82)		20 (4–29)	
Liver metastasis Timing					
Synchronous	6	4 (2–9)	**0.035**	4 (2–8)	0.085
Metachronous	29	28 (10–47)		26 (12–58)	
Tumor size, cm					
< 4.5 cm	21	39 (10–71)	0.07	19 (9–42)	0.376
> 4.5 cm	14	18 (6–29)		18 (5–35)	
Resection margin					
Radical resection (R0)	30	28 (12–51)	**0.001**	28 (12–58)	**0.014**
Irradical resection (R1/R2)	5	6 (3–10)		4 (3–9)	
Number of metastases					
Solitary	22	27 (8–47)	0.653	28 (9–51)	0.967
Multiple	13	19 (8–40)		19 (5–79)	
Grading of RCC					
Low (G1/G2)	24	40 (18–71)	**0.002**	44 (18–71)	**0.001**
High (G3/G4)	11	8 (5–19)		8 (4–19)	
T-stage					
T1/T2	16	44 (12–79)	**0.027**	29 (15–71)	0.071
T3/T4	19	18 (6–39)		18 (4–51)	
Disease-free intervall					
< 12 months	17	28 (5–79)	0.753	28 (5–79)	0.501
> 12 months	18	27 (10–40)		19 (9–58)	

TKI Tyrosinkinase InhibitorTherapy, *ECOG* Eastern Cooperative Oncology Group
The bold data specifies a staticial significance *p*-values < 0.05

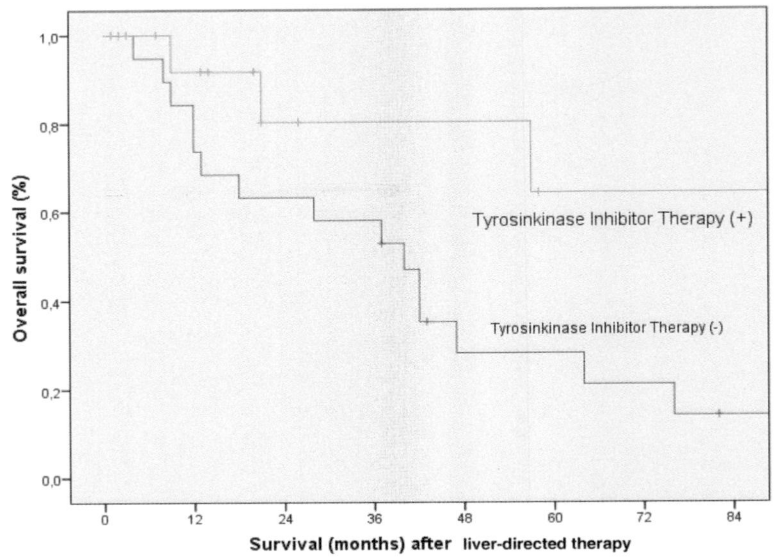

Fig. 3 Kaplan-Meier overall survival curve representing follow-up after liver-directed therapy according to immediate postoperative tyrosinkinase inhibitor therapy ($p = 0.032$)

of synchronous extrahepatic disease such as factors related to tumor biology might help to decide to operate or not.

Overall, approximately 70 % (25/35) of our patients experienced disease recurrence after surgical resection of first metastatic lesions. Our results are consistent with previous studies which have shown that large numbers of patients experience disease recurrence after metastasectomy with excellent cancer-specific overall survival. Johansen et al. reported that disease recurrence was observed in 66.7 % of patients, with complete response achieved by targeted therapy alone or no evidence of disease with additional metastasectomy after a median follow up of 12 months [35]. More recently, Park et al. reported about disease recurrence in 60.4 % of patients received immediate postoperative targeted therapy after metastasectomy or not over a median follow-up of 12 months [27]. These results confirmed the fact that some residual cancer cells might remain after the complete resection of metastatic lesions.

Some clinical trials showed that advanced RCC is often resistant to most systemic therapies, and shows limited response to immunotherapy [8, 16]. Recently, several randomized controlled trials have shown that TKI like sorafenib, sunitinib or pazopinib, and other targeted therapeutical agents are correlated with improvements in PFS and OS [20, 21, 36, 37]. These new drugs have dramatically changed the treatment and prognosis of patients with MRCC, and give the opportunity to perform metastatic resection in a new and expended population of patients as more response has been noted. However, cure is rare with TKI alone and complete remission after TKI treatment occurs in only 1–3 % of cases [18, 19]. Whereas, partial response could be achieved in 10–39 % of patients, and ceiling of the overall survival was 18.8 months (range 7.8 to 43.2 depending of the risk factors) [35, 38, 39]. Therefore, metastasectomy remains an important treatment for MRCC and the growing evidence of long-term response with TKI therapy has been stimulating multimodal approaches in the last years.

However, there is currently low experience with the role of systemic TT after surgical treatment of metastatic lesions in patients with RCC and experience is based on case reports and small series [8, 22, 26, 40]. Reliable data examining patients with RCCLM following liver resection are completely missing. The largest series was published recently by Park et al. who examined the efficacy of adjuvant targeted therapy after complete resection of metastatic lesions in 53 patients with MRCC; however none of the patients had RCCLM. 19 (35.9 %) of the patients received immediate postoperative targeted therapy. Of the 34 who did not receive immediate postoperative targeted therapy, 27 (79.4 %) experienced disease recurrence. Immediate postoperative targeted therapy was associated with better median progression free survival (not reached versus 20.0 months, $p = 0.017$), but not cancer-specific survival [27]. According to the missing available data, prospective, randomized multicentre clinical trials (RESORT Study and SMAT-AN 20/04 of the Working Group of Urological Oncology (AUO)) were initiated within the last years to studying the effects and benefits of targeted adjuvant therapy following metastasectomy [18, 41, 42].

Table 4 Univariate analysis of potential prognostic factors for overall Survival ($n = 35$ patients) following primary tumor resection and liver directed therapy (LDT) , respectively

Variables	n	Follow-Up Liver-directed therapy Median Time (months) with IQR	*p-value*	Follow-Up Primary Tumor Resection Median Time (months) with IQR	*p-value*
Gender					
Male	24	42 (21–98)	0.7	96 (34–130)	0.4
Female	11	37 (12–68)		62 (63–126)	
Targeted therapy					
TKI+	16	98 (57–133)	**0.032**	151 (126–202)	**0.003**
TKI–	19	40 (12–64)		61 (25–103)	
ECOG					
0	29	57 (37–98)	**0.001**	103 (79–151)	**<0.001**
> 1	6	12 (9–18)		15 (13–34)	
Age					
< 65 years	18	64 (35–98)	0.07	96 (34–151)	0.31
> 65 years	17	40 (12–57)		63 (79–126)	
Tumor distribution					
unilobular	28	98 (21–76)	0.911	126 (25–151)	0.8
multilobular	7	42 (12–98)		86 (54–126)	
Synchronous Extrahepatic Disease					
Yes	7	21 (9–37)	0.312	63 (54–126)	0.727
No	28	47 (28–98)		86 (61–159)	
Liver metastasis Timing					
Synchronous	6	9 (8–12)	**0.006**	15 (8–63)	**0.006**
Metachronous	29	47 (28–98)		96 (54–151)	
Tumor size, cm					
< 45 mm	21	98 (28–133)	**0.007**	103 (86–151)	**0.007**
> 45 mm	14	37 (12–57)		63 (18–85)	
Resection margin					
Radical resection (R0)	30	47 (21–98)	**0.013**	96 (48–151)	**0.041**
Irradical resection (R1/R2)	5	9 (8–28)		86 (13–92)	
Number of metastases					
Solitary	22	64 (12–98)	0.850	85 (54–153)	0.990
Multiple	13	42 (21–76)		116 (34–130)	
T-stage					
T1/T2	16	47 (37–98)	0.062	126 (62–151)	0.257
T3/T4	19	40 (12–64)		85 (54–103)	
Grading of RCC					
Low (G1/G2)	24	47 (37–133)	0.543	116 (63–126)	0.501
High (G3/G4)	11	28 (9–98)		85 (51–151)	
Disease-free intervall					
< 12 months	17	13 (9–42)	**0.002**	79 (18–96)	0.2
> 12 months	18	64 (42–98)		103 (62–151)	

Table 4 Univariate analysis of potential prognostic factors for overall Survival ($n = 35$ patients) following primary tumor resection and liver directed therapy (LDT) , respectively *(Continued)*

Histology					
Clear cell	25	47 (40–98)	0.821	96 (51–151)	0.498
Non clear cell	10	42 (18–132)		85 (54–116)	
Surgical complications					
Yes	10	28 (21–40)	0.996	85 (49–118)	0.104
No	25	47 (13–98)		151 (54–202)	

TKI Tyrosinkinase nhibitorTherapy, *ECOG* Eastern Cooperative Oncology Group
The bold data specifies a staticial significance *p*-values < 0.05

Nevertheless, there are some limitations to our study. Firstly, it concerns a small patient sample and due to the retrospective nature of our study it is susceptible to bias in data selection and survival analysis. Although our results show significant differences in overall survival (OS) and progression-free survival (PFS), we could not find significant differences in disease-free survival (DFS), which at first sight might seem astonishing. The three outcome variables are very distinct from each other and may not readily be compared as they include different patients. Also, regarding the trends in the data, the follow up might have been to short to show differences in terms of DFS. Unfortunately, the sample size was too small to allow a final answer to our hypotheses.

Secondly, there are no comparative studies in this highly selected patient population which examine patients with MRCC without surgical intervention who were treated with targeted therapy. Thirdly, there were no standard protocols for the clinical decision making process concerning the choice of given targeted agents as well as the timing of restarting or discontinuating the targeted therapy. This fact is especially mirrored in our study because of the long observation period of 23 years. For our first patients TKI therapy was not yet available. During the next period, several publications about the use of TKI in different clinical settings influenced the decision of our interdisciplinary tumor board to use or avoid additional TKI after surgery, respectively. Furthermore, in patients with R1 resection and higher tumor stages the decisions in favour of using TKI were influenced more positively compared to lower tumor stages. Therefore differences in survival might also be due to some selection bias. Of interest, data on patient Quality of Life (QoL) might be an important addition in future studies for the results of our analysis.

Conclusions

The present data suggest that a surgical approach of MRCC to the liver in combination with adjuvant TKI therapy should be carefully considered case-by-case, taking into account patient QoL in order to optimize the management of these patients. However, future prospective studies, preferably with randomized design and larger populations, are needed do increase the quality of evidence regarding the role of (liver-)metastasectomy with integration of TKI therapy in the (neo)/-adjuvant setting. Moreover, a careful balance of the benefit/risk ratio must be shared among a multidisciplinary team to tailor treatments individually and with the patient. Therefore, prognostic models and algorithms might indeed help in deciding which patients benefit from (liver-) metastasectomy as an additive tool in the multimodal therapeutical setting of MRCC.

Abbreviations

CT, computed tomography; DFI, disease-free interval; DFS, disease-free survival; ECOG, eastern cooperative oncology group; FFP, fresh frozen plasma; HR, hazard ratio; ICU, intensive care unit; IQR, interquartal range; KPS, karnofsky performance scale; LDT, liver-directed therapy; MRCC, metastasic renal cell carcinoma; OS, Overall Survival; PFS, progression-free survival; QoL, quality of life; RBCC, red blood cell concentrate; RCC, renal cell carcinoma; RCCLM, renal cell carcinoma liver metastases; TKI, tyrosinkinase inhibitor; TT, Targeted Therapy

Acknowledgements

We acknowledge support from the German Research Foundation (DFG) and University of Leipzig within the program of Open Access Publishing.

Funding

This work was supported by the German Research Foundation (DFG) and Leipzig University within the program of Open Access Publishing. The funders had no role in study design, data collection and analysis, decision to publish, or preparation of the manuscript.

Authors' contributions

HMH, FT, GW, and MB were responsible for the study conception and design; HMH, FT, GW, MHM, UL, GA, CL and CB were responsible for data acquisition; HMH, FT GW, MS, HMT, UL and MB analyzed and interpreted the data; HMH, FT and GW drafted the manuscript; and MHM, MS, DU, CL and HMT critically revised the manuscript. All authors read and approved the final manuscript.

Competing interests

The authors declare that they have no competing interests.

Author details

[1]Department of Visceral, Transplantation, Vascular and Thoracic Surgery, University Hospital of Leipzig, Liebigstrasse 20, 04103 Leipzig, Germany. [2]Department of General, Visceral and Transplant Surgery, Campus Virchow, Charité-Universitätsmedizin Berlin, Augustenburger Platz 1, Berlin, Germany. [3]Department of Urology, University of Leipzig, Leipzig, Germany. [4]Division of Infectious Diseases and Tropical Medicine, Department of Gastroenterology and Rheumatology, Leipzig University Hospital, Leipzig, Germany.

References

1. Siegel R, Ma J, Zou Z, Jemal A. Cancer statistics, 2014. CA Cancer J Clin. 2014;64:9–29.
2. Bex A, Powles T, Karam JA. Role of targeted therapy in combination with surgery in renal cell carcinoma. Int J Urol. 2016;23:5–12.
3. Ferlay J, Steliarova-Foucher E, Lortet-Tieulent J, Rosso S, Coebergh JWW, Comber H, Forman D, Bray F. Cancer incidence and mortality patterns in Europe: estimates for 40 countries in 2012. Eur J Cancer. 2013;49:1374–403.
4. Mickisch GHJ, Garin A, Van Poppel H, De Prijck L, Sylvester R. Radical nephrectomy plus interferon-alfa-based immunotherapy compared with interferon alfa alone in metastatic renal-cell carcinoma: A randomised trial. Lancet. 2001;358:966–70.
5. Bianchi M, Sun M, Jeldres C, Shariat SF, Trinh QD, Briganti A, Tian Z, Schmitges J, Graefen M, Perrotte P, Menon M, Montorsi F, Karakiewicz PI. Distribution of metastatic sites in renal cell carcinoma: A population-based analysis. Ann Oncol. 2012;23:973–80.
6. Staehler MD, Kruse J, Haseke N, Stadler T, Roosen A, Karl A, Stief CG, Jauch KW, Bruns CJ. Liver resection for metastatic disease prolongs survival in renal cell carcinoma: 12-year results from a retrospective comparative analysis. World J Urol. 2010;28:543–7.
7. Russo P. Multi-modal treatment for metastatic renal cancer. The role of surgery. World J Urol. 2010;28:295–301.
8. Kim DY, Karam J a, Wood CG. Role of metastasectomy for metastatic renal cell carcinoma in the era of targeted therapy. World J Urol. 2014; 32:631–42.
9. Dabestani S, Marconi L, Hofmann F, Stewart F, Lam TBL, Canfield SE, Staehler M, Powles T, Ljungberg B, Bex A. Local treatments for metastases of renal cell carcinoma: a systematic review. Lancet Oncol. 2014;15:549–61.
10. Aloia TA, Adam R, Azoulay D, Bismuth H, Castaing D. Outcome following hepatic resection of metastatic renal tumors: the Paul Brousse Hospital experience. HPB. 2006;8:100–5.
11. Ruys AT, Tanis PJ, Iris ND, van Duijvendijk P, Verhoef C, Porte RJ, van Gulik TM. Surgical treatment of renal cell cancer liver metastases: a population-based study. Ann Surg Oncol. 2011;18:1932–8.
12. Schmelzle M, Eisenberger CF, Am Esch JS, Matthaei H, Krausch M, Knoefel WT. Non-colorectal, non-neuroendocrine, and non-sarcoma metastases of the liver: Resection as a promising tool in the palliative management. Langenbecks Arch Surg. 2010;395:227–34.
13. Hatzaras I, Bischof DA, Fahy B, Cosgrove D, Pawlik TM. Treatment options and surveillance strategies after therapy for hepatocellular carcinoma. Ann Surg Oncol. 2014;21:758–66.
14. Santoni M, De Tursi M, Felici A, Lo Re G, Ricotta R, Ruggeri EM, Sabbatini R, Santini D, Vaccaro V, Milella M. Management of metastatic renal cell carcinoma patients with poor-risk features: current status and future perspectives. Expert Rev Anticancer Ther. 2013;13:697–709.
15. Pal SK, Haas NB. Adjuvant Therapy for Renal Cell Carcinoma: Past, Present, and Future. Oncologist. 2014;19:851–9.
16. McDermott DF. Immunotherapy of metastatic renal cell carcinoma. Cancer. 2009;115:2298–305.
17. Sternberg CN, Davis ID, Mardiak J, Szczylik C, Lee E, Wagstaff J, Barrios CH, Salman P, Gladkov OA, Kavina A, Zarbá JJ, Chen M, McCann L, Pandite L, Roychowdhury DF, Hawkins RE. Pazopanib in locally advanced or metastatic renal cell carcinoma: Results of a randomized phase III trial. J Clin Oncol. 2010;28:1061–8.
18. Coppin C, Kollmannsberger C, Le L, Porzsolt FWT. Targeted therapy for advanced renal cell cancer (RCC): a Cochrane systematic review of published randomised trials. BJU Int. 2011;108:1556–63.
19. Husillos Alonso A, Carbonero García MGEC. Is there a role for systemic targeted therapy after surgical treatment for metastases of renal cell carcinoma? World J Nephrol. 2015;4:254–62.
20. Motzer RJ, Hutson TE, Tomczak P, Michaelson MD, Bukowski RM, Rixe O, Oudard S, Negrier S, Szczylik C, Kim ST, Chen I, Bycott PW, Baum CM, Figlin RA. Sunitinib versus Interferon Alfa in Metastatic Renal-Cell Carcinoma. N Engl J Med. 2007;356:115–24.
21. Escudier B, Eisen T, Stadler WM, Szczylik C, Oudard S, Siebels M, Negrier S, Chevreau C, Solska E, Desai AA, Rolland F, Demkow T, Hutson TE, Gore M, Freeman S, Schwartz B, Shan M, Simantov R, Bukowski RM. Sorafenib in Advanced Clear-Cell Renal-Cell Carcinoma. N Engl J Med. 2007;356:125–34.
22. De Lichtenberg TH, Hermann GG, Rørth M, Højer Larsen M-J, Mansourvar Z, Holm ML, Scheike T. Overall survival after immunotherapy, tyrosine kinase inhibitors and surgery in treatment of metastatic renal cell cancer: outcome of 143 consecutive patients from a single centre. Scand J Urol. 2014;48:379–86.
23. van der Poel HG, Roukema JA, Horenblas S, van Geel AN, Debruyne F. Metastasectomy in renal cell carcinoma: A multicenter retrospective analysis. Eur Urol. 1999;35:197–203.
24. Kwak C, Park YH, Jeong CW, Lee SE, Ku JH. Metastasectomy without systemic therapy in metastatic renal cell carcinoma: Comparison with conservative treatment. Urol Int. 2007;79:145–51.
25. Alt AL, Boorjian SA, Lohse CM, Costello BA, Leibovich BC, Blute ML. Survival after complete surgical resection of multiple metastases from renal cell carcinoma. Cancer. 2011;117:2873–82.
26. Karam JA, Rini BI, Varella L, Garcia JA, Dreicer R, Choueiri TK, Jonasch E, Matin SF, Campbell SC, Wood CG, Tannir NM. Metastasectomy after targeted therapy in patients with advanced renal cell carcinoma. J Urol. 2011;185:439–44.
27. Park YH, Jung JW, Lee BK, Lee S, Jeong SJ, Byun SSLS. Targeted therapy after complete resection of metastatic lesions in metastatic renal cell carcinoma. Int J Urol. 2015;22:153–7.
28. Daliani DD, Tannir NM, Papandreou CN, Wang X, Swisher S, Wood CG, Swanson DA, Logothetis CJ, Jonasch E. Prospective assessment of systemic therapy followed by surgical removal of metastases in selected patients with renal cell carcinoma. BJU Int. 2009;104:456–60.
29. Tosco L, Van Poppel H, Frea B, Gregoraci G, Joniau S. Survival and impact of clinical prognostic factors in surgically treated metastatic renal cell carcinoma. Eur Urol. 2013;63:646–52.
30. Thelen A, Jonas S, Benckert C, Lopez-Hänninen E, Rudolph B, Neumann U, Neuhaus P. Liver resection for metastases from renal cell carcinoma. World J Surg. 2007;31:802–7.
31. Langan RC, Ripley RT, Davis JL, Prieto PA, Datrice N, Steinberg SM, Bratslavsky G, Rudloff U, Kammula US, Stojadinovic A, Avital I. Liver directed therapy for renal cell carcinoma. J Cancer. 2012;3:184–90.
32. Hatzaras I, Gleisner AL, Pulitano C, Sandroussi C, Hirose K, Hyder O, Wolfgang CL, Aldrighetti L, Crawford M, Choti MA, Pawlik TM. A multi-institution analysis of outcomes of liver-directed surgery for metastatic renal cell cancer. HPB. 2012;14:532–8.
33. Motzer RJ, Mazumdar M, Bacik J, Berg W, Amsterdam A, Ferrara J. Survival and prognostic stratification of 670 patients with advanced renal cell carcinoma. J Clin Oncol. 1999;17:2530–40.
34. Cornejo KM, Dong F, Zhou AG, Wu C-L, Young RH, Braaten K, Sadow PM, Nielsen GP, Oliva E. Papillary renal cell carcinoma: correlation of tumor grade and histologic characteristics with clinical outcome. Hum Pathol. 2015;46:1411–7.
35. Johannsen M, Staehler M, Ohlmann CH, Flörcken A, Schmittel A, Otto T, Bex A, Hein P, Miller K, Weikert S, Grünwald V. Outcome of treatment discontinuation in patients with metastatic renal cell carcinoma and no evidence of disease following targeted therapy with or without metastasectomy. Ann Oncol. 2011;22:657–63.
36. Motzer RJ, Escudier B, Oudard S, Hutson TE, Porta C, Bracarda S, Grünwald V, Thompson JA, Figlin RA, Hollaender N, Urbanowitz G, Berg WJ, Kay A, Lebwohl D, Ravaud A. Efficacy of Everolimus in Advanced Renal Cell Carcinoma: A Double-Blind, Randomised, Placebo-Controlled Phase III Trial. Lancet. 2008;372:449–56.
37. Ciccarese C, Massari F, Santoni M, Heng DYC, Sotte V, Brunelli M, Conti A, Cheng L, Lopez-Beltran A, Scarpelli M, Cascinu S, Tortora G, Montironi R. New molecular targets in non clear renal cell carcinoma: An overview of ongoing clinical trials. Cancer Treat Rev. 2015;41:614–22.
38. Heng DYC, Xie W, Regan MM, Harshman LC, Bjarnason GA, Vaishampayan UN, Mackenzie M, Wood L, Donskov F, Tan MH, Rha SY, Agarwal N, Kollmannsberger C, Rini BI, Choueiri TK. External validation and comparison with other models of the International Metastatic Renal-Cell Carcinoma Database Consortium prognostic model: A population-based study. Lancet Oncol. 2013;14:141–8.
39. Bex A, Fournier L, Lassau N, Mulders P, Nathan P, Oyen WJPT. Assessing the response to targeted therapies in renal cell carcinoma: technical insights and practical considerations. Eur Urol. 2014;65:766–77.
40. Lee CY, Bae MK, Park IK, Kim DJ, Lee JG, Choi JS, Han K-HH, Chung KY. Surgical resection for pulmonary metastasis from hepatocellular carcinoma: Analysis of prognosis in relation to primary control. J Surg Oncol. 2010;101:239–43.
41. Procopio G, Verzoni E, Biondani P, Grassi P, Testa I, de BF GE. Rationale and protocol of RESORT, a randomized, open-label, multicenter phase II study to evaluate the efficacy of sorafenib in patients with advanced renal cell carcinoma after radical resection of the metastases. Tumori. 2014;100:28–30.

27

Posttraumatic venous gas in the liver – a case report and review of the current literature

René Fahrner[1*], Falk Rauchfuss[1], Hubert Scheuerlein[1,2] and Utz Settmacher[1]

Abstract

Background: There are numerous causes of hepatic gas formation that range from serious pathologies to incidental findings, including mesenteric infarction, liver abscess, inflammatory bowel disease or minimally invasive hepatic interventions.

Case presentation: We report a case of a 50-year-old man who was admitted to the emergency room after a car accident. The clinical examination and further diagnostics revealed a craniocerebral injury with a fracture of the skull, concomitant soft tissue lesions and subarachnoidal bleeding. Furthermore, a blunt thoracic trauma with hemopneumothorax due to rib fractures was treated with a chest tube. No obvious abdominal pathology was seen. While in the operating theatre for the surgical revision of the cranial soft tissue lesions, a femoral venous catheter was inserted without any complications. A routine ultrasound of the abdomen six hours after the trauma revealed unclear hepatic gas formation. A contrast-enhanced computer tomography (CT) scan of the abdomen was performed, and the gas formation was found to be localized within the left hepatic vein. Afterwards, there was no specific treatment of the hepatic venous gas formation, as no alterations of liver function or liver enzymes were seen. The further course of the patient was uneventful regarding the gas formation in the liver, and another ultrasound two days later revealed no further gas in the liver.

Conclusions: The placement of a femoral venous catheter is a risk factor for gas formation in liver veins. No further treatment is needed in cases with stable liver function. To rule out serious pathologies, diagnostic findings (e.g., ultrasound, CT), clinical history and underlying diseases need to be analyzed carefully after the detection of intrahepatic gas formation. With contrast-enhanced CT, the localization of the gas and its potential causes might be detectable.

Keywords: Abdominal trauma, Gas, Liver vein

Background

There are numerous causes of hepatic gas formation [1]. They range from serious pathologies, such as mesenteric infarction, liver abscess, inflammatory bowel disease, thrombosis of a hepatic artery after liver transplantation, cholecystitis and cholangitis, to incidental findings without any consequences. Furthermore, minimally invasive hepatic interventions (endoscopic retrograde cholangiopancreatography, hepatic artery embolization, tumour ablation, liver biopsy, portal vein embolization) are increasing in frequency, so it is important to rule out these procedures as potential causes of the gas formation in order to detect life-threatening conditions in the patient. Therefore, the patient's history and the radiological findings need to be analyzed carefully. We report here a case of hepatic gas formation after a motor vehicle crash with suspected blunt abdominal trauma and discuss the potential diagnosis.

Case presentation

A 50-year-old man was admitted to the emergency room after a car crash. At the time of admission, the patient was conscious and hemodynamically stable. Therefore, a computer tomography (CT) scan was performed for

* Correspondence:
[1]University Hospital Jena, Division of General, Visceral and Vascular Surgery, Am Klinikum 1, 07740 Jena, Germany
Full list of author information is available at the end of the article

further diagnostics and revealed a craniocerebral injury that involved a fracture of the skull with concomitant soft tissue lesions and subarachnoidal bleeding. In addition, the patient suffered blunt thoracic trauma with hemopneumothorax due to rib fractures, which was treated with a chest tube. No obvious abdominal pathology was seen. The patient was transferred to the operating theatre for surgical revision of the soft tissue lesions. During general anesthesia, a femoral venous catheter was inserted without any procedural complications. Postoperatively, the patient was monitored in the intensive care unit. At our institution, a repeated ultrasound of the abdomen is performed six hours after the trauma to rule out free abdominal liquid or lesions of the parenchymatous organs, because it has been shown that repeated ultrasound examinations decrease the rate of false negative results and increase the sensitivity to detect intraabdominal liquid [2, 3]. In our patient, an unclear hepatic gas formation in the liver veins was seen but still no free liquid. For further differentiation and localization of the gas formation, a contrast-enhanced CT scan of the abdomen was performed. Here, the gas formation was localized in the left hepatic vein (Fig. 1 a/b, black arrow). In addition, the central venous catheter in the inferior vena cava was visible without hematoma or gas formation (Fig. 1 b, white arrow), and no additional abdominal pathology was noted.

There was no specific treatment administered for the hepatic venous gas formation. The further course of the patient was uneventful regarding the gas formation in the liver, and an additional ultrasound to check for further gas formation two days later revealed no more gas in the liver. No changes in liver function or liver enzymes were seen.

Discussion und conclusions

Gas formation within the hepatic veins is rarely seen in routine CT scans, and only a few cases have been reported so far. The largest published investigation of patients with gas formation in the liver vein analyzed 235 CT scans of intensive care unit patients and found that 5% of the CT scans showed gas formation in the hepatic veins [4]. All patients with gas in their hepatic veins in this study had received a femoral venous catheter. Therefore, the authors concluded that a femoral venous catheter is one of the most important risk factors for this complication. Further, they recommended performing a multiplanar reconstruction of the liver vascular structures to identify the localization of the gas formation. Portal venous gas [5, 6], pneumobilia [7] or gas in the liver artery [8] were considered as differential diagnoses and lead to further diagnostics and therapy. In postmortem studies, cardiac gas embolism, putrefaction processes, and open skull fractures due to craniocerebral injury or gunshot injury to the head were associated with gas in the hepatic veins [9–11]. In addition, gas embolism in the hepatic vein during laparoscopic liver surgery has been reported [12–14]. As interventional therapies of the liver, such as endoscopic retrograde cholangiopancreatography, hepatic artery embolization, tumour ablation, liver biopsy, and portal vein embolization, are increasing in number, post-interventional complications with gas within the liver are seen more frequently.

In this report, the further course of the patient was uneventful, and a subsequent ultrasound revealed no more gas in the liver, and no changes in liver function were detected. Most likely, the detection of hepatic venous gas formation in our patient was a coincidence related to the placement of the femoral venous catheter and the open skull fracture. This might explain why the initial CT scan was unremarkable and showed no pathology of the liver.

It has been shown that focused abdominal sonography after blunt abdominal trauma is a reliable and sensitive technique in the hands of experienced investigators [3, 15]. In the case of negative findings, repeated examinations

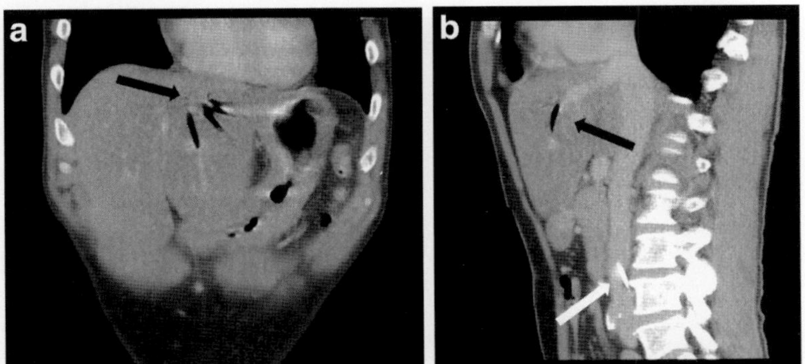

Fig. 1 Contrast-enhanced CT scan of the abdomen several hours after a car crash with suspected blunt abdominal trauma showing gas formation within the left liver vein (black arrow **a**, **b**). Furthermore, the central venous catheter is seen in the vena cava inferior (white arrow, **b**)

may help decrease the rate of false negative results and increase the sensitivity to detect free abdominal liquid [2, 3, 15]. Intravascular abdominal gas after blunt abdominal trauma is rarely seen and is postulated to be a transient finding that can often be treated non-surgically [16, 17]. In total, posttraumatic hepatic gas formations have been reported more frequently within the portal venous system than within the hepatic venous system.

Portal venous gas in combination with pneumatosis intestinalis might be a sign of intestinal ischemia but might also occur after blunt abdominal trauma or abdominal surgery [5, 6, 17, 18]. In this patient, there was no evidence of intestinal ischemia from the clinical examination or the CT scan. Pneumobilia is reported as a consequence of blunt abdominal trauma [7], but in our patient, this pathology was not supported by the localization of the gas formation. Infectious and abscess-forming complications after liver transplantation [8] or liver abscess [19] with gas in the hepatic artery are rare, and they were not considered reasonable diagnoses in our patient due to the short-time follow-up. As the patients' history was uneventful until the car crash, complications of minimally invasive interventions to the liver were also not reasonable.

The causes of hepatic gas formation might range from serious pathologies to incidental, harmless findings. Therefore, it is important to analyze and clarify the underlying cause of hepatic gas formation when it is identified. Multiplanar reconstructions of the vascular structures of the liver by CT scan have been recommended as a means of identifying the exact localization of the gas formation within the liver. Depending on the diagnosis, further treatment may be necessary. Gas formation within the hepatic veins is rare and usually harmless, as in our case, without the need for medical or surgical treatment.

Abbreviations

CT: Computer tomography

Acknowledgements

Not applicable.

Funding

There was no funding for this study.

Authors' contributions

Study concept and design: RF, FR, HS, US. Acquisition of data: RF, FR, HS, US. Analysis and interpretation of data: RF, FR, HS, US. Drafting of manuscript: RF. Critical revision of manuscript: FR, HS, US. All authors have read and approved the final version of this manuscript.

Competing interests

The authors declare that they have no conflict of interest.

Author details

[1]University Hospital Jena, Division of General, Visceral and Vascular Surgery, Am Klinikum 1, 07740 Jena, Germany. [2]St. Vincenz Hospital, Division of General and Visceral Surgery, Am Busdorf 2, 33098 Paderborn, Germany.

References

1. Shah PA, Cunningham SC, Morgan TA, Daly BD. Hepatic gas: widening spectrum of causes detected at CT and US in the interventional era. Radiographics : a review publication of the Radiological Society of North America, Inc. 2011;31(5):1403–13.
2. Hoffmann R, Nerlich M, Muggia-Sullam M, Pohlemann T, Wippermann B, Regel G, Tscherne H. Blunt abdominal trauma in cases of multiple trauma evaluated by ultrasonography: a prospective analysis of 291 patients. J Trauma. 1992;32(4):452–8.
3. Nunes LW, Simmons S, Hallowell MJ, Kinback R, Trooskin S, Kozar R. Diagnostic performance of trauma US in identifying abdominal or pelvic free fluid and serious abdominal or pelvic injury. Acad Radiol. 2001;8(2):128–36.
4. Galbois A, Cazejust J, Arrive L, Boelle PY, Ait-Oufella H, Baudel JL, Alves M, Margetis D, Offenstadt G, Guidet B, et al. Femoral venous catheter: a misleading cause of gas in the liver. Crit Care Med. 2011;39(11):2447–51.
5. Khalaf N, Mittal S. Hepatic portal venous gas: an ominous sign of mesenteric ischemia. Clinical gastroenterology and hepatology : the official clinical practice journal of the American Gastroenterological Association. 2014;12(6): xxix–xx.
6. Hashimoto A, Fuke H, Shimizu A, Shiraki K. Hepatic portal venous gas caused by non-obstructive mesenteric ischemia. J Hepatol. 2002;37(6):870.
7. Barnes SL, Badrudduja M, Bernard AC, Boulanger BR. Pneumobilia after blunt trauma: a self-limited condition? J Trauma. 2006;60(3):637–9.
8. Shaked A, McDiarmid SV, Harrison RE, Gelebert HA, Colonna JO 3rd, Busuttil RW. Hepatic artery thrombosis resulting in gas gangrene of the transplanted liver. Surgery. 1992;111(4):462–5.
9. Egger C, Bize P, Vaucher P, Mosimann P, Schneider B, Dominguez A, Meuli R, Mangin P, Grabherr S. Distribution of artifactual gas on post-mortem multidetector computed tomography (MDCT). Int J Legal Med. 2012;126(1):3–12.
10. Jackowski C, Sonnenschein M, Thali MJ, Aghayev E, Yen K, Dirnhofer R, Vock P. Intrahepatic gas at postmortem computed tomography: forensic experience as a potential guide for in vivo trauma imaging. J Trauma. 2007; 62(4):979–88.
11. Sapienza D, Bottari A, Gualniera P, Asmundo A, Perri F, Gaeta M. Post mortem CT of intrahepatic gas distribution in twenty-seven victims of a flood: patterns and timing. Legal Med. 2017;29:18–21.
12. Otsuka Y, Katagiri T, Ishii J, Maeda T, Kubota Y, Tamura A, Tsuchiya M, Kaneko H. Gas embolism in laparoscopic hepatectomy: what is the optimal pneumoperitoneal pressure for laparoscopic major hepatectomy? Journal of hepato-biliary-pancreatic sciences. 2013;20(2):137–40.
13. Eiriksson K, Fors D, Rubertsson S, Arvidsson D. High intra-abdominal pressure during experimental laparoscopic liver resection reduces bleeding but increases the risk of gas embolism. Br J Surg. 2011;98(6):845–52.
14. Kawahara T, Hagiwara M, Takahashi H, Tanaka M, Imai K, Sawada J, Kunisawa T, Furukawa H. Cerebral infarction by paradoxical gas embolism during laparoscopic liver resection with injury of the hepatic vessels in a patient without a right-to-left systemic shunt. The American journal of case reports. 2017;18:687–91.
15. Tsui CL, Fung HT, Chung KL, Kam CW. Focused abdominal sonography for trauma in the emergency department for blunt abdominal trauma. Int J Emerg Med. 2008;1(3):183–7.
16. Brown MA, Hauschildt JP, Casola G, Gosink BB, Hoyt DB. Intravascular gas as an incidental finding at US after blunt abdominal trauma. Radiology. 1999; 210(2):405–8.
17. Mayet M, Hardcastle TC, Muckart DJ. Benign portal venous gas after blunt abdominal trauma. Injury Extra. 2011;42:189–91.
18. Ginesu GC, Barmina M, Cossu ML, Feo CF, Fancellu A, Addis F, Porcu A. Conservative approach to hepatic portal venous gas: a case report. Int J Surg Case Rep. 2017;30:183–5.
19. Jun CH, Yoon JH, Wi JW, Park SY, Lee WS, Jung SI, Park CH, Joo YE, Kim HS, Choi SK, et al. Risk factors and clinical outcomes for spontaneous rupture of pyogenic liver abscess. J Dig Dis. 2015;16(1):31–6.

Preliminary experience with laparoscopic common bile duct exploration

Asaad F. Salama[1,2], Mohamed E. Abd Ellatif[3,4*], Hesham Abd Elaziz[1], Alaa Magdy[3], Hisham Rizk[1,6], Magdy Basheer[3], Wisam Jamal[1,6], Ibrahim Dawoud[3] and Ayman El Nakeeb[5]

Abstract

Background: Herein we present our experience with laparoscopic common bile duct exploration (LCBDE) in managing common bile duct stones.

Methods: Data of 129 consecutive patients who underwent laparoscopic cholecystectomy (LC) and LCBDE done at our institutes from April 2011 through June 2016 were prospectively recorded and retrospectively reviewed.

Results: Since 2011, 3012 laparoscopic cholecystectomy were performed at our institutes, intraoperative cholangiogram (IOC) was done in 295 (9.8%) patients which detected choledocholithiasis in 129 (4.3%) of them. LCBDE was successful to clear the common bile duct (CBD) in 123/129 (95.4%). Six patients underwent postoperative endoscopic retrograde cholangiopancreatography (ERCP) because of incomplete CBD clearance (4 cases), symptomatic stenosed papilla (2 cases). LCBDE was performed in 103 patients via trans-cystic approach and choledochotomy one in 26 patients. In the choledochotomy group, seven patients had primary closure of the CBD, CBD was closed over T-tube in nine patients whereas the remaining 10 patients the CBD was closed over antegrade inserted stent. The median time of hospital stay was 4 (range; 1–15) days. No patients showed retained CBD stones with mean follow up was 9 ± 3.4 months.

Conclusion: LCBDE is a safe and cost effective option for CBD stones in short-term outcome and can be performed provided proper laparoscopic expertise and facilities are available.

Keywords: Laparoscopic, Choledocholithiasis, Cholelithiasis

Background

Approximately 9–16% of patients who have gall bladder stone harbor common bile duct stones [1, 2]. Open cholecystectomy with CBD exploration and clearance was the standard treatment of CBD stone associated with gall bladder stone [3, 4]. With increasing experience in laparoscopy and as laparoscopic cholecystectomy (LC) became the standard treatment for gall bladder stone, management of CBD stones strategy has been changed and endoscopic retrograde cholangiopancreatography (ERCP) got the upper hand in this field preceded with or followed by LC (two stage procedure) [5]. It has been reported that endoscopic sphinctrotomy has up to 15% morbidity rates and 1% mortality rates and it also increase the cost cause of two stage procedure and it may cause recurrent ductal stones and stenosis of the papilla with cholangitis. Accordingly and in addition to the surge in laparoscopic experience, LCBDE becomes a potential option for managing CBD simultaneously with LC (one stage procedure) [6].

We aimed in this retrospective study to evaluate our initial experience in using LC and LCBDE as a single stage procedure for management of CBD stones with gall bladder in situ.

Methods

From April 2011 to June 2016, we performed 3012 laparoscopic cholecystectomy at our institutes (Theodore Bilharz Research Institute, Egypt, Mansura University Hospital-Egypt, Hafer Albatin Central Hospital, KSA, University of Jeddah-KSA, Al-Jahra hospital, Kuwait). Two hundred ninety-five patients had the indications to undergo intraoperative cholangiogram which documented presence of CBD

* Correspondence: surg_latif@hotmail.com
[3]Department of Surgery, Mansoura University Hospital, Gihan El Sadat St., Mansoura 35511, Dakahlia, Egypt
[4]Department of Surgery, Hafr Elbatin Central Hospital, Hafr Elbatin, Kingdom of Saudi Arabia
Full list of author information is available at the end of the article

stones in 129 patients. These 129 patients' data were prospectively collected and enrolled in this study.

Patients' selection

Patients with history of classic biliary pain and jaundice had underwent routine preoperative preparation including complete blood count (CBC), coagulation profile, kidney functions, liver function tests (LFTs), abdominal ultrasonography and routine pre-anaesthetic evaluation to determine ASA status. Magnetic resonance cholangiopancreatectomy (MRCP) was done in 31 patients. Intraoperative cholangiogram (IOC) was performed for patients with gall bladder stones who had one or more of the following; classic biliary pain, history of biliary pancreatitis, unexplained LFTs abnormalities, and radiologic evidence of dilated biliary tree or CBD stones. LCBDE was done if there were abnormal intraoperative cholangiogram findings (one or more) such as filling defect, wide diameter biliary tree or abnormal passage of contrast into the duodenum. This study was approved by institutional research board (IRB). An informed consent was obtained from all patients after been provided with information about their disease, the current updated treatment options and possibility of conversion to conventional one, T-tube insertion and postoperative ERCP if indicated.

On June 2016, the 129 patients' data sheets were retrospectively reviewed in respect to their preoperative, operative notes and postoperative data. Preoperative data include; age, gender, body mass index (BMI), ASA status, liver function tests (LFTs), ultrasonography and magnetic resonance cholangiopancreatectomy (MRCP) if done. Operative data include; operative time, transcystic or transcholedochal approach. Postoperatively, the hospital stay, wound infection, LFTs abnormalities or pancreatitis were all looked for as well as bile leak, cholangitis, bleeding and follow up data for stone recurrence.

Operative technique

All patients received prophylactic antibiotic and DVT prophylaxis according to the local policy. The procedure was done in supine position with adjustable operative bed to allow fluoroscopic C- arm for imaging the patient's right upper quadrant. The procedure was carried out using a 4-trocars laparoscopic cholecystectomy technique. After dissecting the Calot's triangle, the cystic artery was clipped and transected. A clip was applied on the gall bladder side of the cystic duct to prevent stone slippage either into CBD or the operative field while the cranial side was left connected with the CBD. A small diameter catheter was introduced through a small nick in the cystic duct down to the CBD to flush it and to do intraoperative cholangiogram to look for filling defect, its size, site, and number and free passage of contrast into the duodenum or any anatomical variation if any.

Transcystic clearance (103 patients)

After dilating the cystic duct and on a guide wire, the CBD stones were extracted by flushing or with help of Dormia basket or balloon catheter to pull stones into the intra-abdominal cavity to be retrieved. A complete stone clearance was confirmed by completion cholangiogram or choledechoscope. The CBD side of the cystic duct was clipped and the gall bladder was removed in the usual manner (Figs. 1 and 2).

Choledochotomy approach (26 patients)

This approach was used either after failed trial of cannulation of cystic duct or failed stone extraction through cystic duct, in three patients, we employed it without trying the trans-cystic technique because they were post failed ERCP due to big impacted stones. IOC was done through CBD puncture with lumber needle which showed CBD stones. In these cases we converted to choledochotomy in which the CBD was exposed and a vertical ductotomy was done on the anterior surface of the duct below the junction between cystic duct and CBD (Fig. 3). The techniques for stone clearance are

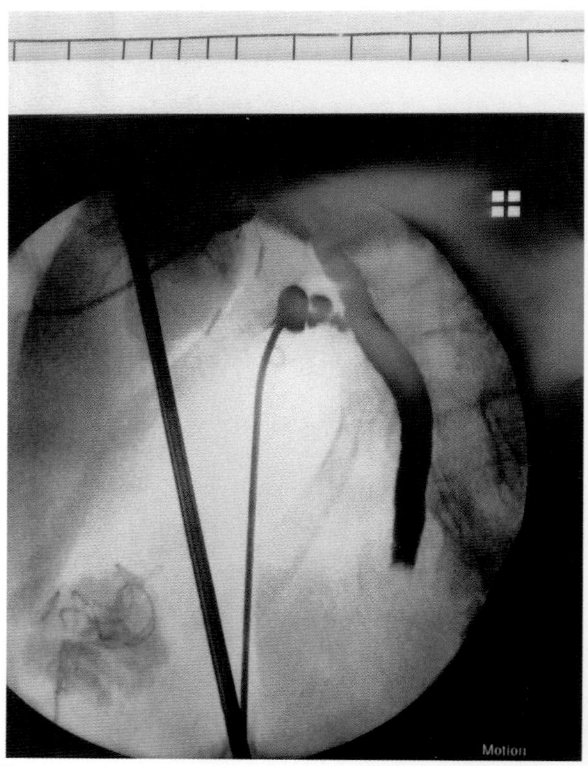

Fig. 1 intraoperative cholangiogram showing a filling defect that prevents passage of contrast into the duodenum

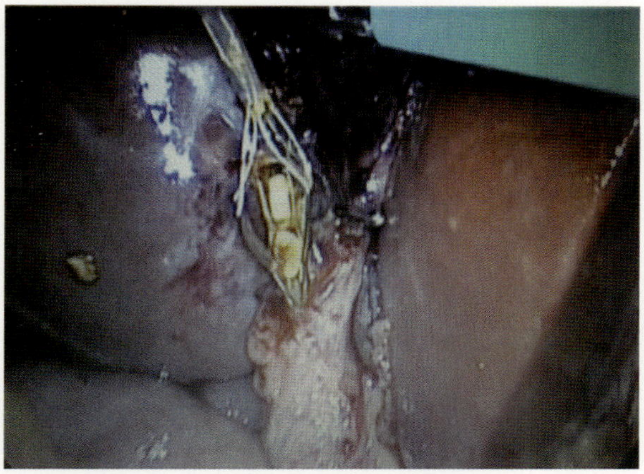

Fig. 2 Trans-cystic stone extraction by Dormia basket

identical to the trans-cystic approach. Through the choledochoscope, flushing with saline was done under pressure to facilitate clearance of small stones. Dormia basket and/or balloon catheter can be also used to pull stones to the abdominal cavity then to be retrieved outside (Fig. 4). The choledochotomy was closed over a T-tube in nine cases and over an antegrade stent in 10 cases; the stent was inserted through the site of cholodotomy under guidance of fluoroscopy for removal by ERCP later. Primary closure of the CBD was done in the remaining seven patients with absorbable suture. External tube drains were used only when we perform choledochotomy technique and not used in trans-cystic technique.

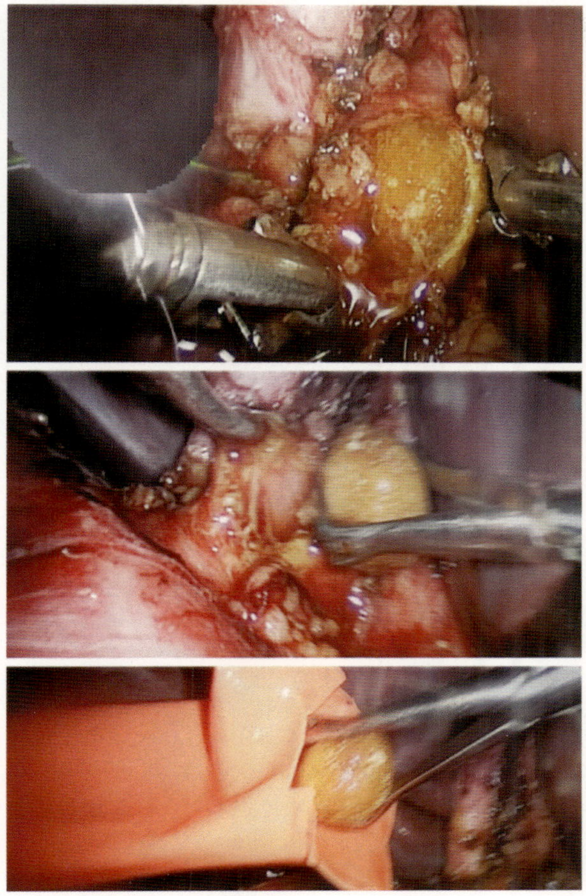

Fig. 3 Choledocotomy technique and extraction of big CBD stone

Statistics

All data were prospectively collected in designed sheets and were reviewed retrospectively for statistical purposes. Continuous variables were compared using a Student *t*-test or Mann-Whitney test, as appropriate. Chi-square test was used for comparing categorical variables. $P < 0.05$ was considered statistically significant. Data are expressed as mean (SD). Statistical analysis was performed using a commercially available software package (SPSS version 11.5 for Windows; SPSS Inc, Chicago, IL).

Results

From April 2011 to June 2016, we performed 3012 laparoscopic cholecystectomy at our institutes. 295 (9.8%) out 3012patients have undergone intraoperative cholangiogram and 129 (4.3%) were diagnosed to have choledocholithiasis. Male to female ratio was 43/86, with mean age of 37 ± 8 years (range 27 to 57 years) (Table 1). Transcystic exploration was done in 103 patients. Transcholedochal route was performed in 26 patients, 13 patients had too big CBD stones to be extracted through cystic duct, and 11 had failed cannulation of the cystic duct while in three patients choledochotomy was employed from the start due to post failed ERCP clearance of big impacted stones. In transcholedochal LCBDE group (26 patients), primary closure of CBD was done in seven patients, nine patients had CBD closed over T-tube whereas 10 patients closed over stent. All patients survived the operation with 0% conversion rate to open surgery. Six patients underwent postoperative ERCP because of incomplete CBD clearance (4 cases), symptomatic stenosed papilla (2 cases). The duration of the operation was 126 min (range, 102–140 min) in both trans-cystic and choledochotomy techniques. Intraoperative blood loss was minimal (less than 10 ml) with no intraoperative complications (Table 2).

During patients' stay, patients' assessment was done clinically and by laboratory evaluation. Transient colic pain occurred in two patients with elevated liver enzymes. One was managed conservatively and the other patient had sustained severe biliary colic for 2 days after her operation and sent for higher hospital to do ERCP which revealed very tight papilla without any CBD stones, sphincterotomy cured the problem. A transient increase in the LFTs (AST & ALT) was observed in three patients, it went back to

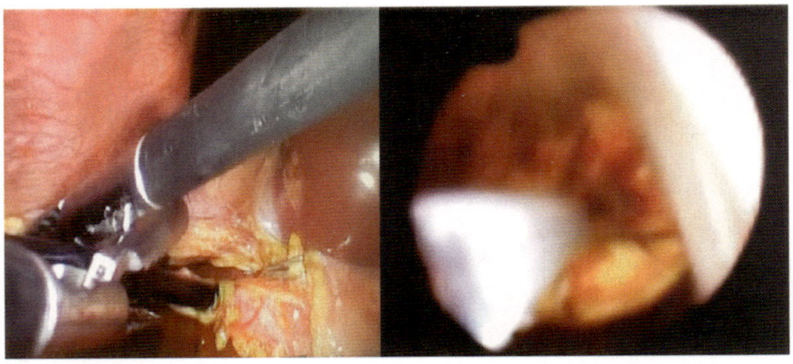

Fig. 4 Intraoperative trans-cystic Choledocoscope

normal on postoperative day 3 with no treatment (Table 3). All patients had an uneventful postoperative period and were discharged home with median hospital stay of 4 (range;1–15 days). In trans-cystic approach group, the patients were discharged home on day 3–4 postoperatively once we were completely assured that the operation. If T-tube was inserted, a post-operative cholangiogram was done after 7–10 days and if free, the tube was clamped and left in place for total 14 days. No haemobilia, abdominal bleeding, or pancreatitis occurred in our series.

Upon discharge, patients were instructed for first follow up after 1 week to have stitches and T-tube removed provided cholangiogram was unremarkable. Schedule of follow up was then given for patients every 6 months during the first year and annually thereafter. Clinical evaluations and liver function tests were done every visit and additional imaging studies were requested if needed. In one patient, T-tube was removed on day 11 post-operatively, but she developed bile leak after removal which necessitated 2 extra days admission, had been treated conservatively and discharged home in good condition. Another patient, female 37 years old, in choledochotomy group with T-tube closure, the catheter 6 Fr failed to pass through the papilla. The average T-tube drainage was around 400 ml bile and her postoperative cholangiogram showed tight papilla with no residual stones, she had been sent to another hospital to have ERCP which revealed no residual stones and sphincterotomy was sufficient. Her T-tube was clamped for one more week and removed after normal cholangiogram. Three patients developed wound infection

Table 1 Patients' characteristics and preoperative parameters

Variable	Patients $N = 129$
Age	37 ± 8 years (range 27 to 57 years)
Gender (female/male)	93/36
Weight	69 ± 13 (59–126 kg)
Height	157 ± 15 (149–178 cm)
BMI	29 ± 6 (23–46)
ASA	
ASA I	76 (59%)
ASA II	47 (36.4%)
ASA III	6 (4.6%)
Hx of biliary pain	59 (45.7%)
Hx of jaundice	9 (7%)
Hx of pancreatitis	13 (10%)
Mean bilirubin	1.003 ± 0.003 (0.3–3.2 mg)
Mean ALP	175 ± 19 (71–396 U)
Mean ALT	209 ± 32 (31–702 U)
Mean ALT	195 ± 29 (29–560 U)
Mean CBD diameter	7.3 ± 1.7 (4–19 mm)

ALP alkaline phosphatase, *ALT* Alanine transaminase, *AST* Aspartate transaminase, *hx* history, *ASA* American Society of Anesthesiologists

Table 2 Operative outcomes

Variable	Patients $N = 129$
Lap. Cholecystectomy	3012
IOC	295 (9.8%)
LCBDE	129 (4.3%)
Trans-cystic	103 (78.8%)
Trans-choledochotomy	26 (21.2%)
T-tube	10
Stent	9
Primary closure	7
Operative time	126 (range, 102–140 min)
LC	39 ± 13 (25–59 min)
Trans-cystic	40 ± 16 (37–63 min)
Trans-choledochotomy	59 ± 19 (47–109 min)
Mean No. of CBD stones	2.4 ± 1.6 (1–7)
Mean size of stones	4.2 ± 1.3 (3–15 mm)
Mean blood loss	10 ± 3.6 (5–50 ml)
Blood transfusion	0

IOC intraoperative cholangiogram, *CBD* common bile duct, *LCBDE* laparoscopic CBD exploration, *LC* laparoscopic cholecystectomy

Table 3 Postoperative outcomes

Variable	Patients $N = 129$
Return to oral intake	6 ± 2.3 (4–19 h)
Return to activity	17 ± 5.3 (6–29 h)
Hospital stay	4 (range;1–15 days)
-Trans-cystic	2 (range;1–3 days)
-Trans-choledochectomy	6 (range; 4–15 days)
Mean postop. bilirubin	0.6 ± 0.03 (0.4–3.2 mg)
Mean post-op. ALP	129 ± 18 (74–293 U)
Mean post-op. ALT	113 ± 11 (23–174 U)
Mean post-op. AST	159 ± 19 (19–163 U)
Mean T-tube cholangiogram	5.2 ± 3 (4–8 days)
T-tube removal	15.7 ± 4 (13–25 days)
Complications (I,II)	
-Pancreatitis (II)	0
-Cholangitis (II)	0
-Hemobilia (II)	0
-Accidental T-tube displacement (II)	0
-Transient liver enzymes elevation (I)	3 (2.3%)
-Wound infection (II)	3 (2.3%)
-Choleperitoneum (II)	1 (0.76%)
-Pneumonia (II)	0
-Biliary colic (II)	2 (1.5%)
-Abdominal bleeding (II)	0

ALP alkaline phosphatase, *ALT* Alanine transaminase, *AST* Aspartate transaminase, * Dindo-Clavien classification

(umbilical port) that was treated conservatively. There were no mortalities and all procedures had been completed laparoscopically with no conversion to open.

The mean follow up was 9 ± 3.4 months (2–39 months). No patients showed retained CBD stones by clinical, laboratory and imaging studies. We used the Dindo-Clavien classification to stratify the severity of operative and postoperative complications [7].

Discussion

If 9–16% of patients who have cholelithiasis harbour concomitant CBD choledocholithiasis, so it is a considerable problem that requires a proper strategy to solve. Options are many, starting from open cholecystectomy with open CBD exploration to laparoscopic cholecystectomy with pre- or post-operative ERCP then laparoscopic cholecystectomy with LCBDE. The introduction of laparoscopic CBD exploration has made it possible to avoid the drawbacks of both two-stages procedure (laparoscopic cholecystectomy plus pre- or post-operative ERCP) and also the drawbacks of the open CBD exploration [8, 9]. LCBD were not commonly used by surgeons till very late after introduction of laparoscopic cholecystectomy. The reasons for this delay are because it needs instrumental difficulties as well as the rely of most of surgeons on the alternative interventional methods especially ERCP because LCBDE is technically demanding and needs high level of experience [10, 11].

In this study, we present our preliminary experience of LCBDE in our institutes with success rate of 95.4% (123/129) which are comparable to the results of ERCP & open CBD exploration with less morbidity and mortality and hopefully the success rate will increase with increasing experience [12, 13].

The trans-cystic approach is technically easier, feasible, and less invasive with better patients' satisfaction. Surgeons usually try it first but it has its limitations and indications e.g. dilated cystic duct, small stones (preferably single stone) and there should be no stent in the CBD [3, 11–13]. We performed this approach in 103/129 (79.8%) patientswith success rate of 98/103 (95%) which is almost comparable to others. Whenever this approach is difficult or impossible, we converted to trans-choledochal one. The choledochotomy approach is technically demanding and needs advanced laparoscopic experience [6, 14, 15]. 29/129 (20.2%) patients have been undergone LCBDE through transcholedochal route with 28/29 (96.6%) success rate. We performed this choledochotomy approach after failed trials of trans-cystic route either due to failed cannulation or failed stone extraction through cystic duct. Choledochotomy technique was our first choice without trying the trans-cystic technique in three patients with failed ERCP due to impacted big stone in the CBD.

We routinely used intraoperative cholangiogram before stone extraction for confirmation the presence of stones and after to make sure of complete clearance of the CBD. Choledocoscope is a very helpful tool in CBD exploration, in both direct visualization of the intraluminal stones and also in removing them by the aid of Dormia basket or Fogarty's vascular catheter [8, 16–18]. We used the choledocoscope in most of our cases to confirm the complete clearance of the CBD and to inject saline for washout of stone fragments and debris.

In our study we closed the choledocotomy over T-tube in 10/26 cases (38.5%). Closure over T-tube provides biliary decompression especially when there was concern about retained fragments or tiny stones, it enables us for imaging the biliary system postoperatively and it provides an access through which any retained stones can be removed. T-tube has its disadvantages, it might make a way for bacteraemia, accidental premature dislodgment, obstruction and it might be associated with bile leak and peritonitis at its removal. Closure over stent was used in 9/26 cases (34.6%) which provides safe closure of choledochotomy as it provides biliary decompression same as T-tube does without its disadvantages, however, it needs follow up ERCP to remove it later. Finally, primary closure without stent was used in 7/

26 cases (26.9%) and wehave no bile leakage in our cases and we have no intra-abdominal collections as well.

However, the length of stay for the laparoscopic cholecystectomy is generally short (from 1 to 3 days), it is longer for laparoscopic CBD exploration 1–7 days in most of studies [12, 18–20]. In our study, the length of stay depended upon the technique employed; it was 1–3 days in trans-cystic group and longer (4–15 days) in choledocotomy one especially when we used T-tube to close the choledocotomy.

In most of studies the mortality of laparoscopic CBD exploration is 0 to 1% in the hands of experienced biliary surgeons. This rate is similar to the incidence found in open CBD exploration [21–25]. In our study, we have no reported mortality cases, which may be attributed to improved preoperative preparation, improved anaesthesia and selection of cases.

Our study has some limitations, it is a retrospective study and showed a wide heterogeneity among the surgeons' experience in performing this LCBDE. The sample size of patients enrolled in this study is relatively small. This study represents our initial experience in preforming LCBDE, this represents a limitation per say. We recommend for another study to be done in a prospective way and to enrol a much larger sample size.

Laparoendoscopic rendezvous is a promising alternative and has many pros; it provides selective cannulation of CBD and avoids both inadvertent cannulation of pancreatic duct with subsequent accidental injection of the contrast under pressure into the pancreatic duct [26]. We had six patients underwent postoperative ERCP, 4 because of incomplete CBD and two cases due to symptomatic stenosis of the papilla. Some hospitals at which this study was conducted are lacking for ERCP services. ERCP is crucial because it is the cornerstone for LCBDE, it provides an alternative optionfor patients with CBD stones synchronous with gall bladder stones and relieved stenosis when present as shown in our study. Therefore a limitation in our study is the lack of access of ERCP for the six patients due to unavailability in hospitals (two patients) and gastroenterologists (four patients). However, if available, Laparoendoscopic rendezvous would have been an excellent intervention for these six patients.

Conclusion

Laparoscopic CBD exploration is an effective single stage procedure for the treatment of GB and CBD stone in one session making use of the benefits of minimally invasive approach and avoiding the drawbacks of ERCP as well as open CBD approach. LCBDE can be performed after proper training and adequate equipment and laparoscopic facilities.

Abbreviations

ASA: American Society of Anesthesiologists; BMI: Body mass index; CBD: Common bile duct; DVT: Deep vein thrombosis; ERCP: Endoscopic retrograde cholangiopancreatography; GB: Gall bladder; IOC: Intraoperative cholangiogram; LC: Laparoscopic cholecystectomy; LCBDE: Laparoscopic common bile duct exploration; LFTs: Liver function tests; MRCP: Magnetic resonance cholangiopancreatectomy

Acknowledgements

Not applicable.

Authors' contributions

AFS, MEAE, HAE, HR, AM, WJ, MB, ID, AE performed the research, AFS, MEAE, ID, MB and AE analyzed the data, HAE, HR, AM, WJ designed the research, and AFS, MEAE wrote the paper. All authors read and approved the final manuscript.

Competing interests

The authors declare that they have no competing interests.

Author details

[1]Department of Surgery, Theodore Bilharz Research Institute, Cairo, Egypt. [2]Department of Surgery, Al-Jahra Hospital, Jahra, Kuwait. [3]Department of Surgery, Mansoura University Hospital, Gihan El Sadat St., Mansoura 35511, Dakahlia, Egypt. [4]Department of Surgery, Hafr Elbatin Central Hospital, Hafr Elbatin, Kingdom of Saudi Arabia. [5]Gastroenterology Surgical Center, Mansoura University, Mansoura, Egypt. [6]Department of Surgery, University of Jeddah, Jeddah, Kingdom of Saudi Arabia.

References

1. Nahrwold D. The biliary system. In: Sabiston X, editor. Textbook of surgery. Philadelphia: WE Saunders; 1986.
2. Way LW, Admirand WJ, Dunphy JE. Management of choledocholithiasis. Ann Surg. 1972;176:347–59.
3. Petelin JB. Laparoscopic common bile duct exploration: Lessons learned from > 12 years experience. Surg Endosc. 2003;17(11):1705–15.
4. Escat J, Fourtanier G, Maigne C, Vaislic C, Fournier D, Prevost F. Choledochoscopy in common bile duct surgery for choledocholithiasis: a must. Am Surg. 1985;51(3):166–7.
5. Fink AS. Current dilemmas in management of common duct stones. Surg Endosc. 1993;7:285–91.
6. Newman KD, Powell DM, Holcomb III GW. The Management of Choledocholithiasis in Children in the Era of Laparoscopic Cholecystectomy. J Pediatr Surg. 1997;32(7):1116–9.
7. Clavien PA, Barkun J, de Oliveira ML, et al. The Clavien-Dindo classification of surgical complications: five-year experience. Ann Surg. 2009;250(2):187–96.
8. Petelin JB. Laparoscopic common bile duct exploration. Surg Endosc. 2003;17(11):1705-715.
9. Traverso LW, Roush TS, Koo K. CBD stones-outcomes and costs. Laparoscopic transcystic techniques other than choledochoscopy. Surg Endosc. 1995;9(11):1242–4.
10. Liberman MA, Phillips EH, Carroll BJ, Fallas MJ, Rosenthal R, Hiatt J. Cost-Effective Management of Complicated Choledocholithiasis: Laparoscopic Transcystic Duct Exploration or Endoscopic Sphincterotomy. J Am Coll Surg. 1996;182:488–94.
11. Phillips EH. Laparoscopic transcystic duct common bile duct exploration—outcome and costs. Surg Endosc. 1995;9(11):1240–2.
12. Topal B, Aerts R, Penninckx F. Laparoscopic common bile duct stone clearance with flexible choledochoscopy. Surg Endosc. 2007;21(12):2317–321.
13. Hanif F, Ahmed Z, Samie MA, Nassar AHM. Laparoscopic transcystic bile duct exploration: the treatment of first choice for common bile duct stones. Surg Endosc. 2010;24(7):1552–556.
14. Traverso LW. A cost-effective approach to the treatment of common bile duct stones with surgical versus endoscopic techniques. In: Berci G, Cuschieri A, editors. Bile Ducts and Bile Duct Stones. Philadelphia: WB Saunders; 1996. p. 154–60.

15. Perissat J, Huibregtse K, Keane FV, Russell CG, Neoptolemos JP. Management of bile duct stones in the era of laparoscopic cholecystectomy. Br J Surg. 1994;81:799–810.
16. Petelin J. Laparoscopic approach to common duct pathology. Surg Laparosc Endosc. 1991;1:33–41.
17. Hunter J. Laparoscopic transcystic common bile duct exploration. Am J Surg. 1992;163:53–8.
18. Carroll BJ, Phillips EH, Daykhovsky L, Grundfest WS, Gersham A, Fallas M, et al. Laparoscopic choledochoscopy: an effective approach to the common duct. J Laparoendosc Surg. 1992;2:15–21.
19. Sackier JM, Berci G, Pas-Partlow M. Laparoscopic transcystic-choledochotomy as an adjunct to laparoscopic cholecystectomy. Am Surg. 1991;57:323–6.
20. Jacobs M, VCerdeja JC, Goldstein HS. Laparoscopic choledocho-lithotomy. Jnl Laparoendosc Surg. 1991;1(2):79–82.
21. Quattlebaum JK, Flanders HD. Laparoscopic treatment of common bile duct stones. Surg Laparosc Endosc. 1991;1(1):26–32.
22. Appel S, Krebs H, Fern D. Techniques for laparoscopic cholangiography and removal of common duct stones. Surg Endosc. 1992;6:134–7.
23. Dion YM, Morin J, Dionne G, Dejoie C. Laparoscopic cholecystectomy and choledocholithiasis. Can J Surg. 1992;35:67–74.
24. Fanning NF, Horgan PG, Keane FBV. Evolving management of common bile duct stones in the laparoscopic era. J R Coll Surg Edinb. 1997;42:389–94.
25. Heili MJ, Wintz NK, Fowler DL. Choledocholithiasis: Endoscopic versus Laparoscopic Management. Am Surg. 1999;65:135–8.
26. Baloyiannis I, Tzovaras G. Current status of laparoendoscopic rendezvous in the treatment of cholelithiasis with concomitant choledocholithiasis. World J Gastrointest Endosc. 2015;7(7):714–9.

A case report of simultaneous orthotopic liver transplantation and jejunectomy

Guoyong Chen[1†], Sidong Wei[1†], Zhongwu Zou[2], Jianjun Sun[1], Gaofeng Tang[1], Jianbin Chen[1] and Shaotang Zhou[3*]

Abstract

Background: Liver transplantation (LT) accompanied by jejunectomy to treat patients with acute or chronic hepatic cirrhosis with thrombosis in the portal system is extremely rare.

Case presentation: A 47-year-old man presented with hematemesis and melena, and a diagnosis of decompensated cirrhosis, chronic portal vein thrombosis (PVT) and secondary gastro-esophageal variceal hemorrhage was made. Coagulants were administered, but portal vein thrombi occurred rapidly, and gastrointestinal bleeding recurred shortly thereafter. The patient underwent LT, phlebothrombectomy and a partial jejunectomy. His recovery from a fistula was uneventful, and follow-up visits over 70 months were unremarkable.

Conclusion: Liver transplantation and partial jejunectomy is a feasible and effective surgical option for select patients with end-stage liver disease accompanied by acute portal venous thrombosis.

Keywords: Acute-on-chronic, End-stage liver disease, Portal vein thrombosis, Liver transplantation, Phlebothrombectomy, Jejunectomy

Background

Chronic portal vein thrombosis (PVT) is a vascular disease that commonly occurs in end-stage liver disease patients waiting for liver transplantation (LT), and it causes challenges for transplant specialists. Nearly three decades ago, advanced cirrhosis and PVT were contraindications for liver transplantation because of surgical technique limitations. In 1985, Shaw et al. first reported using a venous graft conduit to bypass the thrombotic segmental vessel to successfully overcome surgical limitations during LT [1].

More clinical cases were subsequently reported about this entity because of imaging technology progress, such as ultrasound, computerized tomography and magnetic resonance that can detect disease alone or in combination before transplantation [2]. Its prevalence in orthotopic liver transplantation candidates ranged from 2.1 to 21 % [3–5].

Thrombi in the main portal vein can extend to different splanchnic veins because of predisposing factors. Based on how rapidly PVT and collateral veins develop, PVT was clinically classified as either acute or chronic [6–8]. If there is a lack of collateral veins, thrombosis develops quickly and results in congestive ischemia and subsequent gut necrosis, which are typical clinical presentations of acute PVT. However, chronic PVT, which is more common, is almost asymptomatic and develops over months or years. Yerdle et al. graded 4 forms of chronic PVT based on the extent of occlusion and mesenteric veins involved [9], and many surgical strategies had been subsequently developed to revascularize the maintain blood flow to the transplanted liver [10–12]. There have been no cases of LT candidates with acute PVT that is accompanied by intestinal necrosis. Here, we present the first case of a patient with acute-on-chronic PVT with intestinal necrosis that occurred during LT that was used to treat end-stage liver cirrhosis.

Case presentation

A 47-year-old male patient was admitted with esophagogastric hemorrhage secondary to portal hypertension derived from decompensated cirrhosis. At the initial

* Correspondence: zsun7379@yahoo.com
†Equal contributors
[3]Center of Hepatopancreaticobiliary Surgery and Liver transplantation, 100 Xisihuang Middle Road, Fengtai District, Beijing 100039, China
Full list of author information is available at the end of the article

consultation, his chief complaint was hematemesis and two episodes of melena. His past medical history was viral hepatitis B with HBsAg + and HBcAb + for more than 10 years, and his surgical history included splenectomy and periesophagogastric devascularization for portal hypertension, hypersplenism and splenomegaly, and cholecystectomy for gallstones one year before, at a different hospital. His vital signs were as follows: temperature, 36.7 °C; blood pressure, 120/68 mmHg; respiratory rate, 20; and heart rate, 84. He had scleral icterus in both eyes. Physical examination showed negative chest and cardiac findings. Tenderness and rebound pain was marked, and shift dullness was remarkable. His blood work results were as follows: white blood cell count, 16.6×10^9/l; red blood cell count, 2.47×10^{12}/l; platelet cell count, 183×10^9/l; and hemoglobin, 67 g/l. Stool hemoccult test results were positive (+++). His liver function profile was as follows: total bilirubin, 84 μmol/l; ALT, 319; AST, 347; albumin, 32.3 g/l; C-reactive protein, 107 mg/l; alpha-fetoprotein, normal; carcinoembryonic antigen concentration test, normal; and amylase, unremarkable. The patient's coagulopathy parameters were as follows: PT, 19.3 s; PT%, 43.6 %; fibrinogen, 1.4 g/l; APTT, 120.9 s; and TT, 21.3 s.

Paracentesis fluid revealed serosanguinous ascites, and bacterial culture showed that no bacteria were present. Enhanced computerized tomography results showed hepatic nodular regeneration, moderate ascites, a dilated bowel, and emboli in the portal vein and the superior mesenteric vein that extended to the distal and tributary veins (Fig. 1). Melena and hematemesis reoccurred after administering coagulants including thrombase and tranexamic acid, which were administered for a few days. The patient was moved to transplant surgery to await a donated liver.

Two days later, the liver from a 35-year-old deceased male with ABO-compatibility was available, and liver transplantation and thrombectomy were planned. After entry into the abdominal cavity, approximately 2.5 l of ascites was removed using suction. The abdominal cavity was explored; the liver had several nodules, the spleen and gall bladder had been excised, complete occlusion of the portal vein and the superior mesenteric vein (Grade III-IV) was found, and two segments of the proximal jejunum were purplish-black in color. A short distal vein arcade was fully occluded, and there was intestinal necrosis with intestinal tone and no perforation (Figs. 2 and 3). Ascites culture results were negative, which suggested that there was no bacterial translocation. Intraoperative ultrasound confirmed the permeability of the superior mesenteric artery, which had a palpable pulse. Further histology results showed nodular hyperplasia that excluded small cancer. Orthotopic LT was then performed using a piggy-back caval anastomosis, and portal vein eversion was then conducted to remove the thrombi in the portal and superior mesenteric veins. These veins were cavernous, with numerous small thrombi that were flushed out via blood flow. Portal venous blood flow was restored and confirmed intra-operatively using a Doppler ultrasonic flow meter (data not shown), and 25 units of plasma and packed red cells were transfused. Approximately 100 cm of gangrenous jejunum was subsequently resected from Treitz's ligament, and an end-to-end anastomosis of the jejunum was performed to maintain intestinal continuity. The patient recovered fully, although a fistula occurred, which resolved upon draining.

Medications such as the following were administered: immunosuppressive therapy to treat immune rejection, potent broad-spectrum antibiotics to treat potential infection, anti-coagulant agents to treat re-embolism, and lamivudine and immunoglobulin to prevent hepatitis B viral infection recurrence. The allograft functioned well, and ALT, AST and bilirubin levels decreased daily, while albumin levels increased. Thirteen days after OLT, a fistula occurred in the anastomosis, and laparoscopic

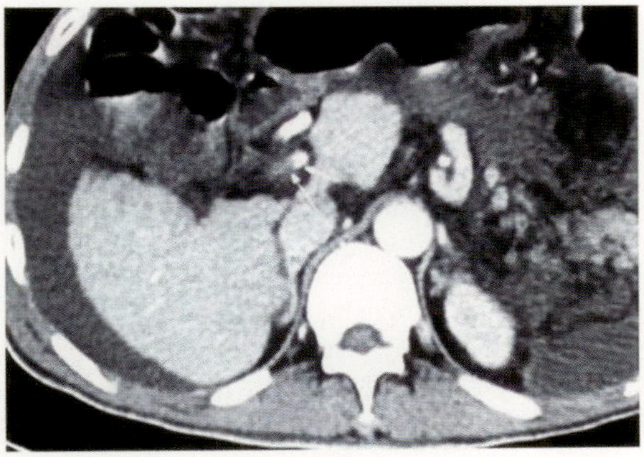

Fig. 1 Computerized tomography scan showed ascites, cirrhosis, emboli in portal vein system (arrows)

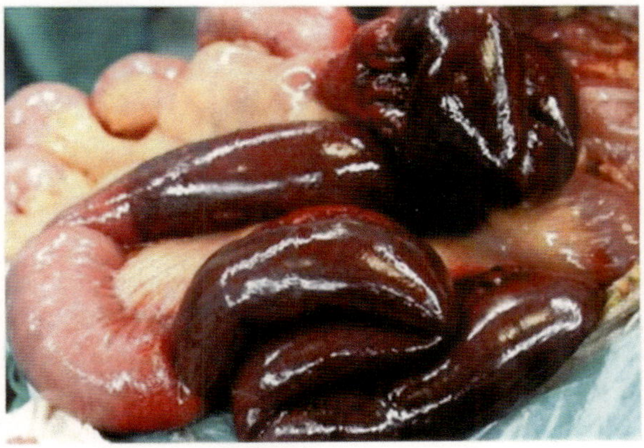

Fig. 2 Appearance of the to-be excised jejunum

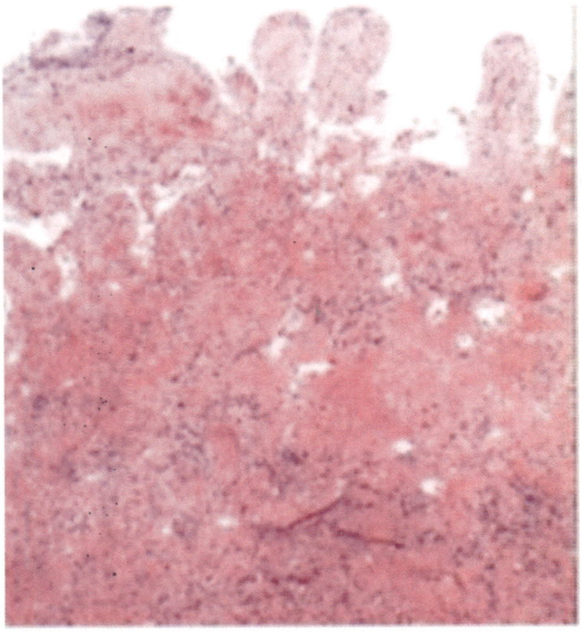

Fig. 3 H&Estain ng showed necrosis in the intestinal wall

surgery was performed again to allow suction and access to the abdominal cavity. A 4-cm mushroom-shaped tube was inserted into the near jejunum to allow drainage, and a feeding tube was also inserted into the distal intestine. After about 3 weeks, the patient was recovering well. Seventy months after surgery, the patient's allograft was functioning well and his medical history has been uneventful.

Discussion

We report the case of a cirrhosis patient with acute-on-chronic PVT. Chronic PVT is a commonly encountered problem in LT candidates [13], and it is characterized by a slow progression into cavernomatosis transformation and portal hypertension. Refractory ascites, gastrointestinal bleeding and disproportional abdominal pain are the physical findings that clinicians observe, and a diagnosis of chronic PVT is usually made by chance [14]. In a patient with an acquired hypercoagulable or primary pro-thrombotic state, chronic PVT can develop into acute PVT because of precipitating factors including pro-coagulants administered to treat bleeding. Acute PVT also has no specific symptoms and signs; intestinal ischemia and necrosis are typical clinical presentations, while abdominal pain, distention, diarrhea, and bleeding are manifestations. However, PVT it is usually not diagnosed at the early stage or before surgical interventions [15]. For our patient, PVT was diagnosed during laparotomy, not pre-transplant. If the thrombi do not resolve, ischemia and gut necrosis will eventually ensue, resulting in peritonitis and septic shock, which will preclude more complex liver transplantation. Patients with cirrhosis and high-grade PVT were shown to have low survival compared with the patients who were PVT-free (5), and their PVT recurrence rate is unacceptably high [16]. An explanation for why few PVT cases have been reported in LT candidates with acute PVT may be because perforation will probably lead to bacterial translocation, and peritonitis or septic shock will ensue, which will endanger the liver allograft and recipient's life. The risk of recurrence and the mortality rate both remain high after LT for PVT. Additionally, an organ donor is not always available, or other patients on the waitlist are considered to be a higher priority to receive donor organs.

Gastrointestinal bleeding is a common complication of PVT. There is consensus that endoscopic variceal obturation is the first-line treatment option, and that it is beneficial to use anticoagulant drugs if the thrombus extends into the PVT and superior mesenteric vein, even in the event of upper gastrointestinal bleeding when the diagnosis was made. Anticoagulant use is associated with low recurrence and high recanalization [17]. For this patient, thrombi seemed to be diffuse, and thrombectomy was used efficiently to ensure blood flow to the liver graft. This is a simple and useful procedure is usually the first choice, especially for acute thrombi. In the hypercoagulable state, thrombi form in the small vessels arising from the superior mesenteric vein, and predisposing factors involve the large veins. Thrombogenesis initiates compression at the site of the main portal vein, and it then extends distally to the superior mesenteric vein [18]. Thrombi that formed in the short time when they were loosely and sparsely adhered to the venous tunica intima were flushed by blood outflow in our patient. Michael et al. reported that phlebothrombectomy was performed successfully in 90 % of these patients [5]. To our knowledge, this is the first report that details treatment of an LT candidate with PVT followed by acute onset and subsequent intestinal ischemia.

Conclusions

In conclusion, isolated resection of intestinal gangrene without perforation that results from acute PVT may not jeopardize liver transplantation in patients with end-stage cirrhosis. Multidisciplinary collaborations and improved imaging technology are needed to screen and prevent rapid progression of PVT at the early stage, and decisive and aggressive approaches are crucial for favorable outcomes.

Abbreviations

LT: Liver transplantation; PVT: Portal vein thrombosis

Funding
Sponsored by the National Natural Science Foundation of China (No. 81370577).

Authors' contributions
GYC: wrote the draft. SDW: revised and discussed the meaning of the manuscript. ZWZ: collected all reference. JJS: responsible for pathology. GFT and JBC: collected all data of the clinical. STZ: offered the conception, design and finalized the draft. All authors read and approved the final manuscript.

Competing interests
The authors declare that they have no competing interests.

Author details
[1]Center of Hepatopancreaticobiliary Surgery, Henan Provincial People's Hospital, Zhengzhou, Henan 450003, China. [2]Hubei Vocational-Technical College School of Medicine, Xiaogan 432000, China. [3]Center of Hepatopancreaticobiliary Surgery and Liver transplantation, 100 Xisihuang Middle Road, Fengtai District, Beijing 100039, China.

References
1. Shaw Jr BW, Iwatsuki S, Bron K, Starzl TE. Portal vein grafts in hepatic transplantation. Surg Gynecol Obstet. 1985;161:66–8.
2. Condat B, Pessione F, Helene DM, Hillaire S, Valla D. Recent portal or mesenteric venous thrombosis: increased recognition and frequent recanalization on anticoagulant therapy. Hepatology. 2000;32:466–70.
3. Shaked A, Busuttil RW. Liver transplantation in patients with portal vein thrombosis and central portocaval shunts. Ann Surg. 1991;214:696–702.
4. Davidson BR, Gibson M, Dick R, Burroughs A, Rolles K. Incidence, risk, factors, management, and outcome of portal vein abnormalities at orthotopic liver transplantation. Transplantation. 1994;57:1174–7.
5. Englesbe MJ, Kubus J, Muhammad W, et al. Portal vein thrombosis and survival in patients with cirrhosis. Liver Transpl. 2010;16:83–90.
6. DeLeve LD, Valla D-C, Tsao GG. Vascular disorders of the liver. AASLD practice guidelines. Hepatology. 2009;5:1729–64.
7. Ponziani FR, Zocco MA, Chiara C, Emanuele R, Annalisa T, Luca Di M. Portal vein thrombosis: insight into physiopathology, diagnosis, and treatment. World J Gastroente. 2010;16:143–55.
8. Suarez Artacho G, Barrera Pulido L, Alamo Martinez JM, Serrano Diez-Canedo J, Bernal Bellido C, Marı´n Gomez LM. Outcomes of liver transplantation in candidates with portal vein thrombosis. Transplant Proc. 2002;8:3156–8.
9. Yerdel MA, Gunson B, Mirza D, Karayalcin K, Oliff S, Buckels J. Portal vein thrombosis in adults undergoing liver transplantation: risk factors, screening, management, and outcome. Transplantation. 2000;69:1873–81.
10. Stieber AC, Zetti G, Todo S, et al. The spectrum of portal vein thrombosis in liver transplantation. Ann Surg. 1991;213:199–206.
11. Dumortier J, Czyglik O, Poncet G, Blanchet MC, Boucaud C, Henry L. Eversion thrombectomy for portal vein thrombosis during liver transplantation. Am J Transplant. 2002;2:934–8.
12. Molmenti EP, Roodhouse TW, Molmenti H, Jaiswal K, Jung G, Marubashi S. Thrombendovenectomy for organized portal vein thrombosis at the time of liver transplantation. Ann Surg. 2002;235:292–6.
13. Orlando G, De Luca L, Toti L. Liver transplantation in the presence of portal vein thrombosis: report from a single center. Transplant Proc. 2004;36:199–202.
14. Bradbury MS, Kavanagh PV, Bechtold RE, et al. Mesenteric Venous thrombosis: Diagnosis and Noninvasive Imaging. Education exhibit RG. 2002;527–41.
15. Webster GJM, Burroughs AK, Riordan SM. Review article: portal vein thrombosis – new insights into aetiology and management. Aliment Pharmacol Ther. 2005;21:1–9.
16. Huard G, Bilodeau M. Management of Anticoagulation for Portal Vein Thrombosis in Individuals with Cirrhosis: A Systematic Review. Int J Hepatol. 2012;2012:1-6.
17. Sobhonslidsuk A, Reddy KR. Portal vein thrombosis: a concise review. Am J Gastroenterol. 2002;97:535.
18. Kumar S, Sarr MG, Kamath P. Mesenteric venous thrombosis. N Engl J Med. 2001;345:1683–8.

Splenectomy before adult liver transplantation: a retrospective study

LingXiang Kong, Ming Li, Lei Li, Li Jiang, Jiayin Yang* and Lvnan Yan

Abstract

Background: A considerable number of patients with portal hypertension (PHT) have to undergo splenectomy because they do not meet the requirements for liver transplantation (LT) or cannot find a suitable liver donor. However, it is not known whether pre-transplantation splenectomy may create occult difficulties for patients who require LT in future.

Methods: We analyzed 1059 consecutive patients who underwent adult liver transplantation (ADLT). Patients with pre-transplantation splenectomy Sp(+) and without splenectomy Sp(−) were compared using a propensity score analysis to create the best match between groups.

Results: There were no differences between patients in group Sp(+) and group Sp(−) with respect to the main post-operative infections (12.20% vs. 15.85%, $P = 0.455$), and the incidence of major complications (6.10% vs. 10.98%, $P = 0.264$). The post-operative platelet count was significantly higher in group Sp(+) ($P = 0.041$), while group Sp(−) had a higher rate of post-operative thrombocytopenia (91.46% vs. 74.39%, $P = 0.006$) and early allograft dysfunction (EAD) (23.20% vs. 10.98%, $P = 0.038$). The 5-year overall survival rates were similar in groups Sp(−) and Sp(+) (69.7% vs. 67.6%, $P = 0.701$).

Conclusions: Compared with Sp(−), the risk of infection and post-operative complications in group Sp(+) was not increased, while group Sp(−) had a higher rate of post-operative EAD. Moreover, pre-transplantation splenectomy is very effective for the prevention of thrombocytopenia after LT. Pre-transplantation splenectomy is recommended in cases with risky PHT patients without appropriate source of liver for LT.

Keywords: Splenectomy, Liver transplantation, Thrombocytopenia, Early allograft dysfunction

Background

The incidence of PHT with post-hepatitis cirrhosis is higher in China than elsewhere worldwide [1]. Early complications caused by increased portal pressure, such as variceal hemorrhage, can be treated with vein ligation under endoscopy and injection; however, it is mandatory to switch to decompressive shunt procedures if endoscopic therapy fails to control recurrent variceal hemorrhage [2].

With the advent of LT, simple symptomatic treatment is no longer used for end-stage liver disease, but radical treatment by LT is often performed, greatly increasing the survival rate of patients with end-stage liver disease. Liver diseases are frequently accompanied by PHT, and splenectomy is one of the basic means of treatment of this condition. However, given the great number of patients with end-stage liver disease, a considerable number of patients would require splenectomy to reduce portal pressure, because they do not meet the requirements for transplantation or cannot find suitable liver donor. Splenectomy plays a significant role in improving the survival of patients and can create precious time for subsequent treatment. However, it is not known whether splenectomy may create occult difficulties for patients who require LT in future.

In the past, many scholars stated their views with regard to this point. Starzl et al. [3] were the first to suggest the role of splenectomy in the prolongation of allograft survival, as four of their five patients treated with thymectomy and splenectomy maintained their renal function for almost 6 months. Later, Hume et al. suggested that splenectomy, if performed prior to or at the time of transplantation, could improve leukocyte count and permit administration of large

* Correspondence: yangjygyz@163.com
Department of Liver Surgery, West China Hospital of Sichuan University, Chengdu, Sichuan Province, China

doses of azathioprine (AZA). With a view to preventing thrombocytopenia, and when using AZA after transplantation, splenectomy was often considered as a preventive surgery. With the discovery of cyclosporine and is application after liver transplant, preoperative or intraoperative splenectomy for liver transplant patients has become rather controversial, and is no longer a routine surgery. In addition, Troisi et al. [4] observed that massive ascites loss was associated with extremely high portal flow and histologically proven graft congestion. Splenectomy reduces the portal flow, resolving the ascites problem. However, a relative increase in mesenteric blood flow, containing nutrient-rich blood [5], or a reduction in liver congestion can contribute to liver regeneration [6]. Moreover, patients with hepatitis C virus (HCV) are commonly treated with interferons. Hirotaka et al. [7] have suggested that, to complete pre-emptive interferon therapy, which is initiated approximately 2 months after the operation, splenectomy should be performed simultaneously with LT in HCV patients with a platelet count of < 60/L.

At present, even though there are many related reports, there is no consensus on pre-transplantation splenectomy and current LT standards for hepatocarcinoma (HCC) also lack a description of such patients, such as Milan criteria [8], UCSF criteria [9], Hangzhou criteria [10] and BCLC criteria [11]. Therefore, we studied a series of patients at our institution. We here report the results of a retrospective analysis of adult liver transplant patients who had undergone splenectomy.

Methods

In our study, the grafts for LT were from donation after cardiac death. No prisoners were included as donors. The protocol was approved by the Ethics Committee of the West China Hospital of Sichuan University West China Hospital. Written informed consent was obtained from all the recipients prior to their surgery, and all of donations were voluntary and altruistic in all cases, and were in accordance with the ethical guidelines of the Declaration of Helsinki.

Patients

Figure 1 shows the inclusion and exclusion criteria used for establishing the study cohort. Based on the different preoperative intervention methods, they were initially divided into 2 groups: Sp(−)group, which consisted of patients who underwent LT without preoperative splenectomy and the Sp(+), which consisted of those who underwent splenectomy before LT. The indication in our study for splenectomy was progressive, invalidating and/or risky PHT (large splenomegaly, hypersplenism with platelet and/or polymorphonuclear cells count less than 100 Giga/L and 4

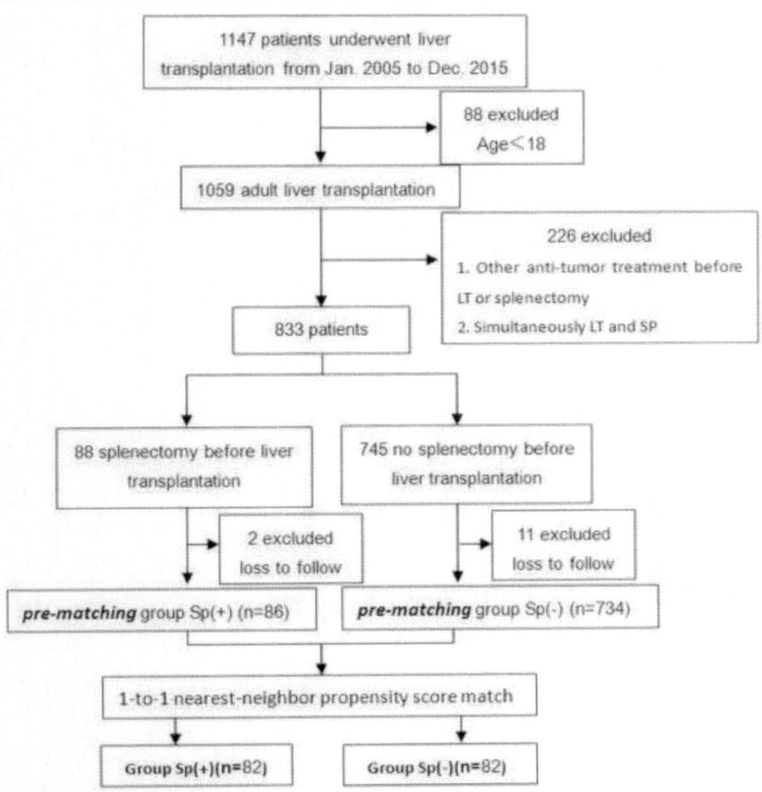

Fig. 1 Flow of study participants. Sp(+), Splenectomy before liver transplantation; Sp(−), No splenectomy before liver transplantation

Giga/L respectively, grade II or more esophageal varices with the presence of red signs or previous bleeding) in patients with preserved liver and lung function [12]. Disease features and perioperative characteristics of patients when they underwent pre-transplant splenectomy were summarized in Additional file 1: Table S1. All patients were treated with only total splenectomy without partial splenectomy or anther surgery. The indication for LT in our study was end-stage liver diseases [13]. All HCC patients in our study were without vascular invasion and extra hepatic metastasis and summarized in Table 1.

To ensure the consistency of baseline data, none of the enrolled patients received any other therapies before surgery. All hepatitis B virus (HBV) DNA-positive patients were treated with anti-viral therapy before and after surgery. They were monitored until Dec. 2015 or until their death, and their medical records were retrospectively reviewed. Clinical and demographic data of donors and recipients were collected from the records of the Chinese Liver Transplant Registry (http://cltr.cotr.cn), and patient demographics, disease features, perioperative course, and long-term outcomes were compared between group Sp(+) and group Sp(−) patients.

Definitions

The Clavien–Dindo complication classification [13] system was used for post-operative complication grading and grade III–IV complications were defined as severe complications. Clinically relevant PHT is defined as the presence of esophageal varices and/or a platelet count of less than 100,000 per mL in association with splenomegaly [14]. EAD defined as the presence of one or more of the following postoperative laboratory: bilirubin ≥10 mg/dL on day 7, international normalized ratio ≥1.6 on day 7,

Table 1 Baseline demographic and disease features characteristics in the two groups

Variables	Before matching		*P* value	After matching		*P* value
	Sp + (*n* = 86)	Sp- (*n* = 734)		Sp + (*n* = 82)	Sp- (*n* = 82)	
Donor						
Age (mean ± SD, years)	34.38 ± 9.46	33.58 ± 9.62	0.465	34.13 ± 9.39	34.94 ± 9.29	0.582
Male (%)	72(83.3%)	611(82.2%)	0.910	69(84.1%)	67(81.7%)	0.836
height (mean ± SD, cm)	166.62 ± 7.48	167.82 ± 6.69	0.121	166.67 ± 7.45	167.10 ± 6.21	0.689
weight (mean ± SD, kg)	61.56 ± 6.45	63.52 ± 7.38	0.019	62.00 ± 6.29	62.10 ± 6.98	0.913
BMI (mean ± SD, kg/m^2)	22.14 ± 1.65	22.50 ± 2.05	0.117	22.28 ± 1.53	22.20 ± 1.85	0.779
Recipient						
Age (mean ± SD, years)	46.34 ± 8.44	44.52 ± 9.90	0.102	46.32 ± 8.39	46.41 ± 9.64	0.945
Male (%)	68(79.1%)	619(84.3%)	0.210	64(78.0%)	67(81.7%)	0.697
Height (mean ± SD, cm)	166.90 ± 7.31	167.48 ± 6.43	0.428	166.856 ± 7.40	167.013 ± 7.06	0.889
Weight (mean ± SD, kg)	61.60 ± 9.55	63.42 ± 10.19	0.114	61.67 ± 9.49	61.15 ± 10.07	0.735
BMI (mean ± SD, kg/m^2)	22.08 ± 2.84	22.56 ± 3.03	0.161	22.11 ± 2.77	21.84 ± 2.81	0.547
HBV (%)	66(76.7%)	574(78.2%)	0.757	62(75.6%)	63(76.8%)	0.854
TB (mean ± SD, μ mol/L)	71.21 ± 98.22	145.73 ± 202.27	0.001	73.54 ± 100.01	83.45 ± 144.73	0.611
ALT (mean ± SD, u/L)	41.54 ± 44.57	29.61 ± 27.63	0.089	36.61 ± 27.09	32.10 ± 22.32	0.363
AST (mean ± SD, u/L)	33.04 ± 35.75	29.65 ± 32.98	0.520	31.81 ± 29.18	29.28 ± 17.80	0.588
Child-Pugh (mean ± SD)	8.71 ± 1.80	8.46 ± 2.13	0.302	8.62 ± 1.76	8.53 ± 1.98	0.751
Child-Pugh <10 (A and B), n (%)	60(69.77%)	531(72.34%)	0.614	58(70.73%)	61(74.39%)	0.600
MELD (mean ± SD)	14.66 ± 6.66	17.54 ± 9.69	0.001	14.82 ± 6.88	14.57 ± 6.50	0.816
Serum AFP > 400 ng/mL (n, %)	14(19.2%)	141(16.3%)	0.511	14(17.1%)	15(18.3)	0.838
Non-tumor (n,%)	53(61.6%)	416(56.7%)	0.380	50(60.97)	49(59.75)	0.873
Number of tumor = 1 (n, %)	27(31.4%)	238(32.4%)	0.395	27(32.9%)	27(32.9%)	1
Number of tumor = 2–3 (n,%)	6(6.98%)	80(10.9%)	0.261	5(6.10%)	6(7.32%)	1
Tumor size < 3 cm (n, %)	25(29.1%)	193(26.3%)	0.581	25(30.5%)	26(31.7%)	0.866
Tumor size > 3 cm (n, %)	8(9.30%)	125(17.0%)	0.080	7(8.54%)	6(7.32%)	0.773
Tumor differentiation grade I, II (n, %)	15(17.4%)	140(19.1%)	0.714	15(18.3%)	14(17.1%)	0.897
Tumor differentiation grade III (n, %)	18(20.9%)	178(24.3)	0.494	17(20.7%)	19(23.2%)	0.706

BMI Body mass index, *HBV* Hepatitis B virus, *AFP* alpha-fetoprotein, *MELD* model for end-stage liver disease, *TB* total bilirubin and alanine or aspartate aminotransferases >2000 IU/L within the first 7 days [15].

Statistical analysis

SPSS 18.0 statistical software (SPSS Inc., Chicago, IL, USA) was used to analyse the relevant data. SPSS 18 did not have a stand-alone function for propensity score analysis, but after the R software and plug-in that could link with the corresponding versions of SPSS and propensity score matching package were installed, propensity score matching could be accomplished by SPSS software [16]. To minimize the influence of other confounders on outcome, we used a propensity score analysis to match Sp(+) patients with Sp(−) patients. Sp(+) patients was matched in a 1:1 ratio with Sp(−) patients using the nearest neighbor matching and based on the variables listed in Table 1. Categorical data were presented as number (per cent) and compared using Pearson chi-Square, Fisher's exact test. Continuous variables were expressed as the mean value ± SD and analyzed using t-test and repeated measure analysis of variance. Overall patient survival was estimated by the Kaplan–Meier method, and differences between two groups were determined by log-rank test. Independent factors for the platelet count and overall survival were analyzed by multiple regression and Cox proportional hazards models, respectively. $P < 0.05$ was considered statistically significant.

Results

Baseline demographic and disease features characteristics

A total of 1147 patients underwent LT between January 2005 and December 2015 at our center. After excluding 11 patients who were lost to follow-up, 734 patients who had not undergone splenectomy before transplantation were retained in pre-matching group Sp(−). After excluding 2 patients who were lost to follow-up, 86 patients who underwent preoperative splenectomy before transplantation were finally included in pre-matching group Sp(+). we used a propensity score analysis to match Sp(+) patients with Sp(−) patients. Sp(+) patients ($n = 82$) was matched in a 1:1 ratio with Sp(−) patients ($n = 82$) using the nearest neighbor matching and based on the variables listed in Table 1.

The baseline characteristics and disease features of Sp(−) and Sp(+) in the pre-match and post-match samples are summarized in Table 1. In the pre-match model, a total of 820 cases were selected to meet the criteria of Sp(+) and Sp(−) group. All cases were 18 years of age or older. In the post-match model, the differences in all variables between Sp(+) and Sp(−) patients were reduced and were therefore not statistically significant. Because period of time after splenectomy may influence the prognosis of LT. We compared the period (≤6 and >6 months) from splenectomy to LT in group Sp(+) (Fig. 2). There is no significant difference of 1-, 3-, and 5-year OS rates between the two groups (71.0% vs.77.4% $P = 0.839$; 71.0% vs. 72.3%, $P = 0.992$; 71.0% vs. 68.6%, $P = 0.973$). The result of single factor analysis with regard to the period from splenectomy to LT related to 5-years OS rates is also not statistically significant ($P = 0.271$).

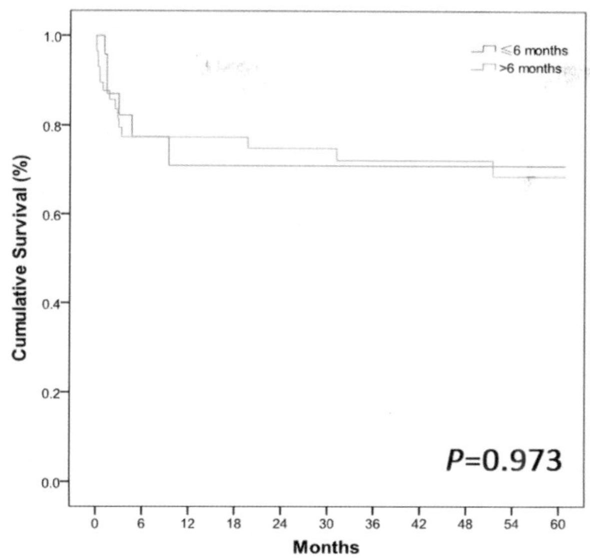

Fig. 2 Group Sp(+) are divided into two groups according to the period (≤6 and >6 months) from splenectomy to liver transplantation. There is no significant difference of 1-, 3-, and 5-year OS rates between the two groups (71.0% vs.77.4% $P = 0.839$; 71.0% vs. 72.3%, $P = 0.992$; 71.0% vs. 68.6%, $P = 0.973$)

Surgical characteristics, post-operative course and survival

Perioperative course post-match samples are summarized in Table 2. There was no significant difference in blood loss during the operation, warm ischemia time and GRWR between group Sp(+) and group Sp(−).

The post-operative course and survival were analyzed using the post-match sample summarized in Table 2. There were no differences between patients in group Sp(+) and group Sp(−) in terms of major infections including lung infection, urinary tract infection, positive blood culture (12.20% vs. 15.85%, $P = 0.455$), the incidence of major complications (Clavien–Dindo ≥ Grade 3; 6.10% vs. 10.98%, $P = 0.264$), and no portal vein thrombosis in both groups. No difference existed between the two groups with regard to 90 days mortality ($P = 0.243$). The length of post-operative hospital stay were similar in group Sp(+) and group Sp(−). In addition, we also analyzed the relationship between group Sp(−) and group Sp(+) with regard to the platelet count and found that group Sp(−) has a higher rate of post-operative thrombocytopenia (91.46% vs. 74.39%, $P = 0.006$), and more EAD than Sp(+) (23.20% vs. 10.98%, $P = 0.038$). The platelet count was significantly higher in group Sp(+) than in group Sp(−) (Fig. 3, $P = 0.041$). Independent

Table 2 Perioperative course and postoperative outcome

Variables	Sp + (*n* = 82)	Sp- (*n* = 82)	*P* value
GRWR (mean ± SD)	1.68 ± 0.52	1.65 ± 0.66	0.739
Warm ischemia time (mean ± SD , min)	5.88 ± 6.95	4.66 ± 4.10	0.171
Intraoperative blood loss (mean ± SD , mL)	1478.29 ± 317.40	1571.95 ± 598.78	0.213
Operation time (mean ± SD , hours)	9.30 ± 2.49	9.07 ± 2.16	0.536
Postoperative major complications (Clavien–Dindo ≥ Grade 3) (%)	5(6.10%)	9(10.98%)	0.264
Postoperative infection (%)	10(12.20%)	13(15.85%)	0.455
Mortality (90 days)	13(15.9%)	8(9.76%)	0.243
Postoperative portal vein thrombosis (%)	0	0	NS
Postoperative thrombocytopenia (%)	61(74.39%)	75(91.46%)	0.006
EAD (%)	9(10.98%)	19(23.20%)	0.038
Length of postoperative hospital stay (mean ± SD, days)	15.34 ± 1.67	15.76 ± 3.24	0.269

GRWR Graft/Recipient's Body Weight Ratio, *EAD* early allograft dysfunction

factors for the platelet count analyzed by multiple regression were summarized in Table 3. Pre-transplantation splenectomy was considered to be a protective independent factor for post-operative thrombocytopenia. ($P = 0.002$)

The mean follow-up for group Sp(+) was 36.1 months, whereas it was 38.4 months in group Sp(−). Fig. 4 shows that 1-, 3-, and 5-year OS rates of 75.0, 70.8 and 67.6%, respectively, in the Sp(+) group vs. 79.7, 71.7 and 69.7%, respectively, in the Sp(−) group ($P = 0.459$, 0.730,0.701 respectively). Independent factors for overall survival were analyzed by Cox proportional hazards models in Table 4. Tumor related factors were considered independent risk factors for overall survival ($P = 0.041$).

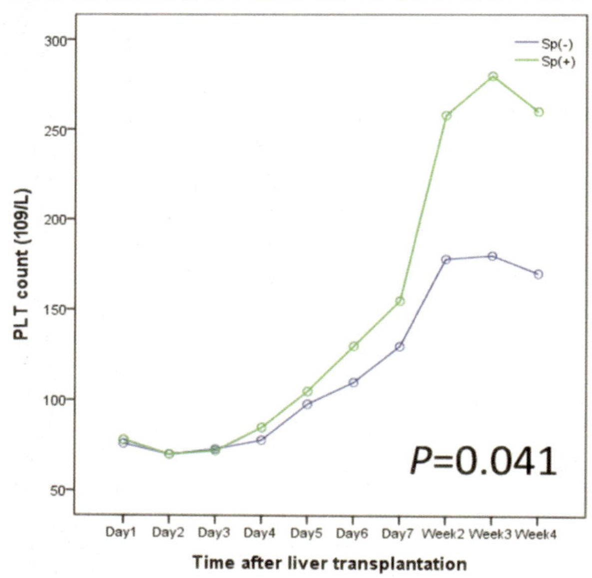

Fig. 3 Platelet count changes after liver transplantation

Discussion

At present, LT is the last choice for many patients with end-stage liver disease. The wait for transplantation is also long due to the shortage of donor organs. Moreover, LT is not feasible for all patients. Therefore, in order to reduce the pressure on the portal vein, many patients with liver disease choose to undergo splenectomy as a bridging therapy prior to LT. Thus, the influence of splenectomy on LT is still worthy of consideration.

First, the most emphasized risk conveyed by pre-transplantation splenectomy is sepsis. By viewing other relevant literature, on follow-up studies of patients who underwent splenectomy for cirrhosis, but never had a LT,

Table 3 Independent variables in the multiple analysis for postoperative thrombocytopenia (post-matched Sp(+) and Sp(−), *n* = 164)

Variables	Relative risk	*P*
Donor		
Male (%)	−0.550	0.416
Age	−0.003	0.896
BMI	0.171	0.265
Recipient		
Male (%)	0.658	0.352
Age	−0.003	0.896
BMI	0.171	0.265
Splenectomy	−0.1644	0.002
MELD score	0.052	0.275
Child-Pugh score	0.153	0.330
Tumor related	−0.125	0.883
HBV	0.634	0.238
GRWR	0.024	0.965
Warm ischemia time	0.049	0.255
Intraoperative blood loss	−0.001	0.229

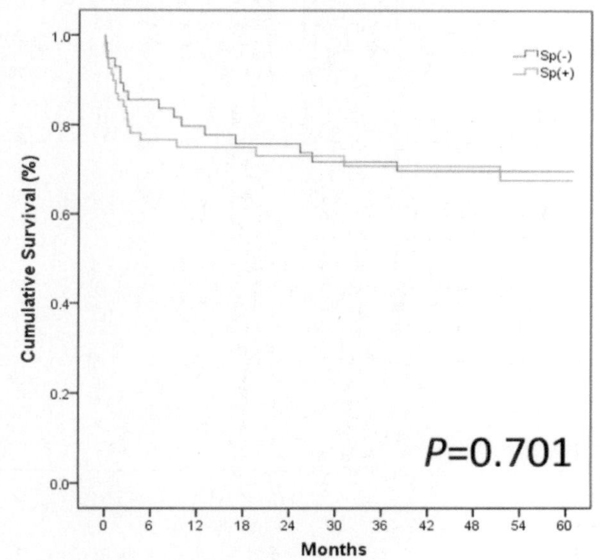

Fig. 4 5-year OS rates of the Sp(−) group and the Sp(+) group

A meta-analysis of follow-up studies involving 19,680 patients showed that the incidence of sepsis among adult splenectomy patients was low, and that a high mortality rate was observed only among children [17]. This meta-analysis thus suggested a low post-operative rate of sepsis after adult splenectomy. Moreover, this is the premise of a low post-operative infection rate in Sp(+) group. Furthermore, for patients who underwent splenectomy and LT synchronously, Samimi et al. [18] reported that synchronous splenectomy resulted in a higher mortality rate, mainly related to septic complications. However, for patients who underwent splenectomy before LT, Jeng et al. [19] and Shimadaet al. [20] found that the risk of infection after LT in patients who had undergone splenectomy remained unchanged. Our results confirm that for the patients who underwent splenectomy before LT (group Sp(+)),the risk of infection was not increased.

Table 4 Independent variables in the Cox analysis for overall survival (post-matched Sp(+) and Sp(−), $n = 164$)

Variables	Relative risk	*P*
Splenectomy	0.191	0.609
Serum AFP	<0.001	0.818
MELD score	−0.038	0.294
Child-Pugh score	0.186	0.157
Tumor related	0.803	0.041
HBV	−0.783	0.054
GRWR	−0.009	0.977
Warm ischemia time	0.006	0.819
Intraoperative blood loss	<0.001	0.478

We further investigated the influence of splenectomy on post-operative complications after LT, based on the Clavien–Dindo complication classification [21]. 21 deaths occurred in the 90 days after operation in either the Sp(−) or Sp(+) group, and no difference existed between the two groups with regard to various grades of post-operative complications and 90 days mortality. Settmacher et al. [22] reported that concomitant splenectomy during LT was associated with a significant and increased risk of venous complications, such as portal vein thrombosis. However, none of our liver transplant patients in whom splenectomy was performed prior to LT developed portal vein thrombosis. This is consistent with the reports of Hirotaka et al. [7] It is interesting that the incidence of one of the post-operative complications of LT, thrombocytopenia, decreased rather than increased in patients who underwent splenectomy. Many studies have found that the platelet count reaches a nadir at days 2–5 post-transplant, but returned to preoperative levels by weeks 1–2 [23–26]. The reason for this remains unclear. Chang et al. [27] have found that persistent thrombocytopenia is an indicator of a higher rate of fungal infections in liver transplant recipients. On the other hand, platelet-derived serotonin has been found to be important for liver regeneration [28]. A retrospective study [29] has shown that transfused platelets are significantly associated with graft regeneration in liver donors. Furthermore, Bleibel et al. [30] recently observed that peripheral platelet count correlated with liver atrophy and predicted long-term mortality in patients on the liver transplant waiting list. Interestingly, splenectomy can increase the number of platelets, yet portacaval or distal splenorenal shunts cannot increase the number of platelets [31–33]. The reason for this may be that platelets participate in splenic destruction, rather than merely pooling in the spleen [34–36]. In our series of 162 post-matched patients, post-operative peripheral platelet levels were significantly higher ($P = 0.041$) in group Sp(+) than in group Sp(−). Therefore, we believe that splenectomy is an effective approach for increasing platelets. Furthermore, EAD is often used as the best choice of the primary outcome after LT. Li et al. [37] have conducted a retrospective study on adult-to-adult living donor liver transplantation (A-A LDLT) and found that an immediate post-operative platelet count of less than 68×10^9/L was an independent risk factor for post-operative EAD. Interestingly, in our study the Group Sp(−) did have more EAD than Sp(+) ($P = 0.038$). As for its reasons, we considered immediate postoperative low platelet mainly affected the recovery of the liver function by liver regeneration, because there was no significant difference between the two groups with regard to post-operative major complications. The results were also confirmed by us in the living donor liver transplantation [37]. But the specific mechanism still remained to be further studied in the laboratory.

We also compared the overall survival rate of patients between the Sp(−) and Sp(+) groups. In the past, there had been many reports on the effects of LT after splenectomy or simultaneous splenectomy in liver transplant patients, but due to the small number of observations, the results were controversial. At present, there is a lack of a corresponding standard for patients who underwent splenectomy prior to liver transplant. In order to verify the effects of splenectomy on liver transplant patients, we here observed 820 patients in a 5-yearfollow-up study. After analyzing the cumulative overall survival rates of groups Sp(+) and Sp(−), we found no significant differences in the 1-, 3-, and 5-year survival rates in the post-match model. Therefore, we concluded that LT may be suitable for the patients who underwent splenectomy. However, well-designed, long-term, randomized, controlled, prospective trials are still necessary to confirm this proposal.

Through the above analysis, pre-transplantation splenectomy is recommended in cases with risky PHT patients without appropriate source of liver for LT. But one thing to note is that as a “re-operation” the splenectomy is often associated with more difficult dissection due to adhesions. We subjectively believed the transplant operation was perhaps more difficult in the splenectomy group. Although the average time spent on Sp(−) was less than group Sp(+), there was no statistic difference between operative times and intraoperative blood loss. Finally, we believe that adhesion does have some effect on group Sp(+), but it is not obvious.

Our study has several limitations. First, we performed our analysis using only about 82 cases in the Sp(+) group. The limited number of patients may underlie the lack of significant differences and a larger multicenter study should investigate this matter further. Second, these data were retrospectively collected and analyzed, and a prospective clinical investigation should be performed to evaluate the role of splenectomy in this context.

Conclusions

The results of the present study suggest that pre-transplantation is a very effective method for the treatment of thrombocytopenia after ADLT. Moreover, compared with Sp(−), the risk of infection and post-operative complications in group Sp(+) is not increased, and group Sp(+) had a lower rate of post-operative EAD. There was no difference in the cumulative survival rates between the two groups. Pre-transplantation splenectomy is recommended in cases with risky PHT patients without appropriate source of liver for LT.

Abbreviations

ADLT: Adult liver transplantation; AFP: Alpha-fetoprotein; AZA: Azathioprine; BCLC: Barcelona Clinic Liver Cancer; BMI: Body mass index; EAD: Early allograft dysfunction; GRWR: Graft/Recipient's Body Weight Ratio; HBV: Hepatitis B virus; HCC: Hepatocarcinoma; HCV: Hepatitis C virus; LT: Liver transplantation; MELD: Model for end-stage liver disease; PHT: Portal hypertension; Sp: Pre-transplantation splenectomy; TB: Total bilirubin; UCSF: University of California San Francisco

Acknowledgements

We thank all patients and staff of our hospital who participated in this study.

Funding

This study was supported by grants from the National Natural Science Fundation of China (no. 81470037).

Authors' contributions

LK, LY, LJ and JY designed the study; LL, ML performed the research and collected the data; LK, ML, LL analyzed and interpreted the data; LK wrote the first draft of the manuscript; All authors edited the manuscript and approved the final draft; The acquisition of funding is from JY.

Competing interests

The authors declare that they have no competing interests.

References

1. Chu H, Han W, Wang L, Xu Y, Jian F, Zhang W, et al. Long-term efficacy of subtotal splenectomy due to portal hypertension in cirrhotic patients. BMC Surg. 2015;15:89.
2. Wolff M, Hirner A. Surgical treatment of portal hypertension. Zentralbl Chir. 2005;130(3):238–45.
3. Starzl TE, Marchioro TL, Talmage DW, Waddell WR. Splenectomy and thymectomy in human renal homotransplantation. Proc Soc Exp Biol Med. 1963;113:929–32.
4. Troisi R, Colle I, Van Vlierberghe H, Hesse UJ, Cuomo O, de Hemptinne B. Splenectomy and liver transplantation. Transplant Proc. 2001;33(1–2):1500–1.
5. Stevenson WC, Sawyer RG, Pruett TL. Recurrent variceal bleeding after liver transplantation–persistent left-sided portal hypertension. Transplantation. 1992;53(2):493–5.
6. Ayalon A, Wiesner RH, Perkins JD, Tominaga S, Hayes DH, Krom RA. Splenic artery aneurysms in liver transplant patients. Transplantation. 1988;45(2):386–9.
7. Tashiro H, Itamoto T, Ohdan H, Fudaba Y, Kohashi T, Amano H, et al. Should splenectomy be performed for hepatitis C patients undergoing living-donor liver transplantation? J Gastroenterol Hepatol. 2007;22(6):959–60.
8. Mazzaferro V, Regalia E, Doci R, Andreola S, Pulvirenti A, Bozzetti F, et al. Liver transplantation for the treatment of small hepatocellular carcinomas in patients with cirrhosis. N Engl J Med. 1996;334(11):693–9.
9. Yao FY, Ferrell L, Bass NM, Watson JJ, Bacchetti P, Venook A, et al. Liver transplantation for hepatocellular carcinoma: expansion of the tumor size limits does not adversely impact survival. Hepatology (Baltimore, Md). 2001;33(6):1394–403.
10. Zheng SS, Xu X, Wu J, Chen J, Wang WL, Zhang M, et al. Liver transplantation for hepatocellular carcinoma: Hangzhou experiences. Transplantation. 2008; 85(12):1726–32.
11. Llovet JM. Updated treatment approach to hepatocellular carcinoma. J Gastroenterol. 2005;40(3):225–35.
12. Louis D, Duc ML, Reix P, Chazalette JP, Durieu I, Feigelson J, et al. Partial splenectomy for portal hypertension in cystic fibrosis related liver disease. Pediatr Pulmonol. 2007;42(12):1173–80.
13. Dindo D, Demartines N, Clavien PA. Classification of surgical complications: a new proposal with evaluation in a cohort of 6336 patients and results of a survey. Ann Surg. 2004;240(2):205–13.
14. Santambrogio R, Kluger MD, Costa M, Belli A, Barabino M, Laurent A, et al. Hepatic resection for hepatocellular carcinoma in patients with Child-Pugh's A cirrhosis: is clinical evidence of portal hypertension a contraindication? HPB. 2013;15(1):78–84.
15. Olthoff KM, Kulik L, Samstein B, Kaminski M, Abecassis M, Emond J, et al. Validation of a current definition of early allograft dysfunction in liver transplant recipients and analysis of risk factors. Liver Transpl. 2010;16(8):943–9.
16. Huang F, Du C, Sun M, Ning B, Luo Y, An S. [Propensity score matching in SPSS]. Nan Fang Yi Ke Da Xue Xue Bao. 2015;35(11):1597–601.

17. Bisharat N, Omari H, Lavi I, Raz R. Risk of infection and death among post-splenectomy patients. J Infect. 2001;43(3):182–6.
18. Cescon M, Sugawara Y, Takayama T, Seyama Y, Sano K, Imamura H, et al. Role of splenectomy in living-donor liver transplantation for adults. Hepato-Gastroenterology. 2002;49(45):721–3.
19. Jeng LB, Lee CC, Chiang HC, Chen TH, Hsu CH, Cheng HT, et al. Indication for splenectomy in the era of living-donor liver transplantation. Transplant Proc. 2008;40(8):2531–3.
20. Shimada M, Ijichi H, Yonemura Y, Harada N, Shiotani S, Ninomiya M, et al. The impact of splenectomy or splenic artery ligation on the outcome of a living donor adult liver transplantation using a left lobe graft. Hepato-Gastroenterology. 2004;51(57):625–9.
21. Clavien PA, Barkun J, de Oliveira ML, Vauthey JN, Dindo D, Schulick RD, et al. The Clavien-Dindo classification of surgical complications: five-year experience. Ann Surg. 2009;250(2):187–96.
22. Settmacher U, Nussler NC, Glanemann M, Haase R, Heise M, Bechstein WO, et al. Venous complications after orthotopic liver transplantation. Clin Transpl. 2000;14(3):235–41.
23. McCaughan GW, Herkes R, Powers B, Rickard K, Gallagher ND, Thompson JF, et al. Thrombocytopenia post liver transplantation. Correlations with pre-operative platelet count, blood transfusion requirements, allograft function and outcome. J Hepatol. 1992;16(1–2):16–22.
24. Richards EM, Alexander GJ, Calne RY, Baglin TP. Thrombocytopenia following liver transplantation is associated with platelet consumption and thrombin generation. Br J Haematol. 1997;98(2):315–21.
25. Chatzipetrou MA, Tsaroucha AK, Weppler D, Pappas PA, Kenyon NS, Nery JR, et al. Thrombocytopenia after liver transplantation. Transplantation. 1999; 67(5):702–6.
26. Lesurtel M, Raptis DA, Melloul E, Schlegel A, Oberkofler C, El-Badry AM, et al. Low platelet counts after liver transplantation predict early posttransplant survival: the 60–5 criterion. Liver Transpl. 2014;20(2):147–55.
27. Chang FY, Singh N, Gayowski T, Wagener MM, Mietzner SM, Stout JE, et al. Thrombocytopenia in liver transplant recipients: predictors, impact on fungal infections, and role of endogenous thrombopoietin. Transplantation. 2000;69(1):70–5.
28. Lesurtel M, Graf R, Aleil B, Walther DJ, Tian Y, Jochum W, et al. Platelet-derived serotonin mediates liver regeneration. Science. 2006;312(5770):104–7.
29. Kim J, Yi NJ, Shin WY, Kim T, Lee KU, Suh KS. Platelet transfusion can be related to liver regeneration after living donor liver transplantation. World J Surg. 2010;34(5):1052–8.
30. Bleibel W, Caldwell SH, Curry MP, Northup PG. Peripheral platelet count correlates with liver atrophy and predicts long-term mortality on the liver transplant waiting list. Transpl Int. 2013;26(4):435–42.
31. Toghill PJ, Green S. Splenic influences on the blood in chronic liver disease. Q J Med. 1979;48(192):613–25.
32. Mutchnick MG, Lerner E, Conn HO. Effect of portacaval anastomosis on hypersplenism. Dig Dis Sci. 1980;25(12):929–38.
33. Lawrence SP, Lezotte DC, Durham JD, Kumpe DA, Everson GT, Bilir BM. Course of thrombocytopenia of chronic liver disease after transjugular intrahepatic portosystemic shunts (TIPS). A retrospective analysis. Dig Dis Sci. 1995;40(7):1575–80.
34. Stein SF, Harker LA. Kinetic and functional studies of platelets, fibrinogen, and plasminogen in patients with hepatic cirrhosis. J Lab Clin Med. 1982;99(2):217–30.
35. Schmidt KG, Rasmussen JW, Bekker C, Madsen PE. Kinetics and in vivo distribution of 111-In-labelled autologous platelets in chronic hepatic disease: mechanisms of thrombocytopenia. Scand J Haematol. 1985;34(1):39–46.
36. Aoki Y, Hirai K, Tanikawa K. Mechanism of thrombocytopenia in liver cirrhosis: kinetics of indium-111 tropolone labelled platelets. Eur J Nucl Med. 1993;20(2):123–9.
37. Li L, Wang H, Yang J, Jiang L, Yang J, Wang W, et al. Immediate postoperative low platelet counts after living donor liver transplantation predict early allograft dysfunction. Medicine. 2015;94(34):e1373.

31

Risk factors for bile leakage after primary closure following laparoscopic common bile duct exploration: a retrospective cohort study

Dongbin Liu*†, Feng Cao†, Jiafeng Liu, Dahua Xu, Yuehua Wang and Fei Li

Abstraction

Background: Primary closure following laparoscopic common bile duct exploration (LCBDE) has been widely adopted because of the efficacy and safety in treatment of common bile duct (CBD) stones. However, the risk factors for bile leakage, the most common complication after primary closure, has not been clarified yet.

Methods: A retrospective cohort study of patients who underwent LCBDE with primary closure after choledochotomy between Feb. 2012 and Jun. 2016 was performed. Risk factors for bile leakage were identified by logistic regression inculding demographic factors, preoperative condition and surgical details.

Results: Between Feb. 2012 and Jun. 2016, a total of 265 LCBDE procedures were applied in our hospital and 141 patients with primary closure were included in this study. Bile leakage occurred in 11.3% (16/141) of these patients, and happened more frequently in patients with slender CBD (<1 *vs* ≥1 cm, 31.6% *vs* 7.0%, $p = 0.04$) and those managed by inexperienced surgeons (initial 70 cases *vs* later cases, 17.1% *vs* 5.6%, $p = 0.04$). After multivariable regression, the diameter of CBD [OR 95% CI, 3.799 (1.081–13.349), $p = 0.04$] and experience of surgeons [OR 95% CI, 4.228 (1.330–13.438), $p = 0.03$] were significantly related to bile leakage.

Conclusion: Slender CBD and inexperienced surgeons were the high risk factors for bile leakage after primary closure following LCBDE.

Keywords: Laparoscopic common bile duct exploration, Primary closure, Bile leakage

Background

Common bile duct (CBD) stone is the strong indication for surgical therapy, especially in patients with obstructive jaundice. With the development of laparoscopic equipment and technology, laparoscopic common bile duct exploration (LCBDE) has been widely used in clinical practice [1–4]. Many previous studies have demonstrated that LCBDE is safe and effective in treatment of CBD stone [2, 4, 5]. After LCBDE, primary closure or T-tube drainage will be applied according to the condition of CBD and experience of surgeon. In 1991, Phillip first reported the technique of LCBDE and T-tube drainage in treatment of CBD calculi encountered during laparoscopic cholecystectomy. On the basis of the experience of open CBD exploration, T-tube drainage has been widely adopted in the past two decades. However, T-tube drainage has many problems, such as fluid and electrolyte disturbance, sepsis, premature dislodgement, bile leakage, prolonged biliary fistula, late bile duct stricture, and possible peritonitis after removal of the T-tube, which accounted for 15% of all patients [6]. These complications and the need of satisfactory follow-up cholangiography prolonged the hospital stay and increased hospital expenses [7].

Primary duct closure after open CBD exploration was first described by Halstead as early as 1917. Since then, the debate between primary closure and T-tube drainage continued even in the era of laparoscopic surgery.

* Correspondence: Liudongbin90266@sohu.com
†Equal contributors
Department of General Surgery, Xuanwu Hospital, Capital Medical University, Beijing 100053, People's Republic of China

In the past decade, numerous studies comparing primary with T-tube were published and revealed the feasibility and safety of primary closure [8–10]. Meta-analysis form Yin demonstrated that among patients with laparoscopic choledochotomy for CBD stones, primary closure of the CBD alone is superior to T-tube drainage in terms of postoperative and biliary-specific complications [11]. However, primary closure following LCBDE is still a technical demanding operation and with a relative high risk of bile leakage. Regardless of the widely use of primary closure after LCBDE, the risk factors for bile leakage is still largely unknown. Therefore, we performed this retrospective study to identify the risk factors for bile leakage after primary closure following LCBDE.

Methods

Patients selection

Patients with CBD stones who were admitted to our center between Feb. 2012 and Jun. 2016 were screened and those who received primary closure after LCBDE were included in this study. In our institution, the indications for primary closure following LCBDE are as follows: (1) CBD stones are confirmed by preoperative MRCP or CT with no intrahepatic bile duct stone; (2) The diameter of CBD is more than 0.8 cm; (3) No obvious inflammatory changes of CBD are detected intraoperatively; (4) No. of stones is less than 5; (5) Function of Oddi sphincter is normal without residual stone which is confirmed by intraoperative flexible choledochoscope. Patients with previous biliary surgery history or converted to open surgery were excluded from this study. This study was approved by the Ethics Committee of Xuanwu hospital.

Operative techniques

After general anesthesia, the patient was placed in the supine position. The pressure of CO_2 in abdominal cavity was maintained at 12 to 14 mmHg. Four trocars were placed in umbilical, medial epigastric, right anterior axillary line and right midclavicular area, respectively. The 10 mm trocar in right midclavicular area was placed for choledochoscope examination. After dissection of the gallbladder, the cystic duct was clipped with Hem-o-lock. Then the dissection continued to expose the cystic duct-CBD junction and the anterior wall of the CBD. The 1.0–1.5 cm longitudinal choledochotomy was made in the anterior surface of the CBD. After the choledochotomy, small stones were washed out by saline irrigation. Then, a flexible choledochoscope was routinely used to examine distal and proximal bile duct. The residual stones were extracted by using a stone basket. For big stones, electrohydraulic lithotripsy was used through the working channel of the choledochoscope. After complete remove the stones, the flexible choledochoscope was preformed to confirm the clearance of the intrahepatic/extrahepatic bile duct and the normal function of Oddi sphincter. Then, primary closure was performed with continuous or interrupted suture using Vicryl 3–0 or 4–0 suture line. Intraoperative cholangiography (IOC) was not performed (Fig. 1).

The definition of bile leakage was as follows: (1) for patients with drainage tube, bile was detected in the

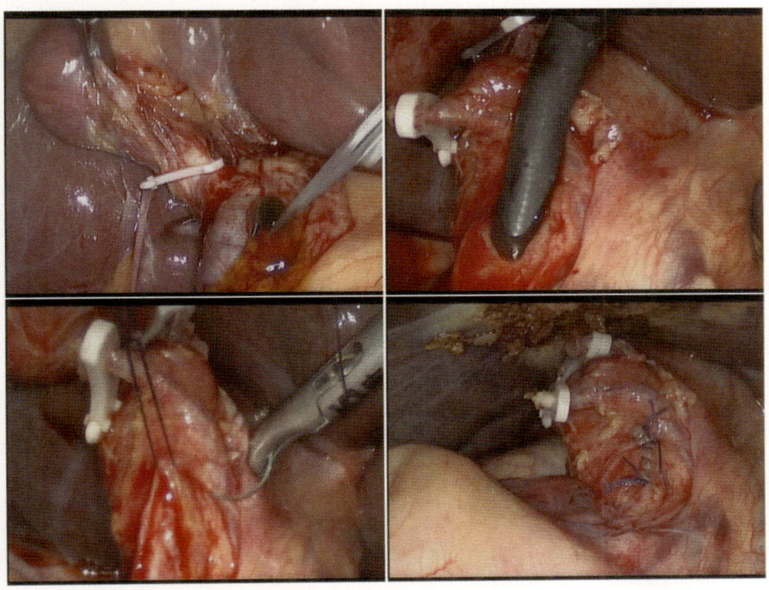

Fig. 1 Intraoperative image of primary closure following LCBDE

drainage for more than 3 days or the volume of drainage containing bile was more than 100 ml/day; (2) for patients without drainage tube, local or general peritonitis was detected and bile was found in ascites by puncture or reoperation.

Possible risk factors

Possible risk factors for bile leakage after primary closure following LCBDE are divided into three groups: demographic factors, preoperative condition and surgical details.

Demographic factors: (1) age; (2) sex; (3) ASA score.

Preoperative condition: (1) serum leukocytes; (2) total bilirubin; (3) diameter of CBD; (4) No. of stones; (5) gallstone.

Surgical details: (1) operative time; (2) total blood loss; (3) method of suture; (4) length of choledochotomy; (5) surgeon's experience.

Statistics

The data is expressed as means ± SD or median (range). For pairwise comparisons of groups, we used the chi-square test or Fisher exact test for categorical variables and Student t test for quantitative variables. The logistic regression analysis was used to identify variables associated with risks for bile leakage after primary closure following LCBDE. All variables with univariable $p < 0.1$ were considered for the multivariable model. Results were presented as odds ratios (ORs) with 95% confidence intervals (CI). A P value <0.05 was considered statistically significant. Statistical analysis was performed with SPSS version 18.0 (SPSS Inc., Chicago, IL, USA).

Results

Patients

Between Feb. 2012 and Jun. 2016, 3109 patients with gallstones and 589 with CBD stones were treated in our hospital. Of the patients with choledocholithiasis, 376 patients received surgical therapy with 111 open and 265 laparoscopic procedures, respectively. In laparoscopic operation group, 8 patients converted to open surgery. The data about the patients who successfully received LCBDE was shown in Table 1. The mean diameter of CBD among patients with LCBDE procedure was 1.2 ± 0.3 cm. According to the MRCP or CT finding, there were 1.7 ± 1.3 stones detected in CBD. 82.8% (213/257) of the patients were complicated with gallstones. After LCBDE, 141 patients received primary closure and were included in this study. Among these cases, 92.2% (130/141) of patients were presented with abdominal pain and 49.6% (70/141) went to the emergency department. Obstructive jaundice was observed in 90 (64.5%) patients. In the same period, 23 patients with CBD stones received ERCP therapy in our hospital.

Surgical results

No perioperative death occurred during the study period. The overall complication rate was 21.3 (30/141), and biliary-specific complication rate was 12.7% (18/141). According to Dindo-Clavien classification, most of the complications were as grade I, while one patient with uncontrolled bile peritonitis (grade IIIb) received reoperation (Table 2). Residual stones were found in 2(1.4%) patients by following CT and ultrasound examination.

Table 1 Patients characters with CBD stones treated by LCBDE and primary closure after LCBDE

	LCBDE, $n = 257$	LCBDE + primary closure, $n = 141$
Male/Female	122/135	72/69
Age (years), mean ± SD	59.2 ± 15.3	58.9 ± 15.2
ASA score (I/II/III/IV)	41/143/55/18	22/79/32/8
Diameter of CBD (cm), mean ± SD	1.2 ± 0.3	1.1 ± 0.3
No. of stones, mean ± SD[a]	1.7 ± 1.3	1.7 ± 1.2
Length of choledochotomy (cm)	1.2 ± 0.6	1.3 ± 1.2
Primary closure/T-tube drainage	141/116	—
Postoperative bile leakage	20 (7.8%)	16 (11.3%)
Postoperative hemorrhage	8 (3.1%)	5 (3.5%)
Residual stones	10 (3.9%)	2 (1.4%)
Stone recurrence[b]	2 (0.8%)	2 (1.4%)
Bile duct stricture[b]	0	0
Duration of drainage placement (days)	4.0 ± 2.0	3.8 ± 2.0
Death	0	0

ASA American Society of Anesthesiologists
[a]according to the MRCP or CT finding, data available in 176 patients in LCBDE and 96 patients in primary closure group, respectively
[b]The median follow-up time was 34 (range 1–76) months

Table 2 Complication after primary closure following LCBDE

Dindo-Clavien classification	Complication	No. of patients	Management
Grade I	Bile leakage Wound infection	10 7	Observation
Grade II	Bile leakage Fluid collection Pneumonia	5 4 2	Antibiotics
Grade III IIIa IIIb	Infected collection Bile leakage	1 1	Percutaneous drainage Reoperation

Follow-up

The median follow-up time was 34 (range 1–76) months, stone recurrence was detected in 2 (1.4%) patients. Repeated LCBDE followed by T tube drainage was performed in these two cases. No bile duct stricture was found during the follow-up period.

Fisk factors for bile leakage

Bile leakage occurred in 11.3%(16/141) of the patients with primary closure following LBCDE. Then, the patients were divided into two groups, bile leakage group and no bile leakage group. Most possible risk factors, such as age, ASA score, total bilirubin, operative time, total blood loss and et al were comparable between two groups. However, bile leakage occurred more frequently in patients with slender CBD (<1 *vs* ≥1 cm, 31.6% *vs* 7.0%, $p = 0.037$) and managed by inexperienced surgeons (initial 70 cases *vs* later cases, 17.1% *vs* 5.6%, $p = 0.036$) (Table 3).

The influences of age, sex, ASA score, serum leukocytes, total bilirubin, diameter of CBD, No. of stones, gallstone, operative time, total blood loss, method of suture, length of choledochotomy and surgeon's experience on bile leakage after primary closure following LCBDE were summarized in Table 4. The slender CBD and inexperienced surgeons were associated with high risk of bile leakage in univariate analysis. Factors that affected bile leakage at the $p < 0.10$ level of significance by univariate analysis were included in a multivariate regression model. After adjusting for these variables, slender CBD [OR 95% CI, 3.799 (1.081–13.349), $p = 0.04$] and inexperienced surgeons [OR 95% CI, 4.228 (1.330–13.438), $p = 0.03$] were found to affect bile leakage.

Discussion

In the era of mini-invasive surgery, laparoscopic cholecystectomy (LC) has been the standard therapy for symptomatic gallstones. However, debate continues

Table 3 Possible risk factors for bile leakage after primary closure following LCBDE

	Bile leakage ($n = 16$)	No bile leakage ($n = 125$)	*P* value
Demographic factors			
Male/Female	7/9	65/60	0.534
Age (years) (≥70/<70)	4/12	29/96	0.873
ASA score (I + II/III + IV)	9/7	92/33	0.154
Preoperative condition			
Serum leukocytes (≥10/<10 × 10^9/L)	2/14	23/102	0.564
Total bilirubin (≥23/<23 umol/L)	5/11	72/53	0.054
No. of stones (≥3/<3)	5/11	33/92	0.681
Diameter of CBD (<1/≥1 cm)	6/10	13/113	0.037
Gallstone (Yes/No)	12/4	97/28	0.799
Surgical details			
Operative time (≥2/<2 h)	2/14	28/97	0.793
Total blood loss (≥50/<50 ml)	1/15	23/102	0.250
Method of suture (continuous/interrupted)	13/3	106/19	0.713
Length of choledochotomy (≥1.5/<1.5 cm)	4/12	14/111	0.131
Surgeon's experience (initial 70 cases/later cases)	12/4	58/67	0.036

ASA American Society of Anesthesiologists

Table 4 Results of Univariable and Multivariable Regression for bile leakage after primary closure following LCBDE

Risk factors	Univariable regression		Multivariable regression	
	OR (95% CI)	*P* value	OR (95% CI)	*P* value
Sex (male/Female)	0.718 (0.252–2.048)	0.53		
Age (years) (≥70/<70)	1.103 (0.331–3.683)	0.87		
ASA score (I + II/III + IV)	2.168 (0.748–6.289)	0.15		
Serum leukocytes (≥10/<10 × 10^9/L)	0.634 (0.135–2.982)	0.56		
Total bilirubin (≥23/<23 umol/L)	0.335 (0.110–1.020)	0.05	0.587 (0.146–2.132)	0.23
No. of stones (≥3/<3)	1.267 (0.410–3.921)	0.68		
Diameter of CBD (<1/≥1 cm)	3.604 (1.092–11.898)	0.04	3.799 (1.081–13.349)	0.04
Gallstone (Yes/No)	0.871 (0.298–2.546)	0.80		
Operative time (≥2/<2 h)	0.838 (0.222–3.153)	0.79		
Total blood loss (≥50/<50 ml)	0.296 (0.037–2.353)	0.25		
Method of suture (continuous/ interrupted)	1.287 (0.335–4.951)	0.71		
Length of choledochotomy (≥1.5/<1.5 cm)	2.643 (0.749–9.324)	0.13		
Surgeon's experience (initial 70 cases/later cases)	3.356 (1.026–10.974)	0.04	4.228 (1.330–13.438)	0.03

regarding the best treatment for managing cholecystocholedocholithiasis, and a consensus has not been reached [12, 13]. In clinical practice, three major procedures, LC + endoscopic retrograde cholangiopancreatography (ERCP)/endoscopic sphincterotomy (EST)/ endoscopic papillary balloon dilation (EPBD), LC+ laparoscopic transcystic common bile duct exploration exploration (LTCBDE) and LCBDE were applied for treatment of cholecystocholedocholithiasis.

The role of ERCP in diagnosis of CBD stones has been replaced by MRCP, however, it is widely used to remove CBD stones in one-stage or staged procedures. EST is associated with serious short-term complications, including bleeding, post-ERCP pancreatitis (PEP), and perforation of the digestive tract. In addition, EST may increase the incidence of long-term complications such as biliary infection due to the dysfunction of the Oddi's sphincter after the procedure [14–16]. In order to preserve (at least partly) the function of the sphincter of Oddi and avoid post-EST bleeding, EPBD is more and more used in treatment of CBD stones. Actually, choledocholithiasis is the only indication for EPBD reported in large controlled series. Unfortunately, the recent RCTs failed to demonstrate the advantages of EPBD over EST in terms of post-operative complications including PEP, bleeding and perforation [17, 18]. The rate of complete stone removal and utilization of endoscopic mechanical lithotripsy in EST group was comparable with EPBD group [19]. Meta-analyses also showed similar efficacy and overall safety (less bleeding but more PEP in EPBD) between the two treatments [20]. In patients with cholecystocholedocholithiasis, ERCP with stone extraction might be performed selectively before, during or after cholecystectomy. However, as discussed by Costi et al., there were several limitations about ERCP therapy [21]. Firstly, performing ERCP before surgery raised questions regarding patient selection, but no consensus has reached even in the recent guidelines from US and Europe [13, 22]. Secondly, performing ERCP contextually to LC implied organizational problems concerning the availability of an endoscopist in the operating theater whenever needed. Finally, performing ERCP after surgery would raise the dilemma of managing CBD stones whenever ERCP failed to retrieve them because a third procedure would then be needed.

LTCBDE was firstly preformed by Stoker in 1995 [23]. Recent report from Zhu demonstrated that in their 708 patients, LTCBDE could be successfully applied in more than 90% patients and with high clearance rate (common bile duct stones residual in 13 patients) and low complication rate (postoperative complications in 27 patients). So they conclude that LTCBDE with or without microincision and/or lithotripsy is a safe and effective approach in treatment of CBD stones [24]. However, the ability to remove stones is restricted by the diameter of cystic duct, even with application of electrohydraulic lithotripsy. In patients with many CBD stones or slender cystic duct, LTCBDE may lead to the high rate of stones retained [25, 26]. To avoid these limitations, LCBDE was used to access to a common bile duct without causing damage to the biliary sphincter and also with the high clearance rate. Several RCTs have revealed the effectiveness and safety of LCBDE comparing with LC+ ERCP/EST. The clearance rate form these studies reached 88% to 100%, which was as effective as EST procedure, without increased in the morbidity and mortality rates. Moreover, LCBDE might result in shorter hospitalizations and lower costs [27–29]. The meta-analysis also revealed that no statistically significant difference in stone clearance [risk ratios (RR) = -0.10, 95% confidence intervals (CI): -0.24 to 0.04, $p = 0.17$], postoperative morbidity (RR = 0.79, 95% CI: 0.58 to 1.10, $p = 0.16$), mortality (RR = 2.19, 95% CI: 0.33 to 14.67, $p = 0.42$), and length of hospital stay (MD = 0.99, 95% CI: -1.59 to 3.57, $p = 0.45$) [30], which was in accordance with the cochrane systematic review [31]. However, in the recent RCT comparing single-stage LCBDE and cholecystectomy versus two-stage endoscopic stone extraction followed by laparoscopic cholecystectomy, significantly greater number of patients with severe complications were detected in staged group (≥grade III: 11.7% vs 0%, $p = 0.0004$), although the overall morbidity was comparable between the two groups (23.8% vs. 22.6%, $p = 1.0$) [32]. In our cases series ($n = 265$), the technique successful rate was 97.0% (257/265), and only 10 (3.9%) patients was observed with residual stones. Bile leakage was most common complication (7.8%, 20/257), followed by residual stones and postoperative hemorrhage (3.1%, 8/257). In our hospital, ERCP was not the first choice in treatment of CBD stones. The reasons were as follows: (1) one-stage operation was as safe and efficacy as staged approach, even in patients with high medical risk [27], but an experienced endoscopist might not be available when needed; (2) ERCP was a costly procedure in China; (3) possibility of serious complications and the bad relationship between doctors and patients now [33] hindered the endoscopist's enthusiasm, especially when there was no strong evidence proving the advantage of ERCP procedure in treatment of CBD stones; (4) surgeons with advanced laparoscopic skills were easy to obtain in our hospital. So, we preferred LCBDE + LC to treat cholecystocholedocholithiasis because of the efficacy, safety and low cost.

After LCBDE, both T-tube drainage and primary closure are widely used in clinical practices. Several comparative studies and meta-analysis have demonstrated that primary closure is at least as effective and safe as T-tube drainage [8, 34, 35], even in emergency operation [36] and elderly patients [37]. Long-term outcome also shown that primary closure after LCBDE had a low incidence of recurrent stones, and no biliary strictures [5]. Thus, primary closure after LCBDE with choledochoscopy is considered to be a safe and effective alternative to T-tube drainage. However, primary closure after LCBDE is still a technique demanding procedure and bile leakage is the most frequently postoperative complication.

The incidence of bile leakage after primary closure following LCBDE varied dramatically [38–40]. It might be attributed to the different definition of bile leakage after biliary surgery among centers. Only few papers explained the definition of bile leakage they used [41]. In our hospital, bile leakage occurred in about 11.3% of patients with primary closure. Although most of them (62.5, 10/16) was mild (Dindo-Clavien GradeI), it seems higher than previously reported. We believed it might be resulted from the stricter criteria we used when comparing with the ISGLS definition [42].

Bile leakage negatively influences the postoperative recovery and patient might need additional imaging study and even reoperation. However, the risk factors for bile leakage after primary closure following LCBDE has not been fully discussed. In our study, we found that the surgeon's experience was the most important risk factor for bile leakage [OR 95% CI, 4.228 (1.330–13.438), $p = 0.03$]. In experienced hands, the incidence of bile leakage decreased significantly form 15.7% to 7.0% ($p = 0.04$). The data form LC, LCBDE and LCTBDE also revealed the importance of surgeon's experience for decreasing the complication rate [24, 26, 43]. Another factor affecting the incidence of bile leakage was the diameter of CBD, which was in accordance with Hua's study [40]. In patients with slender CBD, bile leakage occurred more frequently (<1 *vs* ≥1 cm, 31.6% *vs* 7.0%, $p = 0.04$). Possible reasons for this tendency were as follows: (1) the wall was thin in patients with slender CBD, and the bile could leak from the needle pinprick; (2) when suturing, surgeons might stitch too little tissue because of the fear of CBD stricture; (3) after suturing, transient stenosis of CBD might occur due to the tissue edema, and pressure increased within the biliary tree, then bile leakage occurred. So, in these cases, transcystic biliary drainage should be considered to reduce the pressure within the biliary tree.

In our cases series, one patient received reoperation due to the uncontrolled bile peritonitis. We found intraoperatively that the first suture was too far away from the superior edge of bile duct incision. So in the following cases, we usually preform the first suture above the superior edge of incision to avoid bile leakage resulting from excessive traction in following sutures. Absorbable sutures were used in our hospital to avoid CBD stricture and stone recurrence. In the follow-up period (median 34 moths, range 1–76 months), no CBD stricture was observed and 2 patients experienced stone recurrence.

Despite the limitations of retrospective study design and limited case volume, it was the initial try to detect the risk factors for bile leakage after primary closure following LCBDE. We found that slender CBD and inexperienced surgeons were associated with high bile leakage risk independently in primary closure after LCBDE. However, we believed that primary closure after LCBDE was safe in selected patients preformed by experienced hands.

Conclusion

Slender CBD and inexperienced surgeons were the high risk factors for bile leakage after primary closure following LCBDE.

Acknowledgements
None.

Funding
None.

Authors' contributions
DL designed the studies. FC, JL, DX, and YW performed data acquisition and analysis. DL, FC and FL performed statistical analysis and data interpretation. DL and FC prepared the manuscript. All authors read and approved the final manuscript.

Competing interests
The authors declare that they have no competing interest.

References
1. Darkahi B, Liljeholm H, Sandblom G. Laparoscopic Common Bile Duct Exploration: 9 Years Experience from a Single Center. Front Surg. 2016;3:23.
2. Aawsaj Y, Light D, Horgan L. Laparoscopic common bile duct exploration: 15-year experience in a district general hospital. SURG ENDOSC. 2016; 30(6):2563–6.
3. Gupta N. Role of laparoscopic common bile duct exploration in the management of choledocholithiasis. World J Gastrointest Surg. 2016; 8(5):376–81.
4. Qiu J, Yuan H, Chen S, Wu H. Laparoscopic common bile duct exploration in cirrhotic patients with choledocholithiasis. Surg Laparosc Endosc Percutan Tech. 2015;25(1):64–8.
5. Yi HJ, Hong G, Min SK, Lee HK. Long-term Outcome of Primary Closure After Laparoscopic Common Bile Duct Exploration Combined With Choledochoscopy. Surg Laparosc Endosc Percutan Tech. 2015;25(3):250–3.
6. Wills VL, Gibson K, Karihaloot C, Jorgensen JO. Complications of biliary T-tubes after choledochotomy. ANZ J SURG. 2002;72(3):177–80.
7. Ha JP, Tang CN, Siu WT, Chau CH, Li MK. Primary closure versus T-tube drainage after laparoscopic choledochotomy for common bile duct stones. Hepatogastroenterology. 2004;51(60):1605–8.
8. Dong ZT, Wu GZ, Luo KL, Li JM. Primary closure after laparoscopic common bile duct exploration versus T-tube. J SURG RES. 2014;189(2):249–54.
9. Muzaffar I, Zula P, Yimit Y, Jaan AT, Wen H. Randomized comparison of postoperative short-term and mid-term complications between T-tube and primary closure after CBD exploration. J Coll Physicians Surg Pak. 2014;24(11):810–4.
10. Ambreen M, Shaikh AR, Jamal A, Qureshi JN, Dalwani AG, Memon MM. Primary closure versus T-tube drainage after open choledochotomy. ASIAN J SURG. 2009;32(1):21–5.
11. Yin Z, Xu K, Sun J, Zhang J, Xiao Z, Wang J, Niu H, Zhao Q, Lin S, Li Y. Is the end of the T-tube drainage era in laparoscopic choledochotomy for common bile duct stones is coming? A systematic review and meta-analysis. ANN SURG. 2013;257(1):54–66.
12. Overby DW, Apelgren KN, Richardson W, Fanelli R. SAGES guidelines for the clinical application of laparoscopic biliary tract surgery. SURG ENDOSC. 2010;24(10):2368–86.
13. Chathadi KV, Chandrasekhara V, Acosta RD, Decker GA, Early DS, Eloubeidi MA, Evans JA, Faulx AL, Fanelli RD, Fisher DA, et al. The role of ERCP in benign diseases of the biliary tract. GASTROINTEST ENDOSC. 2015;81(4):795–803.
14. Easler JJ, Sherman S. Endoscopic Retrograde Cholangiopancreatography for the Management of Common Bile Duct Stones and Gallstone Pancreatitis. Gastrointest Endosc Clin N Am. 2015;25(4):657–75.
15. Trikudanathan G, Arain MA, Attam R, Freeman ML. Advances in the endoscopic management of common bile duct stones. Nat Rev Gastroenterol Hepatol. 2014;11(9):535–44.
16. Karsenti D. Endoscopic management of bile duct stones: residual bile duct stones after surgery, cholangitis, and "difficult stones". J VISC SURG. 2013;150(3 Suppl):S39–46.
17. Seo YR, Moon JH, Choi HJ, Kim DC, Ha JS, Lee TH, Cha SW, Cho YD, Park SH, Kim SJ. Comparison of endoscopic papillary balloon dilation and sphincterotomy in young patients with CBD stones and gallstones. Dig Dis Sci. 2014;59(5):1042–7.
18. Oh MJ, Kim TN. Prospective comparative study of endoscopic papillary large balloon dilation and endoscopic sphincterotomy for removal of large bile duct stones in patients above 45 years of age. Scand J Gastroenterol. 2012;47(8-9):1071–7.
19. Minakari M, Samani RR, Shavakhi A, Jafari A, Alijanian N, Hajalikhani M. Endoscopic papillary balloon dilatation in comparison with endoscopic sphincterotomy for the treatment of large common bile duct stone. Adv Biomed Res. 2013;2:46.
20. Zhao HC, He L, Zhou DC, Geng XP, Pan FM. Meta-analysis comparison of endoscopic papillary balloon dilatation and endoscopic sphincteropapillotomy. World J Gastroenterol. 2013;19(24):3883–91.
21. Costi R, Mazzeo A, Tartamella F, Manceau C, Vacher B, Valverde A. Cholecystocholedocholithiasis: a case-control study comparing the short- and long-term outcomes for a "laparoscopy-first" attitude with the outcome for sequential treatment (systematic endoscopic sphincterotomy followed by laparoscopic cholecystectomy). SURG ENDOSC. 2010;24(1):51–62.
22. Testoni PA, Mariani A, Aabakken L, Arvanitakis M, Bories E, Costamagna G, Deviere J, Dinis-Ribeiro M, Dumonceau JM, Giovannini M, et al. Papillary cannulation and sphincterotomy techniques at ERCP: European Society of Gastrointestinal Endoscopy (ESGE) Clinical Guideline. ENDOSCOPY. 2016;48(7):657–83.
23. Stoker ME. Common bile duct exploration in the era of laparoscopic surgery. Arch Surg. 1995;130(3):265–8. 268-269.
24. Zhu JG, Han W, Guo W, Su W, Bai ZG, Zhang ZT. Learning curve and outcome of laparoscopic transcystic common bile duct exploration for choledocholithiasis. Br J Surg. 2015;102(13):1691–7.
25. Jameel M, Darmas B, Baker AL. Trend towards primary closure following laparoscopic exploration of the common bile duct. Ann R Coll Surg Engl. 2008;90(1):29–35.
26. Abellan MI, Qurashi K, Abrisqueta CJ, Martinez IA. Laparoscopic common bile duct exploration. Lessons learned after 200 cases. Cir Esp. 2014;92(5):341–7.
27. Noble H, Tranter S, Chesworth T, Norton S, Thompson M. A randomized, clinical trial to compare endoscopic sphincterotomy and subsequent laparoscopic cholecystectomy with primary laparoscopic bile duct exploration during cholecystectomy in higher risk patients with choledocholithiasis. J Laparoendosc Adv Surg Tech A. 2009;19(6):713–20.
28. Rogers SJ, Cello JP, Horn JK, Siperstein AE, Schecter WP, Campbell AR, Mackersie RC, Rodas A, Kreuwel HT, Harris HW. Prospective randomized trial of LC + LCBDE vs ERCP/S + LC for common bile duct stone disease. Arch Surg. 2010;145(1):28–33.
29. Rhodes M, Sussman L, Cohen L, Lewis MP. Randomised trial of laparoscopic exploration of common bile duct versus postoperative endoscopic retrograde cholangiography for common bile duct stones. LANCET. 1998;351(9097):159–61.
30. Lu J, Cheng Y, Xiong XZ, Lin YX, Wu SJ, Cheng NS. Two-stage vs single-stage management for concomitant gallstones and common bile duct stones. World J Gastroenterol. 2012;18(24):3156–66.
31. Dasari BV, Tan CJ, Gurusamy KS, Martin DJ, Kirk G, McKie L, Diamond T, Taylor MA. Surgical versus endoscopic treatment of bile duct stones. Cochrane Database Syst Rev. 2013;9:D3327.
32. Bansal VK, Misra MC, Rajan K, Kilambi R, Kumar S, Krishna A, Kumar A, Pandav CS, Subramaniam R, Arora MK, et al. Single-stage laparoscopic common bile duct exploration and cholecystectomy versus two-stage endoscopic stone extraction followed by laparoscopic cholecystectomy for patients with concomitant gallbladder stones and common bile duct stones: a randomized controlled trial. SURG ENDOSC. 2014;28(3):875–85.
33. Chinese doctors are under threat. LANCET. 2010;376(9742):657.
34. Podda M, Polignano FM, Luhmann A, Wilson MS, Kulli C, Tait IS. Systematic review with meta-analysis of studies comparing primary duct closure and T-tube drainage after laparoscopic common bile duct exploration for choledocholithiasis. SURG ENDOSC. 2016;30(3):845–61.

35. Gurusamy KS, Koti R, Davidson BR. T-tube drainage versus primary closure after laparoscopic common bile duct exploration. Cochrane Database Syst Rev. 2013;6:D5641.
36. Alhamdani A, Mahmud S, Jameel M, Baker A. Primary closure of choledochotomy after emergency laparoscopic common bile duct exploration. SURG ENDOSC. 2008;22(10):2190–5.
37. Parra-Membrives P, Martinez-Baena D, Lorente-Herce JM, Jimenez-Vega J. Laparoscopic common bile duct exploration in elderly patients: is there still a difference? Surg Laparosc Endosc Percutan Tech. 2014;24(4):e118–22.
38. Cai H, Sun D, Sun Y, Bai J, Zhao H, Miao Y. Primary closure following laparoscopic common bile duct exploration combined with intraoperative cholangiography and choledochoscopy. WORLD J SURG. 2012;36(1):164–70.
39. Wu X, Yang Y, Dong P, Gu J, Lu J, Li M, Mu J, Wu W, Yang J, Zhang L, et al. Primary closure versus T-tube drainage in laparoscopic common bile duct exploration: a meta-analysis of randomized clinical trials. Langenbecks Arch Surg. 2012;397(6):909–16.
40. Hua J, Lin S, Qian D, He Z, Zhang T, Song Z. Primary closure and rate of bile leak following laparoscopic common bile duct exploration via choledochotomy. Dig Surg. 2015;32(1):1–8.
41. Estelles VN, Domingo DPC, Peris TN, Diez AJ, Vazquez TA, Blanes MF. Eleven years of primary closure of common bile duct after choledochotomy for choledocholithiasis. SURG ENDOSC. 2016;30(5):1975–82.
42. Koch M, Garden OJ, Padbury R, Rahbari NN, Adam R, Capussotti L, Fan ST, Yokoyama Y, Crawford M, Makuuchi M, et al. Bile leakage after hepatobiliary and pancreatic surgery: a definition and grading of severity by the International Study Group of Liver Surgery. SURGERY. 2011;149(5):680–8.
43. Conzo G, Amato G, Angrisani L, Bardi U, Belli G, Brancaccio U, Calise F, Celsi S, Corcione F, Cuccurullo D, et al. Hepaticojejunostomy in the treatment of iatrogenic biliary lesions following laparoscopic cholecystectomy. A retrospective study on 51 cases. Hepatogastroenterology. 2007;54(80):2328–32.

32

First right lobe living-donor hepatectomy after sleeve gastrectomy

Aiman Obed[3*], Abdalla Bashir[2] and Anwar Jarrad[1]

Abstract

Background: Obesity presents one of the leading causes of many chronic liver disorders and injuries. Nowadays, non-alcoholic steatohepatitis (NASH) demonstrates a challenging issue for the global health system. NASH can progress to life-threatening conditions such as cirrhosis and hepatocellular or cholangio carcinoma. Currently, NASH cirrhosis is a major indication for liver transplant (LT).

Case presentation: We present the case of a 37 year-old male who has lost 74 kg after undergoing successful laparoscopic sleeve gastrectomy (SG) four years ago. Recently, he underwent right hepatectomy in the course of living-donor liver transplantation for his sick father in our clinic. Before the SG was conducted four years ago, his weight was at 157 kg and his Body Mass Index (BMI) at 49 kg/m^2. At that time, Ultrasound examination showed severe fatty liver changes and intraoperative inspection of the liver was consistent with that observation. At the time of surgery, he weighed 83 kg and his BMI was at 27 kg/m^2. An effective weight reduction after bariatric surgery might protect NASH patients from further deterioration of their medical condition.

Conclusion: To our knowledge, we report the first successful case of a right lobe living-donor hepatectomy in a patient who previously underwent successful laparoscopic sleeve gastrectomy (LSG).

Keywords: First donor, NASH, Liver transplant, Living liver donation, Sleeve gastrectomy

Background

Obesity is associated with many chronic diseases including non-alcoholic fatty liver disease (NAFLD) and non-alcoholic steatohepatitis (NASH). Untreated NASH can progress to fibrosis and cirrhosis. Furthermore, NASH can increase the risk of developing cholangio carcinoma and hepatocellular carcinoma. NASH cirrhosis is becoming a major indication for liver transplant (LT) [1–3].

Weight reduction by bariatric surgery has shown to be an effective way of preventing the progression of NAFLD to chronic liver disease and cirrhosis [4–6]. Additionally, bariatric surgery was found to be feasible and safe in selected cirrhotic patients, liver transplanted patients and in the setting of combined procedures such as liver transplantation [7–10].

Significant weight loss after SG might prevent NASH patients from further deterioration of their liver function.

Herein we report the first right lobe living-donor hepatectomy four years after successful laparoscopic sleeve gastrectomy in a 37 year-old man.

Case presentation

A 37 year-old male who underwent successful laparoscopic sleeve gastrectomy four years ago and who has consequently lost 74 kg was presented to our clinic with other family members willing to provide their sick father with a right lobe for the liver transplantation. Before the SG was done four years ago his weight was at 157 kg and his Body Mass Index (BMI) at 49 kg/m^2. At that time Ultrasound examination showed severe fatty liver changes with diffuse increased hepatic parenchymal echogenicity and also intraoperative inspection of the liver was consistent with that observation. Unfortunately, liver biopsy was not taken. We did not quantify steatosis with other imaging modalities, such as MRI or CT, since the liver donation was not an issue at that time.

At the time of surgery, he weighed 83 kg and his BMI was at 27 kg/m^2. His lowest weight after SG was at 80 kg.

* Correspondence: aimanobed@hotmail.com
[3]Hepatobiliary and Transplant Surgery, Jordan Hospital, Amman, Jordan
Full list of author information is available at the end of the article

Full donor work up including liver biopsy was completed. The liver biopsy showed steatosis in less than 5%, no inflammation, no hepatocyte ballooning and no fibrosis.

He was chosen as an appropriate donor with a total liver volume of 1800 cm^3 and a future remnant liver volume of 900 cm^3. The graft-to-recipient weight ratio (GRWR) was at 0.9%.

Donor work up was completed including extended lab analysis, anesthesia, and cardiac, assessment, psychiatric team and ethical committee evaluation for organ transplantation and was approved for liver donation.

The Liver Transplant Board confirmed the indication for liver transplant and approved the living donor liver transplantation (LDLT). After completing the evaluation, LDLT was performed.

His father suffered from end-stage liver disease secondary to NASH cirrhosis, accompanied by type 2 diabetes mellitus. Evaluations revealed a Child-Pugh stage B, a model for end-stage liver disease (MELD) calculated score of 17 and a body weight at 100 kg.

During the right lobe hepatectomy, only minimal adhesions were found. The liver appeared grossly normal with a sharp left lateral lobe. The left liver lobe was supplied by a branch of the left gastric artery and a smaller branch of the main hepatic artery. The donor common hepatic artery, after the bifurcation of the left HA branch, was recovered with a segment of the gastroduodenal artery (Fig. 1). We chose to perform a right lobe donation, the most commonly performed procedure in our center, since it provides a sufficient liver remnant volume. Additionally, in this particular case the left lobe had two small arteries in comparison with the right lobe that only had a single big right hepatic artery. Also, there were no veins from the right lobe merging into the middle hepatic vein.

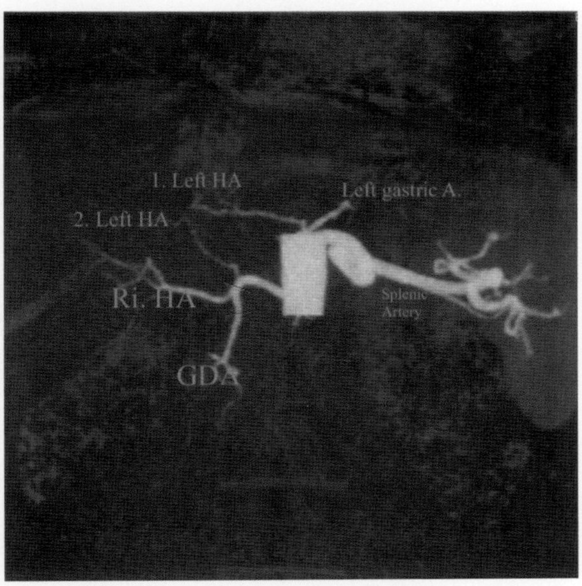

Fig. 1 Preoperative liver triple phase CT- scan showed right hepatic artery arising from celiac trunk with relevant left hepatic artery arising from left gastric artery; short red lines mark the split lines of common hepatic artery and gastroduodenal artery coming out with the right liver lobe

On the recipient side, left and right hepatic arteries were divided and a large anastomosis with branch-patch reconstruction was established. The right hepatic vein and the right portal vein appeared without any abnormalities (Fig. 2). The donor operation time was 3 h and 20 min. The donor didn't receive any blood products and was admitted to our intensive care unit for one day.

The donor had an uneventful recovery. On the first postoperative day, patient ambulation and clear fluid oral intake took place and he was discharged after seven days with normal liver function (Table 1).

Currently, eight months after the right lobe donation procedure, his liver function appears to be normal and his body weight remains stable in comparison to his weight prior to surgery (BMI = 27 kg/m^2).

Graft reperfusion in the recipient was normal and liver biopsy was not required.

Similarly, the recipient had an uneventful postoperative course. Ambulation and reintroduction of oral feeding were started on postoperative day two and he was discharged with normal liver function three weeks after LDLT. His diabetes disappeared after three months.

Discussion and conclusions

Obesity has reached an epidemic level. In many countries the incidence of obesity, defined by a BMI $\geq$ 35 kg/m^2, ranges between 7 and 24% and has even higher prevalences in Europe [11]. It is one of the main contributors to the global burden of the chronic clinical spectrum, including NAFLD. NAFLD includes a variety of liver injuries that range from simple steatosis to non-alcoholic steatohepatitis (NASH) [12].

Weight reduction by bariatric surgery has proved to be an effective way of preventing the progression of NAFLD to chronic liver disease and cirrhosis [4–6]. NASH cirrhosis presents the end stage of the spectrum of NAFLD and is becoming a main indication for LT in the United States. Presently, it is the third most common indication for LT and it is estimated to become the most common indication for LT within the next 1–2 decades.

Bariatric surgery was found to be convincing and safe in selected cirrhotic patients, liver transplanted patients and in the setting of combined procedures such as liver transplantation.

A good percentage of obese patients are disqualified at the time of presentation for LT due to the high risk of combined diseases.

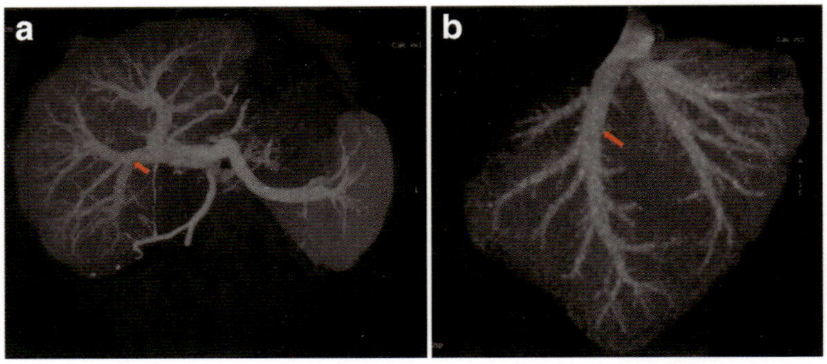

Fig. 2 Preoperative liver triple phase CT-scan showed normal appearance of right hepatic vein (**a**) and right portal vein (**b**)

Obesity is certainly associated with diabetes mellitus, coronary disease and tumors, and might imply significant morbidity and mortality post-LT. There are several surgical strategies to improve the outcome in this group of patients, including bariatric surgery before LT, bariatric surgery after LT and bariatric surgery [13–19] at the time of LT as initially described by Heimbach et al., who reported their expertise of combined LT and gastric sleeve resection (SG) in seven patients with a BMI greater than 35 kg/m^2 [10].

The advantages of combined LT with SG are certainly the reduction to one operative implementation for the patient and the consecutive prevention of a second operation with potentially severe adhesions. Recent studies have demonstrated a significant improvement of NAFLD Activity Score and fibrosis after SG [20].

Significant weight loss after bariatric surgery could help NASH patients to avoid the progression that might require liver transplant.

Even in the absence of published solid data, liver donation after major surgery seems to be feasible. Patients who are willing to donate their liver after successful bariatric surgery should be evaluated. If the donor evaluation reveals no medical contraindication, LDLT could be performed; probably with the same risks that donors without SG in their history would have.

Table 1 Shows postoperative liver function test for seven days

Post-operative day	AST (IU/L)	ALT (IU/L)	Total Bilirubin (mg/dL)
0	159	194	1.4
1	211	178	2.6
2	170	134	1.9
3	100	98	1.7
4	79	88	1.7
5	52	46	1.5
6	43	34	1.3
7	33	29	1.1

In general, all treatments that lead to the increase of the donor pool are welcomed. In absence of the gastric sleeve procedure, our patient would not have been eligible for donation.

The lack of donor biopsy at the time of sleeve gastrectomy demonstrates a study limitation in our case.

To our knowledge, we report the first successful case of a right lobe living-donor hepatectomy in a patient who previously underwent successful laparoscopic sleeve gastrectomy (LSG).

In conclusion, donor hepatectomy and LDLT appear to be safe and feasible operations from donors who underwent SG for obesity. Larger studies are needed to confirm this strategy, especially in the light of donor shortage in the field of liver transplantation.

Abbreviations
BMI: Body Mass Index; GRWR: Graft-to-recipient weight ratio; LDLT: Living donor liver transplant; LSG: Laparoscopic sleeve gastrectomy; LT: Liver transplant; NAFLD: Non-alcoholic fatty liver disease; NASH: Non-alcoholic steatohepatitis; SG: Sleeve gastrectomy

Authors' contributions
AO, AB and AJ analyzed the existing data regarding the treatment of the patient considered, wrote the manuscript, prepared the Figures and analyzed the existing literature on the issue. AO, AB and AJ critically revised the manuscript. All authors read and approved the final version of the manuscript.

Competing interests
The authors declare that they have no competing interests.

Author details
[1]Hepatology, Gastroenterology and Hepatobiliary/Transplant Unit, Jordan Hospital, Amman, Jordan. [2]General and Transplant Surgery, Jordan Hospital, Amman, Jordan. [3]Hepatobiliary and Transplant Surgery, Jordan Hospital, Amman, Jordan.

References
1. Berghofer A, Pischon T, Reinhold T, et al. Obesity prevalence from a European perspective: a systematic review. BMC Public Health. 2008;8:200.
2. Rabin BA, Boehmer TK, Brownson RC. Cross-national comparison of environmental and policy correlates of obesity in Europe. Eur J Pub Health. 2007;17:53–61.

3. Agopian VG, Kaldas FM, Hong JC, et al. Liver transplantation for non-alcoholic steatohepatitis: the new epidemic. Ann Surg. 2012;256:624–33.
4. Luo RB, Suzuki T, Hooker JC, et al. How bariatric surgery affects liver volume and fat density in NAFLD patients. Surg Endosc. 2017 Dec 7. https://doi.org/10.1007/s00464-017-5846-9.
5. Moretto M, Kupski C, da Silva VD, et al. Effect of bariatric surgery on liver fibrosis. Obes Surg. 2012;22(7):1044–9.
6. Mummadi RR, Kasturi KS, Chennareddygari S, et al. Effect of bariatric surgery on nonalcoholic fatty liver disease: systematic review and meta-analysis. Clin Gastroenterol Hepatol. 2008;6(12):1396–402.
7. Dallal RM, Mattar SG, Lord JL, et al. Results of laparoscopic gastric bypass in patients with cirrhosis. Obes Surg. 2004;14(1):47–53.
8. Woodford RM, Burton PR, O'Brien PE, et al. Laparoscopic adjustable gastric banding in patients with unexpected cirrhosis: safety and outcomes. Obes Surg. 2015;25(10):1858–62.
9. Pestana L, Swain J, Dierkhising R, et al. Bariatric surgery in patients with cirrhosis with and without portal hypertension: a single-center experience. Mayo Clin Proc. 2015;90(2):209–15.
10. Heimbach JK, Watt KDS, Poterucha JJ, Ziller NF, Cecco SD, Charlton MR, et al. Combined liver transplantation and gastric sleeve resection for patients with medically complicated obesity and end-stage liver disease. Am J Transplant. 2013;13(2):363–8.
11. Singhal A, Wilson GC, Wima K, et al. Impact of recipient morbid obesity on outcomes after liver transplantation. Transpl Int. 2015;28(2):148–55.
12. Shaker M, Tabbaa A, Albeldawi M, et al. Liver transplantation for nonalcoholic fatty liver disease: new challenges and new opportunities. World J Gastroenterol. 2014;20(18):5320–30.
13. Safwan M, Collins KM, Abouljoud MS. Outcome of liver transplantation in patients with prior bariatric surgery. Liver Transpl. 2017;23(11):1415–21. https://doi.org/10.1002/lt.24832.
14. Kumar S, Khandelwal N, Kumar A, et al. Simultaneous living donor liver transplant with sleeve gastrectomy for metabolic syndrome and NASH-related ESLD-first report from India. Indian J Gastroenterol. 2017;36(3):243–7. https://doi.org/10.1007/s12664-017-0753-5.
15. Butte JM, Devaud N, Jarufe NP, et al. Sleeve gastrectomy as treatment for severe obesity after orthotopic liver transplantation. Obes Surg. 2007;17: 1517–9.
16. Duchini A, Brunson ME. Roux-en-Y gastric bypass for recurrent nonalcoholic steatohepatitis in liver transplant recipients with morbid obesity. Transplantation. 2001;72:156–9.
17. Gentileschi P, Venza M, Benavoli D, et al. Intragastric balloon followed by biliopancreatic diversion in a liver transplant recipient: a case report. Obes Surg. 2009;19:1460–3.
18. Reino DC, Weigle KE, Dutson EP, et al. Liver transplantation and sleeve gastrectomy in the medically complicated obese: new challenges on the horizon. World J Hepatol. 2015;7(21):2315–8. https://doi.org/10.4254/wjh.v7.i21.2315.
19. Dziodzio T, Biebl M, Öllinger R, et al. The role of bariatric surgery in abdominal organ transplantation-the next big challenge? Obes Surg. 2017; 27(10):2696–706. https://doi.org/10.1007/s11695-017-2854-8.
20. Nobili V, Carpino G, et al. Laparoscopic sleeve Gastrectomy improves nonalcoholic fatty liver disease-related liver damage in adolescents by reshaping cellular interactions and hepatic Adipocytokine production. J Pediatr. 2017; https://doi.org/10.1016/j.jpeds.2017.

Table 1 Descriptive statistics of the investigated cohort of 75 patients undergoing surgery for distal cholangiocarcinoma

Variables			n (%)	Mean, Median (min.-max.)	Missing values n(%)
Age (years)			n.a.	65.2, 67 (33–87)	0 (0.0%)
Male gender			62 (82.7%)	n.a.	0 (0.0%)
Preoperative biliary stent			58 (77.3%)	n.a.	5 (6.7%)
Extent of surgery	Local bile duct excision w/o hilus	1 point	7 (9.3%)	3.0, 3 (1–5)	0 (0.0%)
	Local bile duct excision with hilus	2 points	3 (4.0%)		
	Pancreaticoduodenectomy	3 points	54 (72.0%)		
	with hilus resection	4 points	5 (6.7%)		
	with portal vein resection	5 points	6 (8.0%)		
Duration of operation (min)			n.a.	238.1, 230 (130–490)	0 (0.0%)
Grading	G1	1 point	2 (2.7%)	2.3, 2 (1–3)	0 (0.0%)
	G2	2 points	51 (68.0%)		
	G3	3 points	22 (29.3%)		
pT stages	pT1	1 point	4 (5.3%)	2.6, 3 (1–4)	0 (0.0%)
	pT2	2 points	28 (37.3%)		
	pT3	3 points	36 (48%)		
	pT4	4 points	7 (9.3%)		
pN stages	pN0	0 points	34 (45.3%)	0.6, 1 (0–2)	0 (0.0%)
	pN1	1 point	39 (52%)		
	pN2	2 point	2 (2.7%)		
M1 stage			5 (6.7%)	n.a.	0 (0.0%)
R0 resection			65 (86.7%)	n.a.	0 (0.0%)
Perineural invasion			46 (62.2%)	n.a.	1 (1.3%)
Venous invasion			16 (21.6%)	n.a.	1 (1.3%)
Lymph vessel invasion			22 (29.7%)	n.a.	1 (1.3%)
UICC stages	UICC Ia	1 point	4 (5.3%)	3.6, 4 (1–6)	0 (0.0%)
	UICC Ib	2 points	15 (20.0%)		
	UICC IIa	3 points	9 (12.0%)		
	UICC IIb	4 points	32 (42.7%)		
	UICC III	5 points	9 (12.0%)		
	UICC IV	6 points	6 (8.0%)		
Grading of complications	Clavien-Dindo Grade 0	0 points	25 (33.3%)	1.8, 1 (0–5)	2 (2.7%)
	Clavien-Dindo Grade I	1 point	15 (20.0%)		
	Clavien-Dindo Grade II	2 points	7 (9.3%)		
	Clavien-Dindo Grade III	3 points	11 (14.7%)		
	Clavien-Dindo Grade IV	4 points	9 (12.0%)		
	Clavien-Dindo Grade V	5 points	6 (8.0%)		
Complications leading to surgical intervention			19 (26.0%)	n.a.	2 (2.7%)
Observed overall survival in months			n.a.	29.1, 19 (0–145)	2 (2.7%)
Observed disease-free survival in months			n.a.	20.8, 13 (3–143)	47 (62.7%)
Hospital mortality			6 (8.0%)	n.a.	1 (1.3%)
Hospital stay in days			n.a.	29.8, 25 (7–102)	2 (2.7%)
ICU stay in days			n.a.	7.3, 3 (1–94)	17 (22.7%)
Days between onset of symptoms and date of surgery			n.a.	54.9, 34 (8–334)	36 (48.0%)

Table 1: Shown are descriptive statistics of the investigated cohort of 75 patients. The extent of surgery was scaled from 1 (local bile duct excision without resection of the perihilar bile ducts) to 5 points (pancreaticoduodenectomy including partial portal vein resection). This scale was used to calculate the variable *"extent of surgery graded in points multiplied by histological venous invasion"* as displayed in Table 2

tomography for verification of tumor extent with successful detection of the lesions in two patients.

Biopsies were performed in 33 patients (44.0%) whereas brush cytologies were performed in 39 patients (52.0%). Hereby the diagnosis was verified in 49.3% of the patients.

Preoperative biliary stenting via ERCP (internal drainage) as a consequence of relevant cholestasis was performed in 77.3% of the patients ($n = 58$). Percutaneous Transhepatic Cholangio-Drainage (PTCD) was not required in our patient collective. Patients receiving biliary stenting prior to operation showed significantly prolonged duration between onset of symptoms and operation ($p = 0.048$). Preoperative biliary stenting was found to be an independent risk factor for worse overall survival in multivariable Cox regression analysis (HR: 2.530; 95%-CI: 1.146–6.464, $p = 0.020$) (Table 2) (Fig. 1a).

The median time interval between onset of symptoms and operation was 34 days (Table 1).

Surgical results

In ten patients local excisions of the extrahepatic bile ducts were performed which included lymphadenectomy of the hepato-duodenal ligament representing a collective undergoing rather minor extent of surgery.

26 patients underwent pylorus-preserving partial pancreaticoduodenectomy and 28 patients underwent classical partial pancreaticoduodenectomy without preservation of the pylorus.

Six patients underwent additional partial portal vein resection and three patients underwent additional resection of proximal/central extrahepatic bile ducts a in addition to pancreaticoduodenectomy. One patient underwent right trisectorectomy of the liver (Segments 1, 4–8) and perihilar bile duct resection in addition to classical partial pancreaticoduodenectomy.

To analyse the influence of the extent of the surgical approach on patient outcome we graded the aforementioned procedures according to Table 1. Univariable analysis did not show significant influence on survival (Table 2, Fig. 1b). Multivariable analysis however displayed significant influence on survival in case of concomitant venous invasion (HR: 1.209; 95%-CI: 1.017–1.410, $p = 0.032$) (Table 2).

Since resection of the perihilar bile duct bifurcation, due to proximal tumor infiltration of the resection margin, was performed in seven patients we separately analysed postoperative outcome of these cases. Tumor-free resection margins were diagnosed in final histology in four of these seven patients and none developed anastomotic leakage. Median overall survival (28.0 months) was longer as compared to all other patients (16.5), however Cox regression analysis revealed no significant influence on survival ($p = 0.077$).

Segmental portal vein resection due to tumor infiltration, representing a rather extended approach of surgical resection, was performed in six patients in total (8%). Vein reconstruction was achieved by primary suture in five and by insertion of a ringed polytetrafluoroethylene (PTFE) graft in one case. Portal vein thrombosis occurred in one patient and was treated by thrombectomy. Following additional portal vein resection all patients died during follow-up with a lower median overall survival (13.5 versus 21.0 months). Accordingly, Cox regression analysis revealed a negative impact of portal vein infiltration, although not statistically significant ($p = 0.129$).

Negative resection margins (R0) in final histology were achieved in 86.7% of the patients. Residual tumor did not significantly influence overall survival in uni- or multivariable analysis as displayed in Table 2.

Initial intraoperative resection margins revealed residual tumor in 24 patients (32.0%). In eleven of these patients tumor free resection margins could be achieved by further local resection of adjacent tissue and in three patients by an extension of the surgical approach, i.e. pancreatic and hepatic resection respectively.

In the remaining patients further resection was not possible due to infiltration of superior mesenteric artery and/or due to the patients reduced general health condition respectively.

Seven of the ten patients undergoing local excision of the bile duct showed residual tumor in the initial intraoperative resection margins. Residual tumor was localized at the distal resection margin in six patients with simultaneous infiltration of the proximal resection margin in one patient. In one patient residual tumor was detected at the proximal resection margin. Further local resection ultimately led to tumor free resection margins in all but three patients.

Patients with tumor free resection margins in the initial intraoperative frozen sections did not show significantly better outcome regarding recurrence or survival when compared to patients undergoing further local or extended resection in order to achieve tumor free resection margins in final histopathological analysis ($p = 0.092$, $p = 0.903$ respectively).

Histopathological results

Low T-staging depended significantly on a short time period between first symptoms and operation ($p = 0.021$, ordinal regression). However, delayed surgery did not significantly influence tumor stage according to UICC ($p = 0.160$, ordinal regression) or the success of the operation defined as tumor-free resection margins (Odds ratio (OR): 0.995; 0.974–1.017; $p = 0.643$, logistic regression).

Lymph node infiltration (N1/N2), detected in 41 patients (54.7%), was a significant risk factor for worse overall survival in univariable ($p = 0.020$) and multivariable analysis (HR: 2.183; 95%-CI: 1.250–3.841, $p = 0.006$) (Fig. 1c).

Table 2 Shown are the uni- and multivariable Cox regression analysis to identify risk factors for overall survival

Variables (univariable Cox regression analysis)			HR	95%-CI	p-value
Age (years)			1.005	0.980 – 1.032	0.713
Male gender			0.791	0.431 – 1.569	0.482
Preoperative biliary stent			1.412	0.704 – 3.238	0.350
Extent of surgery	Local bile duct excision w/o hilus	1 point	1.034	0.753 – 1.427	0.836
	Local bile duct excision with hilus	2 points			
	Pancreaticoduodenectomy	3 points			
	with hilus resection	4 points			
	with portal vein resection	5 points			
Perihilar bile duct resection			0.439	0.132 – 1.081	0.077
Partial portal vein resection			2.070	0.786 – 4.534	0.129
Duration of operation (min)			0.998	0.994 – 1.001	0.311
Grading	G1	1 point	1.638	0.921 – 2.863	0.092
	G2	2 points			
	G3	3 points			
pT stages	pT1	1 point	1.191	0.855 – 1.656	0.300
	pT2	2 points			
	pT3	3 points			
	pT4	4 points			
pN stages	pN0	0 points	1.717	1.092 – 2.668	**0.020**
	pN1	1 point			
	pN2	2 point			
M1 stage			0.861	0.259 – 2.119	0.769
R0 resection			0.733	0.376 – 1.602	0.411
Perineural invasion			1.913	1.110 – 3.397	**0.019**
Venous invasion			1.932	1.006 – 3.502	**0.048**
Lymph vessel invasion			1.635	0.904 – 2.850	0.102
UICC stages	UICC Ia	1 point	1.119	0.931 – 1.346	0.230
	UICC Ib	2 points			
	UICC IIa	3 points			
	UICC IIb	4 points			
	UICC III	5 points			
	UICC IV	6 points			
Grading of complications	Clavien-Dindo Grade 0	0 points	1.226	1.034 – 1.452	**0.020**
	Clavien-Dindo Grade I	1 point			
	Clavien-Dindo Grade II	2 points			
	Clavien-Dindo Grade III	3 points			
	Clavien-Dindo Grade IV	4 points			
	Clavien-Dindo Grade V	5 points			
Complications leading to surgical intervention			1.302	0.696 – 2.306	0.395

Table 2 Shown are the uni- and multivariable Cox regression analysis to identify risk factors for overall survival *(Continued)*

Variables (univariable Cox regression analysis)	HR	95%-CI	p-value
Variables (final multivariable Cox regression model)			
Preoperative biliary stenting	2.530	1.146 – 6.464	**0.020**
Venous invasion (yes=1, no=0) multiplied by Extent of surgery graded in points	1.209	1.017 – 1.410	**0.032**
Lymph node staging graded in points	2.183	1.250 – 3.841	**0.006**
Perineural invasion	2.118	1.147 – 4.054	**0.016**
Complications graded by Clavien-Dindo	1.395	1.148 – 1.699	**0.001**

Univariable Cox regression analysis identified lymph node staging (N), perineural invasion, venous invasion and grading of complications according to Clavien-Dindo as significant risk factors for worse overall survival
The final multivariable Cox regression model determined preoperative biliary stenting, the extent of surgery in case of positive histological venous invasion, lymph node staging and perineural invasion as well as postoperative complications graded in points according to Clavien-Dindo as independent significant risk factors for survival

In 46 patients (62.2%) histopathological analysis revealed perineural invasion. Univariable ($p = 0.019$) and multivariable analysis (HR: 2.118; 95%-CI: 1.147–4.054, $p = 0.016$) identified perineural invasion as significant risk factor for overall survival (Fig. 1d).

Venous invasion was observed in 16 patients (21.6%) with significant influence on worse overall survival in univariable analysis ($p = 0.048$) (Fig. 1e). Further histopathological results and their influence on patient outcome are displayed in Tables 1 and 2.

Postoperative course and complications

Median postoperative hospital stay was 25 days including a median of 3 days in the ICU. Extended surgery did not significantly prolong postoperative hospital stay nor time spent in the ICU.

Fourty-five patients (60.0%) had complications with varying degrees of severity graded according to Clavien-Dindo (Tables 1 and 3). Univariable ($p = 0.020$) and multivariable analysis (HR: 1.395; 95%-CI: 1.148–1.699, $p = 0.001$) identified the grade of postoperative complications as significant risk factor for worse overall survival (Fig. 1f).

Patients undergoing different extents of surgery as stated above did not experience statistically significant differences regarding rate and severity of postoperative complications.

The most common complications were wound infections with a rate of 21.3%.

Type A pancreatic fistulas were not documented due to missing data on enzyme measurements from abdominal drains. Type B pancreatic fistulas were observed in ten patients (13.3%). Type C pancreatic fistulas were

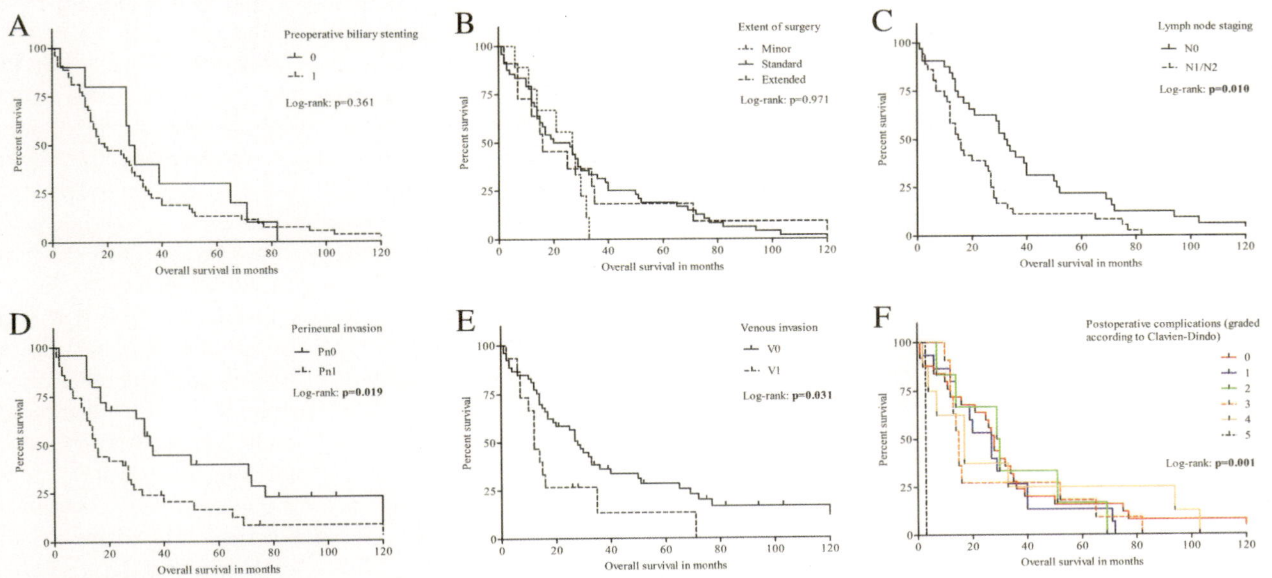

Fig. 1 Survival (Kaplan–Meier) after resection of distal cholangiocarcinoma according to preoperative biliary stenting (**a**), extent of surgery (**b**), lymph node staging (**c**), perineural invasion (**d**), venous invasion (**e**) and postoperative complications graded by Clavien-Dindo (**f**). Shown are all risk factors that were significant in univariable or multivariable Cox regression analysis, respectively. Overall survival in months after resection of distal cholangiocarcinoma depending to the studied factors

Table 3 Complications in patients with distal cholangiocarcinoma after receiving surgical treatment

Complications	number of patients (%)
Wound infection	16 (21.3)
Pancreatic fistula grade B	10 (13.3)
Insufficiency of biliodigestive anastomosis	8 (10.7)
Pancreatic fistula grade C	7 (9.3)
Death within 30 postoperative days	5 (6.7)
Renal insufficiency	5 (6.7)
Delayed gastric emptying	5 (6.7)
Erosion haemorrhage	4 (5.3)
Acute confusional state	3 (4.0)
Pleural effusion	3 (4.0)
Pneumonia	2 (2.7)
Cardiovascular events	2 (2.7)
Urinary tract infection	1 (1.3)
Hepatic insufficiency	1 (1.3)
Thrombosis of portal vein	1 (1.3)
Intrabdominal abscess	1 (1.3)
Postoperativ bleeding	1 (1.3)

Table 3: Number (and frequency) of complications in patients with distal cholangiocarcinoma after receiving surgical treatment

diagnosed in seven patients (9.3%) and total pancreatectomy was performed in six individuals (8.0%).

Eight patients (10.7%) suffered from insufficiency of the biliodigestive anastomosis.

Early mortality, defined as death in the first 30 post-operative days was 6.7% ($n = 5$). Causes of death were cardiac arrest due to cardiac infarction in one patient, sepsis and organ failure after total pancreatectomy due to insufficiency of the pancreatic anastomosis and arterial bleeding in two patients, and organ failure due to severe pneumonia in two further patients.

After local excision of the extrahepatic bile duct three of ten patients suffered from local tumor recurrence while another patient developed liver metastasis in the observation period. Patients undergoing standard pancreatic resection developed tumor recurrence in 21 documented cases ranging from local recurrence ($n = 5$), to lymph node, liver, bone and peritoneal metastases ($n = 16$). Three of eleven patients after extend pancreatic surgery suffered from local recurrence whereas two patients developed distant metastases in liver and peritoneum.

The rate of observed tumor recurrence was not significantly influenced by the extent of surgery.

The median overall survival was 19 months (0–145). Fifty-two (72.0%), 18 (30.0%) and 11 (22.0%) patients survived more than 1, 3 and 5 years, respectively. Thirteen patients (17.3%) were still alive at the time of data analysis.

Discussion

Due to the aforementioned comparatively low incidence of DCC among the general population, especially from Western countries, reports on outcome after surgery, of large patient collectives, are scarce. This data from a single high-volume center was analysed to identify prognostic factors for unfavourable patient outcome.

Interestingly no published data investigated preoperative stenting in patients with DCC and its impact on survival yet. In multivariable analysis we identified preoperative stenting as strongest risk factor for survival. A significantly longer duration between first symptoms and surgery in these patients could provide a clinically plausible explanation for the inferior outcome (Table 2). A prospective trial aiming to elucidate the role of preoperative biliary stenting in patients with pancreatic head cancer showed a significantly higher rate of complications after preoperative stenting [20]. So far similar observations have not yet been reported for DCC. The current study did not find a significant influence of biliary stenting on the rate or severity of postoperative complications. Nonetheless, we are well aware that preoperative conditions, which were not analysed in the current study, like cholangitis or severe biliary obstruction which require prolonged biliary drainage could be an explanation for the inferior postoperative outcome [21].

Survival after surgical treatment in the current study was similar to several previous studies [22–28].

Reported outcomes of patients with DCC after extended pancreatic surgery are extremely scarce. Solely Courtin-Tanguy et al. investigated extended surgery for treatment of DCC and found that combined organ resection was an independent risk factor for worse survival [29]. Interestingly, the present study showed that extended pancreatic resection was not significantly associated with inferior survival except in case of concomitant histological venous invasion as displayed by the identified interaction variable. Previous studies on risk factors for survival have not taken possible multiplicative factor interactions into account [28, 30]. The approach to multivariable Cox regression in this study deploys the previously published methodology for the detection of such factor interactions [18]. However, the displayed factor interaction is not suitable for intraoperative decision making regarding the extent of surgery due to the circumstance that histopathogical results verifying microscopic venous invasion are rarely available pre- or intraoperatively. Instead the prognostic value of venous invasion in patients undergoing extended surgery should be considered within the postoperative therapeutic strategy.

Partial portal vein resection due to macroscopic tumor invasion had no statistically significant influence on survival in Cox regression analysis (Table 2) in this study while several studies described poor survival for patients after portal vein resection, although only Miura et al. were able to show significant influence on survival in multivariable analysis [28, 31, 32]. This discrepancy could be due to the small number of cases in this study since a tendency towards worse survival in patients after partial portal vein resection has been observed. The benefit of portal vein resection therefore remains unclear.

Intraoperative frozen sections were crucial for flexible intraoperative decision making on the extent of resection, achieving tumor-free resection margins and partially led to an extension of the surgical strategy including partial portal vein, additional liver or perhilar bile duct resection. This is emphasized by the fact that the preoperative CT scans in the displayed cohort were not a reliant predictor of tumor extent. CT scans of 22 patients identified no measurable tumor mass although final histology revealed tumor sizes between T stage 1 and 4 in these patients. Even additional MR tomography did not provide significantly better results in preoperative detection of tumor extent. Therefore, in some cases endosonography might help for identification of tumor extent.

Finally patients with stricture of the distal bile duct suspicious of a malignant tumor should be explored surgically even if histology was negative, since 49.3% of preoperative histologies were false negative.

The impact of positive tumor infiltration at the surgical resection margin (R1/2 resection) on postoperative survival following curative resection of DCCs is widely discussed. We found no significant impact of R1/2 resection on overall survival in Cox regression analysis (Table 2). This finding is in line with some of the published series [15, 33–35]. Other studies identified positive resection margins as an independent prognostic factor on overall survival [3, 28]. Interestingly the percentage of R1 or R2 resected patients differs widely between the aforementionend published series from 7.0 to 43.3% [3, 15, 28, 33–37]. Our series shows a comparatively low rate of R1/R2 resections with 13.3%. A comparable retrospective study with 10.5% positive resections margins found no significant difference in survival for these patients in uni- and multivariable analysis [15]. Two published series found rates of 13.4 and 14.0% of R1/2 resected patients, respectively with significant influence on patient survival in uni- but not in multivariable analysis [33, 35]. In contrast series with higher rates of cancer positive resection margins identified R1/2 resections as an independent significant negative prognostic factor on survival in multivariable analysis [28, 38]. This could implicate a correlation of higher rates of positive resection margins with the identification of R1/2 resections as a significant negative prognostic factor in multivariable analysis in some series, which in turn would explain the conflicting results of our and these series [15, 33–35]. As displayed above, further local or extended resection in case of initially positive intraoperative resection margins was performed on a regular basis especially in patients undergoing local excision of bile duct and did not impact recurrence rate or overall survival. Interestingly there is presently no further data on this matter in patients undergoing resection for distal cholangiocarcinoma. Until further clarification the primary goal of surgical resection of DCC should be to achieve R0 resection. We therefore recommend intraoperative frozen sections of the resection margins and when residual disease is detected, additional resection of the bile duct bifurcation or locally infiltrated structures should be performed if technically feasible.

The presence of tumor positive lymph nodes was identified as a significant prognostic factor in multivariable analysis (Table 2) as was reported by different meta-analysis and some multicenter studies [28, 30, 36, 38]. Apart from a German study by Petrova et al., all mentioned publications reported a significant impact of lymph node metastasis on survival in uni- and not in multivariable analysis [28]. The above mentioned German colleagues did not report on the impact of the number of metastatic lymph nodes on survival. This seems to be relevant as Kiriyama et al. demonstrated earlier that the total number of infiltrated lymph nodes influences patients outcome. They found a significant difference when comparing no lymph node metastasis with 1–3 and more than 4 metastases [39]. This correlates well with our findings, as we classified the number of lymph node metastasis according to the newest TNM 8th edition classification for DCC in N0 versus N1 (1–3 positive lymph nodes) versus N2 (≥ 4 positive lymph nodes) resulting in a negative prognostic factor for each grade with a hazard ratio of 2.18 in multivariable analysis.

Postoperative complications graded in points according to Clavien-Dindo had a significant impact on patient outcome (Table 2). The influence of postoperative morbidity on the outcome of patients with DCC was recently observed by Petrova et al. and Andrianello et al.. Aside from direct consequences leading to early death in hospital it is assumed that patients with complicated postoperative course experience delay in the start of adjuvant therapy options (i.e. chemotherapy) resulting in an inferior survival [28, 40]. However the efficiency of adjuvant chemotherapy in patients with cholangiocarcinoma, as currently investigated by the multicenter prospective ACTICCA trial, remains unclear [41].

Conclusion

Preoperative biliary stenting, positive lymph node staging, perineural invasion as well as extended surgery in patients with concomitant venous invasion and postoperative complications should be considered within the perioperative therapeutic strategy. It is important to state that it is difficult to draw definite conclusions from this retrospective study considering the small patient collective undergoing extended surgery, respectively. Therefore it would certainly be beneficial performing multi-center studies with prospective analysis to determine which surgical approach is justifiable regarding optimal patient outcome. In addition the effects of preoperative biliary drainage in patients with DCC and relevant cholestasis on survival should be thoroughly examined in respect of our presented data.

Abbreviations

DCC: Cholangiocarcinoma; EVG: Elastic Van Gieson's; HE: Haematoxylin and eosin; HR: Hazard ratio; ICU: Intensive care unit; OR: Odds ratio; OS: Overall survival; PAS: Periodic acid–Schiff; PTFE: Polytetrafluoroethylene

Funding

There is no funding for the present study.

Authors' contributions

Study conception and design: OB, HS, FV, MoK. Acquisition of data: OB, MiK, HS, MoK, KJO. Analysis and interpretation of data: OB, HS, JG, MoK, KJO. Drafting of manuscript: OB, MiK, HS, MoK, KJO. Critical revision of manuscript: HS, JG, FV, SC, FO, JK. All authors have read and approved the final version of this manuscript.

Competing interests

The authors declare that they have no competing interests.

Author details

[1]Department of General, Visceral and Transplant Surgery, Medizinische Hochschule Hannover, Carl-Neuberg-Strasse 1, 30625 Hannover, Germany. [2]Core Facility Quality Management Transplantation, Integrated Research and Treatment Center Transplantation (IFB-Tx), Hannover Medical School, Hannover, Germany. [3]Department of General, Visceral and Oncological Surgery, Asklepios Klinik Barmbek, Hamburg, Germany.

References

1. Bragazzi M, Carpinale V, Carpino G, Venere R, Semeraro R, Gentile R, Gaudio E, Alvaro D. Cholangiocarcinoma: epidemiology and risk factors. Translational Gastrointestinal Cancer. 2011;1:21–32.
2. Nakeeb A, Pitt HA, Sohn TA, Coleman J, Abrams RA, Piantadosi S, et al. Cholangiocarcinoma. A spectrum of intrahepatic, perihilar, and distal tumors. Ann Surg. 1996;224:463,73. discussion 473-5
3. DeOliveira ML, Cunningham SC, Cameron JL, Kamangar F, Winter JM, Lillemoe KD, et al. Cholangiocarcinoma: thirty-one-year experience with 564 patients at a single institution. Ann Surg. 2007;245:755–62.
4. Kayahara M, Nagakawa T, Ohta T, Kitagawa H, Tajima H, Miwa K. Role of nodal involvement and the periductal soft-tissue margin in middle and distal bile duct cancer. Ann Surg. 1999;229:76–83.
5. Sakamoto Y, Kosuge T, Shimada K, Sano T, Ojima H, Yamamoto J, et al. Prognostic factors of surgical resection in middle and distal bile duct cancer: an analysis of 55 patients concerning the significance of ductal and radial margins. Surgery. 2005;137:396–402.
6. Jang JY, Kim SW, Park DJ, Ahn YJ, Yoon YS, Choi MG, et al. Actual long-term outcome of extrahepatic bile duct cancer after surgical resection. Ann Surg. 2005;241:77–84.
7. Sasaki R, Takeda Y, Funato O, Nitta H, Kawamura H, Uesugi N, et al. Significance of ductal margin status in patients undergoing surgical resection for extrahepatic cholangiocarcinoma. World J Surg. 2007;31:1788–96.
8. Bahra M, Jacob D, Langrehr JM, Neumann UP, Neuhaus P. Carcinoma of the distal and middle bile duct: surgical results, prognostic factors, and long-term follow-up. J Hepato-Biliary-Pancreat Surg. 2008;15:501–7.
9. Todoroki T, Kawamoto T, Koike N, Fukao K, Shoda J, Takahashi H. Treatment strategy for patients with middle and lower third bile duct cancer. Br J Surg. 2001;88:364–70.
10. Valle J, Wasan H, Palmer DH, Cunningham D, Anthoney A, Maraveyas A, et al. Cisplatin plus gemcitabine versus gemcitabine for biliary tract cancer. N Engl J Med. 2010;362:1273–81.
11. Yoshida T, Matsumoto T, Sasaki A, Morii Y, Aramaki M, Kitano S. Prognostic factors after pancreatoduodenectomy with extended lymphadenectomy for distal bile duct cancer. Arch Surg. 2002;137:69–73.
12. Murakami Y, Uemura K, Hayashidani Y, Sudo T, Ohge H, Sueda T. Pancreatoduodenectomy for distal cholangiocarcinoma: prognostic impact of lymph node metastasis. World J Surg. 2007;31:337,42. discussion 343-4
13. Lee HG, Lee SH, Yoo DD, Paik KY, Heo JS, Choi SH, et al. Carcinoma of the middle bile duct: is bile duct segmental resection appropriate? World J Gastroenterol. 2009;15:5966–71.
14. Wakai T, Shirai Y, Tsuchiya Y, Nomura T, Akazawa K, Hatakeyama K. Combined major hepatectomy and pancreaticoduodenectomy for locally advanced biliary carcinoma: long-term results. World J Surg. 2008;32:1067–74.
15. Ebata T, Nagino M, Nishio H, Igami T, Yokoyama Y, Nimura Y. Pancreatic and duodenal invasion in distal bile duct cancer: paradox in the tumor classification of the American joint committee on Cancer. World J Surg. 2007;31:2008–15.
16. Wiltberger G, Krenzien F, Benzing C, Atanasov G, Klein F, Hau HM, et al. Prognostic accuracy of the seventh edition of the TNM classification compared with the fifth and sixth edition for distal Cholangiocarcinoma. Ann Surg Oncol. 2016;23:1320–6.
17. Dindo D, Demartines N, Clavien PA. Classification of surgical complications: a new proposal with evaluation in a cohort of 6336 patients and results of a survey. Ann Surg. 2004;240:205–13.
18. Hosmer DW, Lemeshow S, May S. Applied survival analysis: regression modeling of time to event data. 2nd ed. New York: Wiley-Interscience; 2008.
19. Gwiasda J, Schulte A, Kaltenborn A, Ramackers W, Kleine M, Beetz O, et al. Identification of the resection severity index as a significant independent prognostic factor for early mortality and observed survival >5 and >10 years after liver resection for hepatocellular carcinoma. Surg Oncol. 2017;26:178–87.
20. van der Gaag NA, Rauws EA, van Eijck CH, Bruno MJ, van der Harst E, Kubben FJ, et al. Preoperative biliary drainage for cancer of the head of the pancreas. N Engl J Med. 2010;362:129–37.
21. Rodarte-Shade M, Kahaleh M. Stent placement as a bridge to surgery in malignant biliary obstruction (pancreatic cancer, distal bile duct cancer, and hilar tumors). Gastrointestinal Intervention. 2015;4:21–6.
22. Fong Y, Blumgart LH, Lin E, Fortner JG, Brennan MF. Outcome of treatment for distal bile duct cancer. Br J Surg. 1996;83:1712–5.
23. Zerbi A, Balzano G, Leone BE, Angeli E, Veronesi P, Di Carlo V. Clinical presentation, diagnosis and survival of resected distal bile duct cancer. Dig Surg. 1998;15:410–6.
24. Allen PJ, Reiner AS, Gonen M, Klimstra DK, Blumgart LH, Brennan MF, et al. Extrahepatic cholangiocarcinoma: a comparison of patients with resected proximal and distal lesions. HPB (Oxford). 2008;10:341–6.
25. Hatzaras I, George N, Muscarella P, Melvin WS, Ellison EC, Bloomston M. Predictors of survival in periampullary cancers following pancreaticoduodenectomy. Ann Surg Oncol. 2010;17:991–7.
26. Woo SM, Ryu JK, Lee SH, Yoo JW, Park JK, Kim YT, et al. Recurrence and prognostic factors of ampullary carcinoma after radical resection: comparison with distal extrahepatic cholangiocarcinoma. Ann Surg Oncol. 2007;14:3195–201.
27. Chung YJ, Choi DW, Choi SH, Heo JS, Kim DH. Prognostic factors following surgical resection of distal bile duct cancer. J Korean Surg Soc. 2013;85:212–8.
28. Petrova E, Ruckert F, Zach S, Shen Y, Weitz J, Grutzmann R, et al. Survival outcome and prognostic factors after pancreatoduodenectomy for distal bile duct carcinoma: a retrospective multicenter study. Langenbeck's Arch Surg. 2017;402:831–40.
29. Courtin-Tanguy L, Rayar M, Bergeat D, Merdrignac A, Harnoy Y, Boudjema K, et al. The true prognosis of resected distal cholangiocarcinoma. J Surg Oncol. 2016;113:575–80.

30. Zhou Y, Liu S, Wu L, Wan T. Survival after surgical resection of distal cholangiocarcinoma: a systematic review and meta-analysis of prognostic factors. Asian J Surg. 2017;40:129–38.
31. Miura F, Sano K, Amano H, Toyota N, Wada K, Yoshida M, et al. Evaluation of portal vein invasion of distal cholangiocarcinoma as borderline resectability. J Hepatobiliary Pancreat Sci. 2015;22:294–300.
32. Maeta T, Ebata T, Hayashi E, Kawahara T, Mizuno S, Matsumoto N, et al. Pancreatoduodenectomy with portal vein resection for distal cholangiocarcinoma. Br J Surg. 2017;104:1549–57.
33. Cheng Q, Luo X, Zhang B, Jiang X, Yi B, Wu M. Distal bile duct carcinoma: prognostic factors after curative surgery. A series of 112 cases. Ann Surg Oncol. 2007;14:1212–9.
34. Hernandez J, Cowgill SM, Al-Saadi S, Villadolid D, Ross S, Kraemer E, et al. An aggressive approach to extrahepatic cholangiocarcinomas is warranted: margin status does not impact survival after resection. Ann Surg Oncol. 2008;15:807–14.
35. Qiao QL, Zhang TP, Guo JC, Zhan HX, Zhao JX, Liu YC, et al. Prognostic factors after pancreatoduodenectomy for distal bile duct cancer. Am Surg. 2011;77:1445–8.
36. Ercolani G, Dazzi A, Giovinazzo F, Ruzzenente A, Bassi C, Guglielmi A, et al. Intrahepatic, peri-hilar and distal cholangiocarcinoma: three different locations of the same tumor or three different tumors? Eur J Surg Oncol. 2015;41:1162–9.
37. Iso Y, Kita J, Kato M, Shimoda M, Kubota K. When hepatic-side ductal margin is positive in N+ cases, additional resection of the bile duct is not necessary to render the negative hepatic-side ductal margin during surgery for extrahepatic distal bile duct carcinoma. Med Sci Monit. 2014;20:471–5.
38. Wellner UF, Shen Y, Keck T, Jin W, Xu Z. The survival outcome and prognostic factors for distal cholangiocarcinoma following surgical resection: a meta-analysis for the 5-year survival. Surg Today. 2017;47:271–9.
39. Kiriyama M, Ebata T, Aoba T, Kaneoka Y, Arai T, Shimizu Y, et al. Prognostic impact of lymph node metastasis in distal cholangiocarcinoma. Br J Surg. 2015;102:399–406.
40. Andrianello S, Marchegiani G, Malleo G, Rusev BC, Scarpa A, Bonamini D, et al. Over 700 Whipples for Pancreaticobiliary malignancies: postoperative morbidity is an additional negative prognostic factor for distal bile duct Cancer. J Gastrointest Surg. 2017;21:527–33.
41. Stein A, Arnold D, Bridgewater J, Goldstein D, Jensen LH, Klumpen HJ, et al. Adjuvant chemotherapy with gemcitabine and cisplatin compared to observation after curative intent resection of cholangiocarcinoma and muscle invasive gallbladder carcinoma (ACTICCA-1 trial) - a randomized, multidisciplinary, multinational phase III trial. BMC Cancer. 2015;15:564,015–1498-0.

34

Single-site robotic cholecystectomy: comparison of clinical outcome and the learning curves in relation to surgeon experience in a community teaching hospital

Mohamad Dughayli*, Sergey Shimunov, Sherry Johnson and Fadi Baidoun

Abstract

Background: The aim of this study was to analyze the experience of two surgeons who have different laparoscopic skills and case volume, with single-site robotic cholecystectomy (SSRC) and evaluate their learning curves.

Methods: All SSRCs performed between March 2013 and April 2015 were retrospectively reviewed. The patients were divided among two surgeons based on the surgeon's level of laparoscopic skills and case volume. Surgeon 1 had experience in advanced laparoscopy while surgeon 2 had basic laparoscopic skills. Patients' demographic data, intraoperative and short-term postoperative results were assessed.

Results: The analysis included 102 patients for surgeon 1 and 15 patients for surgeon 2. There were no major or minor complications in either cohort. Operative time was significantly longer for surgeon 2, conversion to laparoscopy rate was 4% for surgeon 1 compared to 20% for surgeon 2, $P = 0.044$, which is statistically significant.

Conclusions: SSRC is an easy and safe procedure that can be quickly learned and performed in a reproducible manner by surgeons with experienced laparoscopic skills and greater case volume.

Keywords: Single-site, Robotic surgery, Cholecystectomy

Background

Laparoscopic cholecystectomy is the most common laparoscopic procedure and is the gold standard for treatment of gallbladder disease. Single-incision laparoscopic cholecystectomies aimed to reduce the number of incisions, and therefore, reduce the risk of surgical site infection, scarring and postoperative pain while allowing earlier return to the patient's activities of daily living. Navarra et al. in 1997 [1] performed the first single-incision laparoscopic cholecystectomy via the trans-umbilical approach. Although promising results have been reported [2] in terms of safety and technique feasibility, others have reported increased complications, bile duct injuries [3–5] and incisional hernia occurrence. The single-incision port approach had significant limitations, mainly associated with instrumentation and proper triangulation [6], image instability, instrument collision, limited range of motion and decrease in the amount of force available at the tips of flexible instruments.

Robotic surgery has become an established alternative to conventional laparoscopy by solving the problems of angulation, improving the ergonomics of single-incision technologies [7], and overcoming the intrinsic limitations of single-incision laparoscopy, as reported by Kroh et al. [8].

Henry Ford Wyandotte Hospital, a community based teaching hospital, initiated its robotic surgery program in March 2013. Our team performed the first operation using the single-site platform for single-incision surgery with the da Vinci Si system (Intuitive Surgical, Sunnyvale, CA). Plans were made to expand the application of this new technology in our teaching hospital. As with most

* Correspondence: mdughay1@hfhs.org
Department of General Surgery, Henry Ford Wyandotte Hospital, 2333 Biddle Avenue, Wyandotte, MI 48192, USA

operative procedures, case volume and the surgeon's expertise are considered to have a major influence on procedure success, learning curve as measured by the total operative time and complication rates. In our hospital, surgeries were performed by two surgeons with different levels of laparoscopic skills and overall surgical experience and case volume. The primary aim of this study was to evaluate whether intraoperative and postoperative measures differ significantly based on a surgeon's previous laparoscopic experience and case volume, with the focus on factors such as operative time as a reflection of the learning curve, conversion to laparoscopy, hospital stay, and previous abdominal surgery. Moreover, the learning curve was noted to be greatly influenced by the surgeon's experience and patient prior surgeries. In this report we assess the learning curve based on two surgeons' experience and case volume.

Methods

This retrospective study was approved by the Henry Ford Health System Institutional Review Board (No. 10555). There were 117 patients who underwent single-site robotic cholecystectomy (SSRC) between March 2013 and April 2015 at our institution. Variables including demographics, operative time, estimated blood loss, length of stay, previous abdominal surgeries, postoperative hemorrhage and operative times among patients with previous abdominal surgeries, a variable generally excluded in previously published SSRC studies, were compared between two surgeons based on the surgeon's level of experience. Surgeon 1 had training in advanced laparoscopy, greater case volume and more than 10 years of experience and surgeon 2 had basic laparoscopic skills, less case volume and was at the beginning of his first 2 years of practice.

The indications of the procedure were chronic cholecystitis, biliary colic, biliary dyskinesia, and gallstone pancreatitis in both inpatient and outpatient settings. Acute cholecystitis diagnosed pre-operatively served as the only exclusion criterion. There were no exclusions based on body mass index or previous abdominal surgery.

Patients were assigned a case identification number sequentially by date of surgery (i.e., Case #1 corresponds with the earliest date in the dataset [March 11, 2013] and Case #117 corresponds to the last date in the dataset [June 1, 2015]). Patient demographic data and information regarding patient comorbidities, indications for surgery, complications, rate of conversion, average length of hospital stay, and total operative time were collected. Operative time was recorded electronically and was measured from the beginning of skin incision until subcuticular skin closure. Data compared for both groups of surgeons included age, sex, body mass index, diagnosis, conversion rate, intraoperative and postoperative complications, and postoperative outcome.

After surgery all patients are seen in the office at 2 weeks, then at 6 weeks for evaluation. Meanwhile patients were counseled regarding signs and symptoms of complications, including developing hernias, and were asked to notify their surgeons regarding any concerns. To assess the learning curve, the operative times were compared between the two surgeons.

Technique

A 2.5-cm vertical incision is made through the umbilicus, carried down to the fascia, and the peritoneum to accommodate the port [9]. A single-site silicon port was used with an 8.5-mm high-definition endoscope. After establishment of the pneumoperitoneum and docking the robot, the camera and two curved single-site cannulas were inserted as well as a 5-mm trocar for the assistant. The robotic surgical system automatically establishes an association between the hands of the surgeon and the ipsilateral tip of the surgical instrument enabling intuitive control.

After exploring the abdominal cavity, the assistant grasped the fundus of the gallbladder to expose the sub-hepatic space. At the console, the surgeon performs the dissection of the gallbladder in a similar fashion to laparoscopic cases. Both the cystic duct and the cystic artery are dissected with the monopolar hook or Maryland dissector and divided between clips (Hem-O-Lock medium-large clips, Teleflex Incorporated, Morrisville, NC). Using electrocautery, further dissection of the gallbladder is continued until its detachment from the liver bed. The single-site port is removed through the umbilical incision along with the specimen, after undocking the robot and removing the instruments and camera. The fascial defect is closed with a running 0-Vicryl (Ethicon Inc., Somerville, NJ) suture and the skin with a 4.0-Vicryl subcuticular continuous suture.

Statistical analysis

All continuous variables are described using means and standard deviations, while all categorical variables are described using counts and percentages. Two-group comparisons are carried out using Wilcoxon rank-sum tests for continuous variables due to the small group sizes and non-Gaussian distributions and using chi-square or Fisher's exact tests as appropriate for categorical variables. Statistical significance is set at $P < 0.05$. All analyses are performed using SAS 9.4 (SAS Institute Inc., Cary, NC).

Results

Between March 2013 and April 2015, 117 SSRC cases were performed by two surgeons based on their laparoscopic skills and experience (Table 1). Surgeon 1 had a larger number of patients ($n = 102$) compared to surgeon 2, who had 15. There were 24 males (24%) and 78 females (76%) in the series of patients for surgeon 1 compared to surgeon

Table 1 Descriptive statistics and univariate surgeon comparisons

Variable	Response	All (*N* = 117)	Surgeon 1 (*N* = 102)	Surgeon 2 (*N* = 15)	*P**
Age	N, Mean ± SD	117, 44.4 ± 17.1	102, 44.6 ± 16.6	15, 43.0 ± 20.8	0.572
Sex	Male	29 (25%)	24 (24%)	5 (33%)	0.522
	Female	88 (75%)	78 (76%)	10 (67%)	
BMI (kg/m2)	N, Mean ± SD	117, 28.7 ± 6.1	102, 28.8 ± 5.6	15, 27.9 ± 8.6	0.185
ASA	N, Mean ± SD	117, 2.0 ± 0.6	102, 2.0 ± 0.5	15, 2.1 ± 0.7	0.548
Preoperative diagnosis	Biliary colic	2 (2%)	0 (0%)	2 (2%)	**0.024**
	Biliary dyskinesia	1 (1%)	1 (7%)	0 (0%)	
	Chronic cholecystitis	41 (35%)	2 (13%)	39 (38%)	
	Gallstone pancreatitis	4 (3%)	0 (0%)	4 (4%)	
	Symptomatic cholelithiasis	69 (59%)	12 (80%)	57 (56%)	

ASA American Society of Anesthesiologists, *BMI* body mass index
*Statistically significant differences between the 2 surgeons are noted with a bold *p*-value

2 who had 5 males (33%) and 10 females (67%). No statistically significant differences were found for patient age mean ± standard deviation 44.6 ± 16.6 years and 43 ± 20.8 years for groups 1 and 2, respectively, $P = 0.572$), body mass index 28.8 ± 5.6 and 27.9 ± 8.6 for surgeons 1 and 2, respectively, $P = 0.185$) or for American Society of Anesthesiologists 1–4 classification using univariate analysis ($P = 0.548$). No other significant differences were found except for preoperative diagnosis of biliary colic, which was 2% for surgeon 2 compared to 0% for surgeon 1 ($P = 0.24$).

Table 2 contains intraoperative and postoperative parameters and all patients were stratified by surgeon experience. Forty-three of surgeon 1's patients (42%) had previous abdominal surgery compared to 2 (13%) of surgeon 2 ($P = 0.045$). Intraoperative cholangiography was not required in any of the cases. Additional ports were required in 6 patients, 3 for surgeon 1 (3%) versus 3 for surgeon 2 (20%, $P = 0.027$). Four of the patients of surgeon 1 (4%) were converted to multiport laparoscopic cholecystectomy compared to 3 (20%) for surgeon 2 ($P = 0.044$). One of surgeon 2's conversions was attributed to the cannulas being too long, which made it technically not safe to proceed with the dissection. Postoperative outcomes were similar between the 2 surgeons; no one had a postoperative hemorrhage or bile leak. The average length of hospital stay in surgeon 1's patients was 1.5 ± 1.3 days as compared to 1 ± 0.0 days for surgeon 2's patients; the variation is due to the that fact some of the patients were admitted to the hospital for other medical conditions.

Table 2 Intraoperative and postoperative parameters - univariate surgeon comparisons

Variable	Response	All (*N* = 117)	Surgeon 1 (*N* = 102)	Surgeon 2 (*N* = 15)	*P**
Operative time (min)	N, Mean ± SD	117, 49.3 ± 17.8	102, 45.0 ± 12.7	15, 78.8 ± 19.5	**< 0.001**
Single incision		109 (93%)	97 (95%)	12 (80%)	0.065
Additional port		6 (5%)	3 (3%)	3 (20%)	**0.027**
Converted to laparotomy		7 (6%)	4 (4%)	3 (20%)	**0.044**
IOC		0	0	0	N/A
Incision length (cm)	1.5	1 (1%)	0 (0%)	1 (25%)	**< 0.001**
	2	2 (2%)	0 (0%)	2 (50%)	
	2.5	103 (97%)	102 (100%)	1 (25%)	
EBL	N, Mean ± SD	117, 6.6 ± 9.7	102, 6.8 ± 10.3	15, 5.0 ± 0.0	> 0.999
Hospital stay		24 (21%)	21 (21%)	3 (20%)	> 0.999
Days post-OR	N, Mean ± SD	25, 1.5 ± 1.2	22, 1.5 ± 1.3	3, 1.0 ± 0.0	0.466
Postoperative hemorrhage		0	0	0	N/A
Previous abdominal surgery		45 (38%)	43 (42%)	2 (13%)	**0.045**
Days between surgeries	N, Mean ± SD	116, 7.0 ± 19.5	101, 5.2 ± 10.9	15, 19.0 ± 46.0	0.910

EBL estimated blood loss, *IOC* intraoperative cholangiography, *OR* operating room, *SD* standard deviation
*Statistically significant differences between the 2 surgeons are noted with a bold *p*-value

Figures 1 and 2 Surgeon 1 had a significantly lower average operative time (45.0 ± 12.7 min) compared to surgeon 2 (78.8 ± 19.5 min, $P < 0.001$) (Table 1 and Figs. 1 and 2). A trend of decreasing operative time that fit a line of regression was observed in the cases performed by surgeon 1, starting at case #40, extending through case #102 (Fig. 2). It was noted that some variations exist with scattered blots above the line due to patients having previous abdominal surgeries (Fig. 2). Unfortunately a learning curve could not be inferred for surgeon 2 due to the smaller number of cases.

Patients with previous abdominal surgeries was another variable found to be significantly higher among surgeon 1's patients (42%) compared to surgeon 2's patients (13%) ($P = 0.045$). On the other hand, when the operative time was stratified by whether or not the patients had a previous abdominal surgery (Table 3), it was shown that the operative time in 59 patients with no previous abdominal surgery was 45.6 ± 12.9 min for surgeon 1 compared to 73.2 ± 13.6 min in 13 patients of surgeon 2, $P < 0.001$. In the series of 43 patients of surgeon 1 who had previous abdominal surgeries, the mean operative time was 44.0 ± 12.6 min as compared to 115.5 ± 2.1 min for surgeon 2's patients with previous abdominal surgeries, $P = 0.019$. In both instances, patients with and without previous abdominal surgeries, the mean operative time is significantly higher for surgeon 2 as compared to surgeon 1. For case volume, the average number of cases performed on a single day was 1.3/day for surgeon 1 and 1.1/day for surgeon 2. The average number of days between procedures is 6.5 days for surgeon 1 vs 38.8 days for surgeon 2. There was no significant difference in patient-related factors such as age and sex. Additionally, the two series of patients for both surgeons did not significantly differ in any of the following: average length of hospital stay ($P > 0.999$), intraoperative complications, postoperative complications, readmissions, or reoperations. None of the patients received a cholangiogram.

Discussion

This study investigated the impact of surgeon experience on the perioperative and postoperative functional outcome of SSRC utilizing a single-site robotic platform technology. The total operative time, a reflection of the learning curve among two surgeons with different laparoscopic skills and case volume, was assessed and compared to the existing literature.

The introduction of the robotic single-site platform in 2011 has resolved the limitations of single-incision laparoscopy. The procedure has become easy to master with robotic assistance with functional results similar to those of conventional laparoscopy [10]. The curved trocars were designed to diminish the triangulation problem and four access cannulas in the trocar eliminate the need for percutaneous suture retraction [11]. The three-dimensional high-definition view provides the additional advantage of better visualization of the Calot's triangle, so the dissection phase of the cystic artery and duct can be performed more

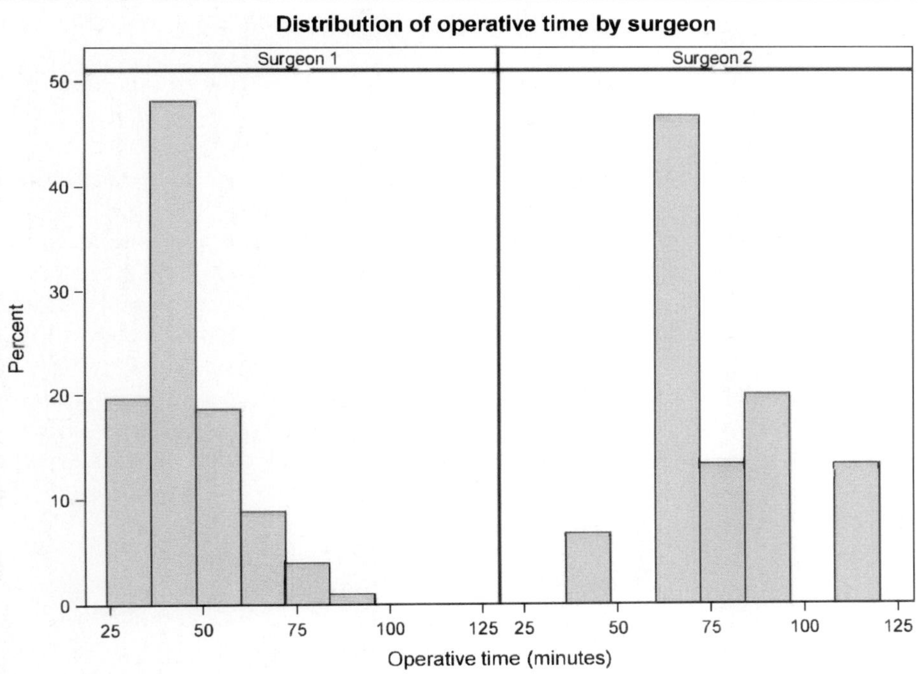

Fig. 1 Distribution of operative times by surgeons 1 and 2

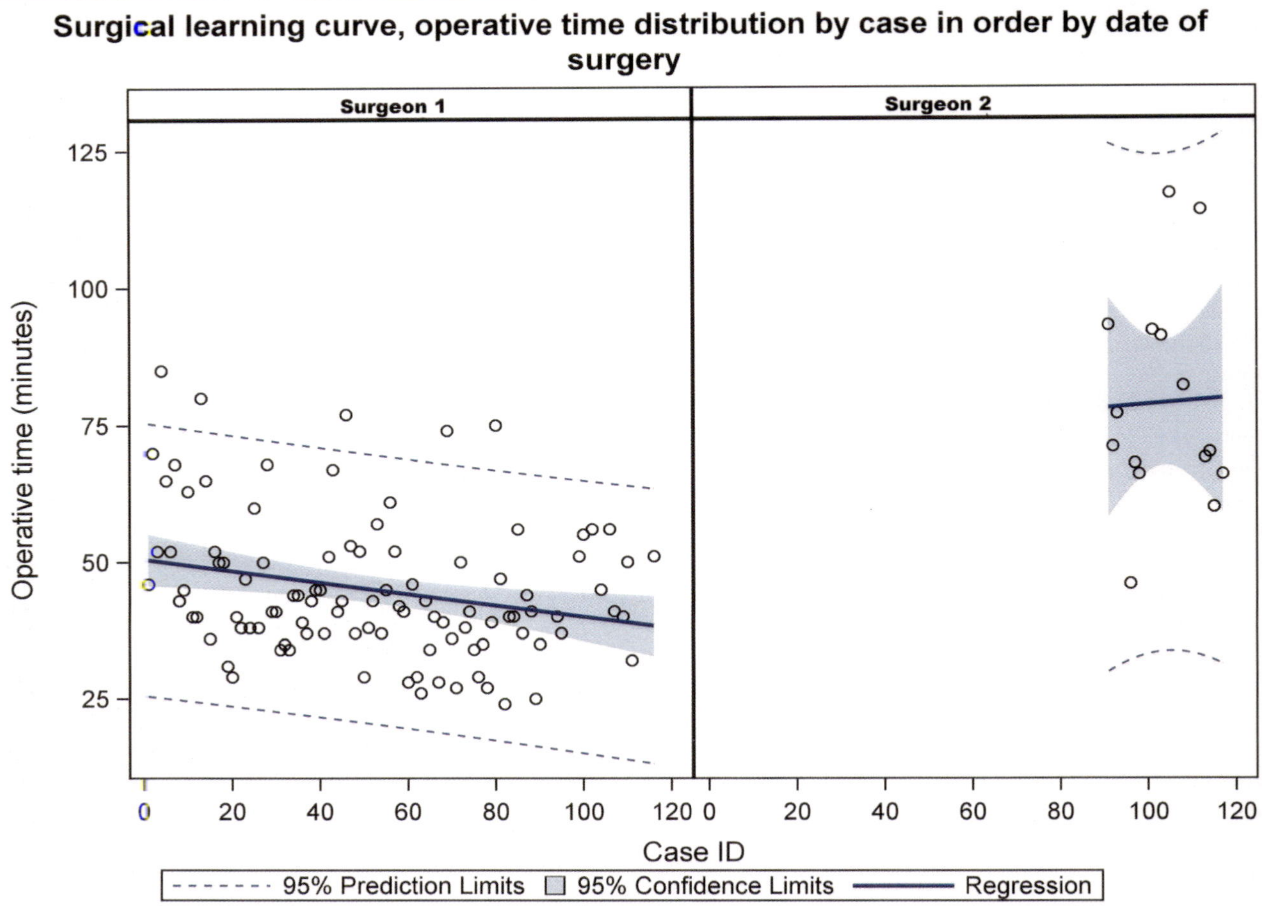

Fig. 2 Surgical learning curve, operative time distribution by case in order by date of surgery

safely. However, the da Vinci Si robotic system has its own limitations; it has a considerable size that limits the space in the operating room for the circulating staff while the arms of the robot limits the access of the bedside assistant [11].

According to Pietrabissa et al. [12], "In surgery an important factor in deciding whether to embrace a new technology for an old problem is the degree of difficulty in mastering the new skill set." Completing the task in a timely manner is the parameter most commonly used to objectively evaluate a learning curve. Four comparative studies on conventional four-port laparoscopic versus multiport robotic cholecystectomy have described reaching equivalent operative times using the robot after a learning curve of 20 to 50 procedures [13–16]. Most reported studies observed a learning curve to be an important component of the total operative time [13, 14]. Although experienced laparoscopic surgeons can safely perform a single-site laparoscopic cholecystectomy in about the same time they do using the four-port technique [15], the steep learning curve and potential complications of this technology [17] might have prevented its implementation on a larger scale. Solomon and colleagues [18] reported a learning curve of approximately 10 cases to master the single-incision laparoscopic cholecystectomy, dropping the average operative time from 110 min to 75 min.

Single-site robotic platform technology provided the surgeon more flexibility, and better visualization allowing surgical skills to be easily mastered and shortening the

Table 3 Operative time by surgeon, stratified by surgery status

Variable	Response	Surgeon 1	Surgeon 2	*P*
Operative time, no previous abdominal surgery	N, Mean ± SD	59, 45.6 ± 12.9	13, 73.2 ± 13.6	< 0.001
Operative time, previous abdominal surgery	N, Mean ± SD	43, 44.0 ± 12.6	2, 115.5 ± 2.1	0.019

SD standard deviation

learning curve. In our observation, the learning curve is highly influenced by the experience of the surgeon, degree of laparoscopic skills, the case volume the surgeon has, the number of cases the surgeon does in one day and the duration of time between procedures.

The aim of this study was to report the experience of two surgeons with different levels of training and experience with SSRC in a community teaching hospital. Study data comprise the initial experience of two surgeons from the same institution who treated 117 patients with varied gallbladder diseases. The demographics of our cohort were similar to the patient population of standard laparoscopic cholecystectomies: mainly women, obese, middle-aged and varied gallbladder diseases. No statistical demographic differences existed between the two surgeon series of patients. There were no complications reported in any of the procedures. None of our cases had unusual bleeding that required a blood transfusion. Furthermore, none of the cases in our series developed a bile leak, bile duct injury, pneumonia, pulmonary embolism, deep vein thrombosis or postoperative sepsis and there were no cases of retained bile duct stones or any that required reoperation (Table 2). Most of the previous studies on SSRC have reported no major complications [19]. Our perioperative outcomes are consistent with the accumulating knowledge with respect to the safety and feasibility of SSRC [20].

The conversion rate in our series was 4% for surgeon 1 compared to 20% for surgeon 2, which was statistically significant ($P = 0.044$). The reasons for conversion to laparoscopy in the series of patients of surgeon 1 included two cases of acute cholecystitis with significant inflammation, one case of the cystic duct tearing and one case where the right arm and the left arm were tangled in which they had to call the support team and did not receive help. The reason for conversion among surgeon 2's patients included two cases of acute cholecystitis with significant inflammation and a case reporting the cannulas being too long, which made the dissection challenging.

To assess the learning curve differences in our series of patients for both surgeons, we compared the total operative times required to complete the procedure safely. The two series had the same inclusion and exclusion criteria.

The overall mean operative time of 49.3 ± 17.8 min remained acceptable and less than what has been reported in the literature, despite the differences that exists between the two surgeons. The total operative time significantly differed between the two surgeons ($P < 0.001$). Surgeon 1, who performed most of the procedures, showed statistically significant progress in their overall operative time due to advanced laparoscopic skills and case volume, in comparison to surgeon 2 who showed a progression in his total operative time, but his results were not significant due to the variability of the measures and the limited amount of data (Figs. 1 and 2). These results of operative time correlates significantly with the case volume, number of cases/day, and the time lapse between the procedures (Table 2).

Some studies [12, 21] have reported longer operative time in patients with acute cholecystitis compared to those without cholecystitis. Khambaty et al. [22] noted that the operative time tended to stabilize after the first 10 cases, finding a decrease from the initial time of 105.3 min to 74.4 min in the 10th case. In this series, the trends in the total operative time with the surgeon experience is demonstrated in Figs. 1 and 2. Surgeon 1 showed a continuous linear regression after 40 cases, while due to limited data it is non-conclusive for surgeon 2. Our hypothesis was that surgical skills would be more easily mastered and the learning curve would be shortened based on the laparoscopic skills of the surgeon, case volume and the number of cases the surgeon performed in a single day as well as the number of days between the procedures.

An expert surgeon in laparoscopic surgery might need a very short training period in SSRC to achieve an observed reduction in the operative time after the first 10 cases. Surgeons entering practice recently having basic laparoscopic skills will require a longer period of training and closed supervision before being able to achieve an acceptable learning curve.

It could easily be argued that the use of the robot for a cholecystectomy is unnecessary and too expensive. However, the robotic technique became widely popular and its use exceeded expectations. We believe that single-site robotic technology could be easily adapted to perform more complex intraabdominal procedures in a timely manner by more experienced surgeons with greater case volumes. Our data show some trends that do not reach statistical significance due to the relatively small sample size for surgeon 2, still this is a single-institutional data collection assessing the feasibility and safety of adopting a new technology, despite differences in surgeons' experience.

However, this study has some limitations that need to be addressed. Since SSRC has been introduced recently, we are progressing in a learning mode and there will probably be some additional adjustments in terms of manipulations and optimization of all parts of the procedure, which could influence future operative times. We recommend that surgeons with basic laparoscopic skills and limited case volume have longer supervised SSRC training.

Other limiting factors included improper documentation of the docking time and console time. These factors further assist in the evaluation of the learning curve. Even though statistical significance was reached for some aspects, the findings represent an analysis of our initial experience with this procedure.

Conclusion

It is recommended that SSRC can be performed with high standards of safety and efficacy, by general surgeons possessing both advanced and basic laparoscopic skills; however, it is advisable for surgeons of limited robotic skills and case volume to have more supervised single-site robotic cases until the learning curve is reached. SSRC provides surgeons with a system that possesses a gradual learning curve, atypical of the steep learning curve associated with learning new surgical procedures. Furthermore, we found that overall surgeon experience in laparoscopic cholecystectomy and amount of practice with SSRC procedures translated to decreased operation times. Future prospective, randomized trials are necessary to evaluate further benefits of this approach with respect to patient quality of life, satisfaction, cosmetics, and the advantage of significantly decreased postoperative pain, overall long- term umbilical sequelae and cost related issues in a community hospital setting.

Abbreviations

SSRC: single-site robotic cholecystectomy

Acknowledgements

Mahan Meredith: Biostatistician, Public health sciences, HFHS.
Stephanie Stebens: Librarian, Sladen Library, HFHS.

Authors' contributions

MD drafted the manuscript and participated in revising it critically for important intellectual content. SS helped in data collection, statistical analysis and study design. SL participated in data collection, statistical analysis and revisions. FB participated in revising the manuscript. All authors read and approved the final manuscript.

Competing interests

The authors declare that they have no competing interests.

References

1. Navarra G, Pozza E, Occhionorelli S, Carcoforo P, Donini I. One-wound laparoscopic cholecystectomy. Br J Surg. 1997;84(5):695.
2. Vidal O, Valentini M, Espert JJ, Ginesta C, Jimeno J, Martinez A, Benarroch G, Garcia-Valdecasas JC. Laparoendoscopic single-site cholecystectomy: a safe and reproducible alternative. J Laparoendosc Adv Surg Tech A. 2009;19(5): 599–602.
3. Hodgett SE, Hernandez JM, Morton CA, Ross SB, Albrink M, Rosemurgy AS. Laparoendoscopic single site (LESS) cholecystectomy. J Gastrointest Surg. 2009;13(2):188–92.
4. Iranmanesh P, Morel P, Wagner OJ, Inan I, Pugin F, Hagen ME. Set-up and docking of the da Vinci surgical system: prospective analysis of initial experience. Int J Med Robot. 2010;6(1):57–60.
5. Podolsky ER, Curcillo PG 2nd. Reduced-port surgery: preservation of the critical view in single-port-access cholecystectomy. Surg Endosc. 2010; 24(12):3038–43.
6. Rivas H, Varela E, Scott D. Single-incision laparoscopic cholecystectomy: initial evaluation of a large series of patients. Surg Endosc. 2010;24(6):1403–12.
7. Seo IY, Rim JS. Bilateral robotic single-site partial nephrectomy. J Laparoendosc Adv Surg Tech A. 2011;21(5):435–8.
8. Kroh M, El-Hayek K, Rosenblatt S, Chand B, Escobar P, Kaouk J, Chalikonda S. First human surgery with a novel single-port robotic system: cholecystectomy using the da Vinci single-site platform. Surg Endosc. 2011; 25(11):3566–73.
9. Escobar PF, Fader AN, Paraiso MF, Kaouk JH, Falcone T. Robotic-assisted laparoendoscopic single-site surgery in gynecology: initial report and technique. J Minim Invasive Gynecol. 2009;16(5):589–91.
10. Konstantinidis KM, Hirides P, Hirides S, Chrysocheris P, Georgiou M. Cholecystectomy using a novel single-site((R)) robotic platform: early experience from 45 consecutive cases. Surg Endosc. 2012;26(9):2687–94.
11. Morel P, Hagen ME, Bucher P, Buchs NC, Pugin F. Robotic single-port cholecystectomy using a new platform: initial clinical experience. J Gastrointest Surg. 2011;15(12):2182–6.
12. Pietrabissa A, Sbrana F, Morelli L, Badessi F, Pugliese L, Vinci A, Klersy C, Spinoglio G. Overcoming the challenges of single-incision cholecystectomy with robotic single-site technology. Arch Surg. 2012;147(8):709–14.
13. Heemskerk J, van Dam R, van Gemert WG, Beets GL, Greve JW, Jacobs MJ, Bouvy ND. First results after introduction of the four-armed da Vinci surgical system in fully robotic laparoscopic cholecystectomy. Dig Surg. 2005;22(6):426–31.
14. Caratozzolo E, Recordare A, Massani M, Bonariol L, Jelmoni A, Antoniutti M, Bassi N. Telerobotic-assisted laparoscopic cholecystectomy: our experience on 29 patients. J Hepato-Biliary-Pancreat Surg. 2005;12(2):163–6.
15. Lai EC, Yang GP, Tang CN, Yih PC, Chan OC, Li MK. Prospective randomized comparative study of single incision laparoscopic cholecystectomy versus conventional four-port laparoscopic cholecystectomy. Am J Surg. 2011; 202(3):254–8.
16. Perez A, Zinner MJ, Ashley SW, Brooks DC, Whang EE. What is the value of telerobotic technology in gastrointestinal surgery? Surg Endosc. 2003;17(5):811–3.
17. Hansen AJ, Augenstein J, Ong ES. Large subcapsular liver hematoma following single-incision laparoscopic cholecystectomy. JSLS. 2011;15(1):114–6.
18. Solomon D, Bell RL, Duffy AJ, Roberts KE. Single-port cholecystectomy: small scar, short learning curve. Surg Endosc. 2010;24(12):2954–7.
19. Marks JM, Phillips MS, Tacchino R, Roberts K, Onders R, DeNoto G, Gecelter G, Rubach E, Rivas H, Islam A, Soper N, Paraskeva P, Rosemurgy A, Ross S, Shah S. Single-incision laparoscopic cholecystectomy is associated with improved cosmesis scoring at the cost of significantly higher hernia rates: 1-year results of a prospective randomized, multicenter, single-blinded trial of traditional multiport laparoscopic cholecystectomy vs single-incision laparoscopic cholecystectomy. J Am Coll Surg. 2013;216(6):1037–47.
20. Vidovszky TJ, Smith W, Ghosh J, Ali MR. Robotic cholecystectomy: learning curve, advantages, and limitations. J Surg Res. 2006;136(2):172–8.
21. Tang B, Hou S, Cuschieri SA. Ergonomics of and technologies for single-port lapaxroscopic surgery. Minim Invasive Ther Allied Technol. 2012;21(1):46–54.
22. Khambaty F, Brody F, Vaziri K, Edwards C. Laparoscopic versus single-incision cholecystectomy. World J Surg. 2011;35(5):967–72.

Long standing biliary colic masking chylous ascites in laparoscopic roux-en-Y gastric bypass

Louai R. Zaidan[1,2], Elhaitham K. Ahmed[1,2], Bachar Halimeh[1], Yasser Radwan[2] and Khalil Terro[1,2*]

Abstract

Background: Chylous ascites is considered to be an intra-abdominal collection of creamy colored fluid with triglyceride content of > 110 mg/dL. Chylous ascites is an uncommon but serious complication of numerous surgical interventions. However, it is a rare complication of LRYGB. An internal hernia limb defect is thought to be the underlying etiology, where the hernia will cause lymphatic vessel engorgement and lymphatic extravasation.

Case presentation: We report a case of a 29 years old male with a 9 year history of laparoscopic Roux en y gastric bypass (LRGYB), presenting with recurrent abdominal pain for 2 months radiating to the right shoulder. Ultrasound examination revealed gallstones and the patient was subsequently admitted for laparoscopic cholecystectomy. Intraoperatively, whitish colored fluid, high in triglycerides content was aspirated. During exploration, an internal hernia limb defect was found and corrected.

Conclusion: Post LRGYB patients with symptoms of recurrent abdominal pain should be suspected for chylous ascites reflecting an internal hernia.

Keywords: LRYGB, Chylous ascites, Internal hernia, Biliary colic, Abdominal pain

Background

Chyloperitoneum is defined as the accumulation of lymphatic fluid in the peritoneum due to leakage/break in the lymphatic system. Three reasons have been thought to cause this accumulation: (1) Obstruction of the vessels by a mass or tumor, leading to exudation through dilated lymphatic vessel's wall or rupture of the vessel. Usually, these patients develop protein losing enteropathy. (2) Formation of a fistula between the lymphatic vessels and the peritoneum or mesentry secondary to adhesions, trauma or surgery. (3) Leakage from the retroperitoneal megalymphatics with or without an evidence of fistula, usually as a consequent of congenital diseases. In order to define ascetic fluid as chyle, the triglyceride content of the fluid must be greater than 110 mg/dl (2 to 8 times higher than plasma levels) and its specific gravity greater than 1.012. It commonly has the appearance of a turbid, milky fluid with no odor [1].

Chylous ascites has been reported to be most commonly due to malignancies in adults. In post-surgical cases, it has been most related to either vascular or lymphatic related operations [1]. However, only five cases have been reported in post-bariatric surgeries, three of which were after Roux en Y gastric bypass, all of them presenting 12–24 months later in in the mid post-op period. [2–5] We are reporting a fourth case of chylous ascites, interestingly presenting 9 years after LRYGB.

Case presentation

A 29-year-old male, with a known surgical history of LRYGB 9 years ago, presented to the emergency department complaining of sharp, severe abdominal pain in the right upper quadrant (RUQ). The pain began two months ago in an intermittent fashion that would occasionally radiate to his right shoulder and progressively became worse with time. The patient did not report any constipation, distension, or vomiting despite feeling

* Correspondence: khaleelterro@gmail.com
[1]Alfaisal University, Riyadh, Saudi Arabia
[2]Specialized Medical Center Hospital, Riyadh, Saudi Arabia

nauseated during these attacks. The pain was not related to any movement or meals and it was moderately relieved by over the counter analgesia.

Ten years ago, the patient was diagnosed with obstructive sleep apnea (OSA), through a sleep study, due to morbid obesity. He then was advised to undergo LRYGB as a treatment. He does have any other medical problems. Family history is notable for diabetes mellitus and hypertension but no history of hyperlipidemia or obesity. His body mass index (BMI) prior to the surgery was 49.3 Kg/m^2. He underwent a successful LRYGB with no complications or readmissions. After the surgery for a year and a half, he followed up with his primary surgeon. During that time, he lost 75 Kg, reaching a BMI of 26.9 Kg/m^2. He then was able to maintain his weight following the operation, but failed to continue to follow up for the past 2 years. In those 2 years, he gained weight, raising his BMI to 29.9 Kg/m^2, after which he modified his diet to reduce his BMI to 23.9 Kg/m^2. This weight reduction was achieved prior to his presentation.

On physical examination, the patient was afebrile with normal vital signs. Examination of his abdomen revealed moderate tenderness over the epigastrium, central abdomen, and right hypochondrium with a positive Murphy's sign. His laboratory investigations, including complete blood count, urine analysis, liver and renal function tests, were all within normal limits. An ultrasound examination revealed two gallstones and upper borderline diameter of common bile duct, raising the suspicion of biliary obstruction.

Correlating his investigation results with his symptoms, he was admitted and scheduled for a cholecystectomy. Formal laparoscopic cholecystectomy was carried out the next morning. During exploration, twisting of the common channel was observed, indicating an internal hernia, although the patient's complaint did not suggest internal hernia in the differential diagnosis. The internal hernia was identified but reduction was not feasible through laparoscopy. Mini midline laparotomy was subsequently done for reduction of the hernia and more detailed exploration. The hernia was through the mesenteric defect between the alimentary limb and the biliopancreatic limbs. Both limbs of the anastomosis were identified and complete reduction of the internal hernia was done, in addition to suturing of the defect found in the mesentery. No other defects were found. The small intestine's mesentery showed prominent whitish colored vessels. Whitish thick fluid was noticed, accumulating in the right paracolic gutter and in Morison's pouch. All of the fluid was then aspirated, measuring a total of 752 mL. Analysis of the fluid showed a triglyceride level of 534 mg/dL and a Lactate Dehydrogenase (LDH) level of 512 U/L. A classic Blake drain 24 F was inserted into the pelvis. The patient passed an uneventful post-operative period. On Postoperative Day (POD) one, fluid collected from the drain was 440 ml, chylous in appearance, while on POD 2–4 the drainage was serous in appearance. The drain was removed on POD 4. The patient was discharged on POD 4 after being able to ambulate independently on his own and eat and drink with no complications.

The patient did not return back for his follow-up visits and when he was called by the team, he confirmed that he has no complains up to this day.

Discussion and conclusion

Obesity is still considered a major burden worldwide. Obesity is defined as a BMI > 30 kg/m2. The World Health Organization (WHO) has reported that in 2016, 13% of the world's adult population were obese, with obesity prevalence doubling between 1975 and 2016 [6]. Obesity is an extensively spread modifiable risk factor for several diseases including diabetes mellitus, cardiovascular disease, joints disease, etc. [7, 8].

Several approaches have been addressed worldwide to treat obesity and prevent its complications. However, lifestyle modifications and medical therapy are not always effective, especially in cases involving morbid obesity. Therefore, bariatric surgery is an indication for treating obesity with a BMI above 40 kg/m2 or a BMI above 35 kg/m2 with comorbidities, according to the latest consensus guideline by the American Society for Metabolic and Bariatric Surgery (ASMBS). Of the various bariatric surgeries, LRYGB is considered the gold standard in treating obesity. Nevertheless, like any surgical procedure, LRGYB has a risk for developing several complications, several of which require repetitive follow-up postoperatively [7–9].

Internal hernia is one of the most common complications of LRYGB [10]. The prevalence of internal hernia has reached up to 14% [11]. Small bowel obstruction is the most feared complication, as it is considered an emergency and is most likely due to an internal hernia [12]. A review by Koppman et al. reported an incidence of small bowel obstruction in 0.6–11% [13]. Ghandi et al. reported that 3.8% of LRYGB patients suffered from small bowel obstruction, with 55% of obstruction cases being a result of internal hernia [14]. Internal hernia is frequently a result of the loss of the mesenteric fat, which provides protection and occupation of space to limit the movement of the small bowel, presenting in a delayed fashion. Moreover, fewer adhesions are formed from laparoscopic surgeries compared to open procedures, allowing more space for small bowel movement [15].

It was reported from a review of several studies that the incidence of internal hernia after a LRYGB was between 0.2–8.6%. The most common presentation was small bowel obstruction symptoms, ranging from 1.8–9.7% after a LRYGB [16].

Typically, patients with internal hernia have a chronic recurrent presentation of colicky abdominal pain, nausea and vomiting. The presence of an internal hernia increases the risk of developing small bowel obstruction as a sequela, usually presenting in a late stage [9].

In our case, the patient presented with the typical symptoms of biliary colic, which was supported by the presence of gallstones on ultrasound. This presentation masked the real patient's problem; an internal hernia leading to chylous ascites.

Internal hernia can occur due to a surgical defect, depending on whether a retrocolic or antecolic approach is utilised. Petersen's defect is the presence of space between the Roux limb and the transverse mesocolon. A second defect might also be present between the biliopancreatic and Roux limbs at the jejunojejunostomy. In cases of retrocolic approach, a third defect in the transverse mesocolon might be created. This is the most common reported site of internal hernia, prompting several surgeons to adopt the antecolic technique to eliminate such defect. In addition, the latter is consistent with an intermittent internal hernia that has the potential to reduce itself spontaneously, which explains the recurrent pain that our patient was having. Review of the literature supports the antecolic technique, as lower rates of herniation were reported when compared to the retrocolic technique. Most of internal hernias can be successfully treated laparoscopically, through the reduction of the herniated limb and the closure of the mesenteric defect. However, due to the fact that laparoscopy procedures possess a lower risk of adhesion formation, this can contribute to the risk of hernias by allowing more intestinal movement around a potential mesenteric space. Thus, laparotomy may help reduce the risk of developing internal hernia, as a result of more adhesions presence. [17].

Up to our knowledge, only three cases of chylous ascites post LRYGB were reported. An average time for presentation with chylous ascites in these cases was 20 months [2, 4, 5]. In our patient, the presentation was after 9 years.

Hidalgo et al. reported a 40-year-old morbid obese patient with comorbidities of exertional dyspnea and joint disease who underwent a LRYGB 15 months prior to his presentation. He presented with mild chronic abdominal pain and nausea. A computed tomography showed intra-abdominal fluid collection. The patient was taken for a diagnostic laparoscopy where a common channel internal hernia was identified and corrected. In addition, milky fluid was extracted and analyzed, with reports showing high triglycerides levels [2].

Hanson et al. reported a 22-year-old woman presenting with severe abdominal pain 2 years after undergoing LRYGB, during which she lost 90lbs. Computed tomography showed a huge collection of mesenteric free fluid, necessitating an urgent operation. Intraoperatively, a mesenteric defect was identified, in which the common channel was fully herniating through. 4 l of free fluid was extracted with the analysis reporting a triglycerides level of 388 mg/dL [4].

Capristo et al. reported a 61-year-old heavy smoker and heavy alcohol drinking man who underwent a LRYGB 18 months prior to the presentation of a sudden weight gain of 5 Kg, abdominal distention and shortness of breath. His BMI was reduced from 41.8 kg/m2 to 31.7 kg/m2. On physical examination, the patient had significant ascites, right pleural effusion and left supraclavicular lymph node enlargement. Paracentesis and thoracentesis evacuated a total of 4.5 L of whitish fluid, high in triglycerides. However, lymph node biopsy, computed tomography and positron-emission tomography revealed a poorly differentiated gastric carcinoma. This finding indicated that the chylous ascites was not related to the LRYGB [5].

These cases along with our case showed that chylous ascites is a manifestation of an internal herniation from a mesenteric defect after a LRYGB. These cases might present with vague or misleading symptoms.

Physicians, including general practitioners and emergency doctors, should have a high index of suspicion for internal hernia for post LRYGB patients, even if they present with mild to moderate symptoms of abdominal colicky pain. A delayed diagnosis of internal hernia increases the risk of developing acute small bowel obstruction. Such cases should be transferred to bariatric surgery if possible or undergo laparoscopic exploration, as it is the most sensitive and specific diagnostic tool, compared to imaging such as Computed Tomography (CT) scan which does not help in diagnosis [18].

In conclusion, our case was about a patient who developed chylous ascites 9 years after he underwent a LRYGB. While the most common cause of chylous ascites in adults is malignancy, it can also be an unusual presentation due to internal herniation that arises from a mesenteric defect post LRYGB. Chylous ascites in these case present with very mild and vague symptoms that might deviate the differential diagnosis away from a possible internal hernia. Thus, chylous ascites should be suspected in all LRYGB patients presenting with mild abdominal symptoms and properly managed accordingly.

Abbreviations

ASMBS: American Society for Metabolic and Bariatric Surgery; BMI: Body Mass Index (Kg/m2); CT: Computed Tomography; LDH: Lactate DeHydrogenase; LRYGB: Laparoscopic Roux-en-Y Gastric Bypass; OSA: Obstructive Sleep Apnea; POD: Post-Operative Day; RUQ: Right Upper Quadrant; WHO: World Health Organization

Acknowledgements

The authors acknowledge the continuous support of the Medical Academic Affairs (MAA) department and the MAA chairman, Dr. Lina Kibbe.

Authors' contributions

YR assisted in diagnosing, operating and maintaining proper health care to the patient. LZ, EA and BH gathered and analysed the data, participated in an extensive literature review and wrote the manuscript. KT is the senior surgeon, who operated on the patient, supervised and contributed to the final version of the case report. All authors read and approved the final manuscript.

Competing interests

The authors declare that they have no competing interests.

References

1. Aalami OO, Allen DB, Organ CH. Chylous ascites: a collective review. Surgery. 2000;128(5):761–78.
2. Hidalgo JE, Ramirez A, Patel S, Acholonu E, Eckstein J, Abu-Jaish W, Szomstein S, Rosenthal RJ. Chyloperitoneum after laparoscopic roux-en-Y gastric bypass (LRYGB). Obes Surg. 2010;20(2):257–60.
3. Nau P, Narula V, Needleman B. Successful management of chyloperitoneum after laparoscopic adjustable gastric banding in 2 patients. Surg Obes Relat Dis. 2011;7(1):122–3.
4. Hanson M, Chao J, Lim RB. Chylous ascites mimicking peritonitis after laparoscopic roux-en-Y gastric bypass for morbid obesity. Surg Obes Relat Dis. 2012;8(1):e1–2.
5. Capristo E, Spuntarelli V, Treglia G, Arena V, Giordano A. Mingrone G. A case report of chylous ascites after gastric bypass for morbid obesity. Int J Surg Case Rep. 2016;31(29):133–6.
6. WHO Obesity and overweight. 2017. http://www.who.int/mediacentre/factsheets/fs311/en/ . Accessed 21 Oct 2017.
7. Mechanick JI, Youdim A, Jones DB, Garvey WT, Hurley DL, McMahon MM, Heinberg LJ, Kushner R, Adams TD, Shikora S, Dixon JB. Clinical practice guidelines for the perioperative nutritional, metabolic, and nonsurgical support of the bariatric surgery patient—2013 update: cosponsored by American Association of Clinical Endocrinologists, the Obesity Society, and American Society for Metabolic & bariatric surgery. Obesity. 2013;21(S1):1.
8. Karlsson J, Taft C, Ryden A, Sjöström L, Sullivan M. Ten-year trends in health-related quality of life after surgical and conventional treatment for severe obesity: the SOS intervention study. Int J Obes. 2007;31(8):1248–61.
9. Geubbels N, Lijftogt N, Fiocco M, van Leersum NJ, Wouters MW, de Brauw LM. Meta-analysis of internal herniation after gastric bypass surgery. Br J Surg. 2015;102(5):451–60.
10. Rodríguez A, Mosti M, Sierra M, Pérez-Johnson R, Flores S, Dominguez G, Sánchez H, Zarco A, Romay K, Herrera MF. Small bowel obstruction after antecolic and antegastric laparoscopic roux-en-Y gastric bypass: could the incidence bereduced? Obes Surg. 2010;20(10):1380–4. https://doi.org/10.1007/s11695-010-0164-5.
11. Abasbassi M, Pottel H, Deylgat B, Vansteenkiste F, Van Rooy F, Devriendt D, D'Hondt M. Small bowel obstruction after antecolic antegastric laparoscopicRoux-en-Y gastric bypass without division of small bowel mesentery: asingle-Centre, 7-year review. Obes Surg. 2011;21(12):1822–7. https://doi.org/10.1007/s11695-011-0462-6.
12. Buchwald H. Bariatric surgery for morbid obesity: health implications for patients, health professionals, and third-party payers. J Am Coll Surg. 2005; 200(4):593–604.
13. Koppman JS, Li C, Gandsas A. Small bowel obstruction after laparoscopicRoux-en-Y gastric bypass: a review of 9,527 patients. J Am Coll Surg. 2008;206(3):571–84. https://doi.org/10.1016/j.jamcollsurg.2007.10.008.
14. Gandhi AD, Patel RA, Brolin RE. Elective laparoscopy for herald symptoms ofmesenteric/internal hernia after laparoscopic roux-en-Y gastric bypass. Surg Obes Relat Dis. 2009;5(2):144–9; discussion 149. https://doi.org/10.1016/j.soard.2008.11.002.
15. Lockhart ME, Tessler FN, Canon CL, Smith JK, Larrison MC, Fineberg NS, Roy BP, Clements RH. Internal hernia after gastric bypass: sensitivity and specificity of seven CT signs with surgical correlation and controls. Am J Roentgenol. 2007;188(3):745–50.
16. Jeannsonne IVL. Internal hernia after Laparascopic gastric bypass: a review of literature. In: Bariatric Times; 2007. http://bariatrictimes.com/internal-hernia-after-laparoscopic-gastric-bypass-a-review-of-the-literature/. Accessed 18 Sep 2017.
17. Steele KE, Prokopowicz GP, Magnuson T, Lidor A, Schweitzer M. Laparoscopic antecolic roux-en-Y gastric bypass with closure of internal defects leads to fewer internal hernias than the retrocolic approach. Surg Endosc. 2008;22(9):2056–61.
18. Paroz A, Calmes JM, Giusti V, Suter M. Internal hernia after laparoscopic roux-en-Y gastric bypass for morbid obesity: a continuous challenge in bariatric surgery. Obes Surg. 2006;16(11):1482–7.

Blunt liver trauma: a descriptive analysis from a level I trauma center

Ibrahim Afifi[1], Sheraz Abayazeed[2], Ayman El-Menyar[3,4*], Husham Abdelrahman[1], Ruben Peralta[1] and Hassan Al-Thani[1]

Abstract

Background: We aimed to review liver injury experience in a level 1 trauma center; namely clinical presentation, grading, management approach and clinical outcomes.

Methods: It is a retrospective analysis to include all blunt liver injury patients who were admitted at the Level 1 trauma center over a 3-year period. Data were compared and analyzed based on the liver injury grades and management approaches.

Results: Blunt liver injury accounted for 38% of the total blunt abdominal trauma cases with a mean age of 31 ± 13 years. Liver injury grade II (44.7%) was most common followed by grade I (28.8%), grade III (19.1%), grade IV (7. 0%) and grade V (0.4%). Blood transfusion was more frequently required in patients with grade IV ($p = 0.04$). Out of 257 patients with blunt liver trauma, 198 were initially treated conservatively, that was successful in 192 (97%), whereas it failed in 6 (3%) patients due to delayed bleeding from hepatic hematoma, associated splenic rupture and small bowel injury which mandate surgical intervention. Fifty-nine patients (23%) underwent emergent surgery in terms of packing, resection debridement, left lobe hepatectomy and splenectomy. Hepatic complications included biloma, pseudoaneurysm and massive liver necrosis. Subanalysis of data using the World Society of Emergency Surgery (WSES) classification revealed 19 patients were categorized as a WSES grade IV who needed surgical intervention without having an initial computerized tomography scanning. The overall mortality was 7.8% which was comparable among the conservative and operative group.

Conclusions: In our center, low grade liver injury in young males prevails. NOM is successful even for high graded injuries. All conservatively treated patients with high-grade liver injuries should be closely monitored for signs of failure of the non-operative management. Introducing the new WSES classification makes clear how is important the hemodynamic status of the patients despite the lesion. However, further larger prospective and multicenter studies are needed to support our findings.

Keywords: Blunt hepatic trauma, Liver injury grades, Management, Complications, Outcome

Background

Over the past two decades, treatment of blunt hepatic injuries has been changed dramatically. A shift has occurred from the operative management (OM) emphasizing non-resection techniques and packing in the 1980s to selective non-operative management (NOM) in the 1990s and currently to NOM with selective operative management that relies on the computerized tomography (CT) scan findings [1]. Abdominal CT scan is an appropriate modality for the accurate diagnosis and grading of liver injuries in hemodynamically stable patients and is considered useful to guiding the management approach [2]. Beside injury grading, CT scan detects active bleeding (i.e., blush, contrast extravasation and venous phase), pseudoaneurysm which is a common cause of failure to NOM, and associated intraperitoneal injuries and also it quantifies the associated hemoperitoneum [3]. The utility of intervention with angioembolization supports liver injury management either primarily as an adjunct to NOM or immediately post packing in

* Correspondence: Aymanco65@yahoo.com
[3]Clinical Research, Trauma & Vascular Surgery, HGH, Doha, Qatar
[4]Clinical Medicine, Weill Cornell Medical College, PO Box 3050, Doha, Qatar
Full list of author information is available at the end of the article

the 'sandwich technique' approach in OM [2, 4]. This change in the management has several potential benefits in terms of early hospital discharge, cost-effectiveness, and minimization of nontherapeutic celiotomies, intra-abdominal complications, and blood transfusion [5]. Selective NOM of blunt hepatic injury is associated with less mortality when compared to operative therapy [6–9]. The current literature supports NOM for all grades of blunt liver injury in hemodynamically stable adults, but inconsistency still exists in terms of the efficacy, patient selection, and management of high-grade injury [7, 10–13]. Operative management is usually considered immediately for the hemodynamically unstable patients with extensive injuries or selectively to treat liver injury-associated complications [14–16]. To date, the OM have limited approaches such as perihepatic packing, resection-debridement, and selective vascular ligation [7, 15]. Improved survival after liver trauma could be attributed to the decline in major venous injuries requiring operative intervention, as well as the widely used hemorrhagic control by angioembolization as adjunct to NOM, improved outcomes with venous injuries and hepatic packing [16].

Hemodynamic instability is the primary indication for OM [14, 17, 18]. The objective of this study is to examine the prevalence, clinical presentation, management and outcomes of patients sustained blunt liver injuries in a small rapidly developing country in the Middle East.

Methods

It is a retrospective chart review study that included all blunt abdominal trauma patients with liver injuries who were admitted and treated at the national Level 1 trauma center in the state of Qatar, from June 2011 and June 2014. Data were extracted from the trauma registry, which is a mature database, in existence since 2007 that is a participant in both the National Trauma Data Bank (NTDB) and the Trauma Quality Improvement Program (TQIP) of the American College of Surgeons-Committee on Trauma (ACS-COT). Inclusion criteria included all blunt liver trauma patients with complete relevant data in adults of both genders (age ≥ 18 years). Patients sustained penetrating abdominal injuries and those who were declared dead at the scene or on arrival were excluded.

Collected data included demographics (age, gender, nationality), mechanism of injury, associated injuries, patient characteristics, Glasgow Coma Score (GCS), Injury severity score (ISS), vital signs (admission blood pressure, heart rate, respiratory rate), laboratory (hemoglobin, hematocrit, platelet count, white blood count, base deficit, International normalized ratio, Alanine Aminotransferase, Aspartate Aminotransferase, and Alkaline Phosphatase) and computed tomography (CT) findings when available, blood transfusion use, blood products transfused, severity of liver injury, ED disposition, management approach and outcomes including length of hospital and Trauma intensive care (TICU) stay,ventilator days, complications and mortality. All patients are resuscitated according to the advanced Trauma Life Support guidelines (ATLS) guidelines [19]. The severity of liver injury is reported using the organ injury scale (OIS) proposed by the American Association for Surgery of Trauma (AAST) and were graded as I-VI based on abdominal CT scan and/or intra-operative findings [20]. Focused Assessment with Sonography for Trauma (FAST) is utilized in the early assessment of all patients to detect the presence or absence of hemoperitoneum. CT scan abdomen was performed in hemodynamically stable patients. Non-operative management was considered in patients who met the following criteria: hemodynamic stability, transfusion of 2 packed red blood cells in relation to liver injury, absence of signs of peritonitis and other abdominal injuries that demand immediate surgery. All patients with high grade liver injury were admitted to the TICU for closed observation and follow-up. This enables early identification of hemodynamic deterioration as indicated and conformed by a significant drop of hemoglobin levels (i.e., acute drop in hemoglobin to a level of 7–8 g/dL).

Planned repeating of abdominal CT scan for higher grades liver injury was not a routine procedure during the study period. On the other hand, hemodynamically unstable patients were candidates for either immediate angioembolization when feasible or surgical treatment depending upon the severity of hepatic injury and degree of instability.

The failure of NOM was defined as need to resort to operative management after a period of watchful observation in TICU weather the reason was related to the liver or associated injuries or demonstration of re-bleeding and need for late angioembolization.

Our protocol for management of liver trauma patients begins with the standard assessment of trauma patients based primarily on their hemodynamic stability status, where unstable patients with positive FAST are directly shifted for operative management (i.e., exploratory laparotomy). On the other hand, stable patients and/or rapid responders to fluid boluses are directed to NOM; starting with an immediate IV enhanced CT scanning of the abdomen within 30–60 min after arrival and subsequent management according to the CT findings. Stable patients with positive FAST are directed to CT scan while the operative theater were kept ready for possible intervention if patient develops hypotension or there is an evidence of active bleeding on abdominal CT and not tolerate a delay to try angioembolization.

Indications of angioembolization included: 1-Presence of arterial blush in the CT scan for either the liver or spleen, if the patient is hemodynamically stable throughout the initial assessment.

2-Post-operative for unstable high-grade liver injury, where damage control perihapatic packing is used then angioembolization before return to OR for definitive repair and closure (Sandwich technique).

3-Evidence of arterial bleeding from associated other injuries (i.e., pelvic fractures, lumbar vessels, or other solid organ injuries).

4-Treatment for pseudoaneurysm and arteriovenous fistula that are diagnosed upon follow up and for rebleeding or hemobilia which occur in some patient as a complication of high grade liver injuries during follow up.

This study was conducted in line with the STROBE checklist (https://www.strobe-statement.org/index.php?id=strobe-home), and has been registered at: http://www.researchregistry.com: Researchregistry3211.

Statistical analysis

Data were presented as proportions, mean ± standard deviation or median as appropriate. Shapiro–Wilk test was the test of normality for continuous variables, whenever applicable. Sample size was not determined priori as we intended to include all liver injury cases during the study period. Blood products transfused, injury severity, and outcomes were compared according to hepatic injury grades using the one-way ANOVA test for continuous variables and Pearson chi-square test for categorical variables. Injury characteristics and outcome of patients with blunt liver injury were also analyzed according to treatment (non-operative versus operative management) using the Student's t test for continuous variables and Pearson chi-square test for categorical variables. The Fisher's exact test was used, if the expected cell frequencies were below 5. Two tailed p-values < 0.05 were considered to be significant. Data analysis was carried out using the Statistical Package for Social Sciences version 18 (SPSS Inc., Chicago, IL, USA).

Results

Patients' demographics and clinical characteristics

Blunt abdominal trauma constituted 15% of the total trauma admissions of each year in our center. During a

Table 1 Demographics, clinical presentation, laboratory, intra-operative findings and complications

Variables	Value	Variables	Value
Age; years (Mean ± SD)	31 ± 13	CT abdomen findings	177 (68.9%)
Males; n (%)	216 (84.0%)	Laceration	99 (38.5%)
Nationality		Liver contusion	81(31.5%)
Qatari; n (%)	46 (18.5%)	Perihepatic fluid	14 (5.4%)
Non-Qatari; n (%)	202 (81.5%)	Blush	8 (3.1%)
History of liver disease	2 (0.8%)	Shattered liver	1 (0.4%)
Vital signs		Intra-operative findings	
Systolic blood pressure (mmHg)	114.5 ± 20.1	Laceration	9 (3.5%)
Diastolic blood pressure (mmHg)	69.7 ± 14.9	Hematoma	6 (2.3%)
Heart rate (beat/min)	97.4 ± 22.8	Lobectomy	1 (0.4%)
Oxygen saturation % (Mean ± SD)	97.7 ± 4.6	Active bleeding	2 (0.8%)
Laboratory parameters		Mesenteric tear	3 (1.2%)
Hemoglobin g/dL	13.0 ± 2.3	Complications	
Hematocrit % (Mean ± SD)	39.8 ± 6.6	Pneumonia	43 (16.7%)
White blood cell count 10^9/L	16.1 ± 6.8	Sepsis	26 (10.1%)
Platelet count 10^9/L	257 ± 79	ARDS	9 (3.5%)
Base excess mEq (Mean ± SD)	−4.8 (−22.4–7.0)	Wound dehiscence	4 (1.5%)
International normalized ratio ((Mean ± SD)	1.15 ± 0.71	Coagulopathy	2 (0.8%)
Alanine Aminotransferase U/L	172 (7–1534)		
Aspartate Aminotransferase U/L	175.5 (10–996)		
Alkaline Phosphatase U/L	69.7 ± 37.4		
Glasgow coma score (Mean ± SD)	12.7 ± 4.2		
Injury severity score(Mean ± SD)	19.6 ± 11.4		
Ethanol intake; n (%)	34 (13.2%)		
Ethanol level mmol/L (Mean ± SD)	39.3 ± 18.5		

3-year study period, there were 257 patients with blunt liver injury (84% males) admitted to the level 1 trauma center which accounted for 38% of the blunt abdominal trauma cases. The mean age of patients was 31 ± 13 years. The most frequent mechanism of injury was motor vehicle collisions (37%), followed by fall from height (15.2%) and pedestrian struck (7.4%).

Table 1 shows demographics, clinical presentation and intra-operative findings of blunt liver injury. The most commonly involved extra-abdominal injuries were chest (51%), head (34.6%), thoracolumbar spine (23.7%) and pelvis (18.3%) (Fig. 1). The frequently associated abdominal injuries were spleen (10.9%), kidney (7.4%), retroperitoneal hematoma (2.7%), and pancreas (2.7%). FAST test was positive in 42 cases. Hollow viscus injuries occurred in a total of 23 patients (8.9%), of which small bowel, large bowel and stomach injuries were identified in 11, 9 and 3 patients, respectively. The mean ISS and GCS were 19.6 ± 11.4 and 13 ± 2.0, respectively. Low GCS and hemodynamic instability were indications for intubation in 57 patients (22.2%). Blood transfusion was required in 27.2% of cases.

Liver injury grading and major findings on initial abdominal CT scan are summarized in Table 1.

Table 2 demonstrates the blood transfused based on liver injury grades. The need for 1–2 units of packed RBCs was more frequent in patients with grade I and II liver injuries. While, significantly more number of PRBCs were transfused to patients with grade IV liver injuries ($p = 0.02$). Massive transfusion defined by transfusion of more than 10 units of packed RBCs was needed in 38.9% of grade IV injuries and less commonly in the lower grades (I-III) due to associated non-hepatic injuries.

A comparison of associated injuries, severity of injury and outcome among different liver injury grades is shown in Table 3. Low GCS, high ISS and mortality rates were comparable among all liver injury grades. Subanalysis of data using World Society of Emergency Surgery (WSES) classification revealed19 patients were categorized as a WSES grade IV who underwent surgical intervention without having initial CT scanning. Table 4 shows the AAST and WSES classification of liver injury.

Management

Table 5 shows the management and outcomes of hepatic injury patients in the study cohort.

Non-operative management

Out of 198 stable patients, conservative management was successful in 192 (97%); Splenic injury was reported in 19 patients (7.4%) and one patient had mesenteric tear in NOM group. The NOM failed in 6 (3%) patients due to delayed bleeding from hepatic hematoma, associated splenic rupture and small bowel injury which mandate an operation. One patient was successfully managed with angioembolization while the remaining five patients were operated successfully.

Operative management

Fifty-nine patients (23%) underwent emergent surgery which included packing (perihepatic and/or intraparenchymal hemostatic packs), resection debridement, left lobe hepatectomy and splenectomy. The primary indications for surgery were hemodynamic instability, peritonism/peritonitis and other associated intra-abdominal injuries that necessitate surgical interventions (Table 5). Operative findings revealed grade III liver injuries in 40 (67.8%), grade IV in 18 (30.5%) patients, and one (1.7%) patient had grade V injury.

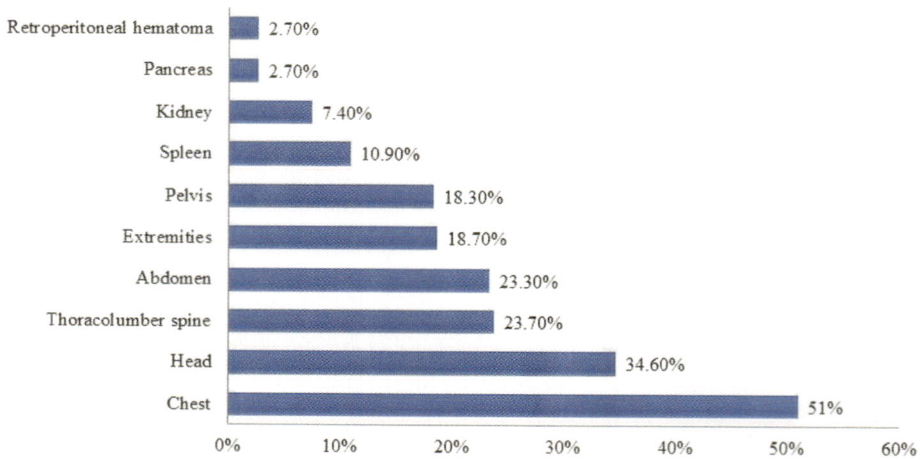

Fig. 1 Associated injuries in blunt liver trauma

Table 2 Blood products transfused based on liver injury grades

	Grade I ($n = 74$)	Grade II ($n = 115$)	Grade III ($n = 49$)	Grade IV-V ($n = 19$)	P
Packed RBC unit					
Not transfused	55 (74.3%)	83 (72.2%)	40 (81.6%)	9 (47.3%)	0.02 for all
1–2	7 (9.5%)	12 (10.4%)	2 (4.1%)	1 (5.6%)	
3–6	4 (5.4%)	7 (6.1%)	4 (8.2%)	2 (11.1%)	
7–10	1 (1.4%)	6 (5.2%)	1 (2.0%)	0 (0.0%)	
> 10	7 (9.5%)	7 (6.1%)	2 (4.1%)	7 (38.9%)	
Fresh frozen plasma unit					
Not transfused	60 (81.1%)	93 (80.9%)	43 (87.8%)	9 (50.0%)	0.05 for all
1–2	3 (4.1%)	6 (5.2%)	0 (0.0%)	0 (0.0%)	
3–6	5 (6.8%)	7 (6.1%)	4 (8.2%)	4 (22.2%)	
7–10	0 (0.0%)	3 (2.6%)	0 (0.0%)	2 (11.1%)	
> 10	6 (8.1%)	6 (5.2%)	2 (4.1%)	4 (21%)	
Platelets units					
Not transfused	61 (82.4%)	100 (87.0%)	44 (89.8%)	10 (53%)	0.08 for all
1–2	3 (4.1%)	1 (0.9%)	0 (0.0%)	1 (5.6%)	
3–6	3 (4.1%)	6 (5.2%)	3 (6.1%)	3 (16.7%)	
7–10	0 (0.0%)	1 (0.9%)	0 (0.0%)	1 (5.6%)	
> 10	7 (9.5%)	7 (6.1%)	2 (4.1%)	4 (22.2%)	

In-hospital complications and outcomes

Overall, pneumonia (16.7%), sepsis (10.1%) and ARDS (3.5%) were the most frequently associated in-hospital complications. Specifically, complications related to liver injury per say include biloma in two cases managed with laparoscopic wash out and drainage. Three cases developed pseudoaneurysm on the NOM group. Massive liver necrosis occurred in one patient after angioembolization and was managed successfully conservatively. The overall mortality rate was 7.8% (20 patients) which was higher but statistically not significant in the OM group (6.6% vs. 12.1%; $p = 0.17$).

Based on the liver injury grades, the mortality was 12.2% in Grade I, 7.8% in Grade II, and 4.1% in Grade III, which is mainly attributed to the severity of associated traumatic brain injuries.

Table 5 demonstrates the injury characteristics and outcome between OM and NOM. The two groups were comparable for severity of injury, associated injuries (spleen, kidney and pelvis) and length of hospital stay. However, the rate of FAST, medications used to control bleeding; AAST grading, WSES classification and TICU length of stay were different in the 2 groups.

Discussion

This is a large descriptive study from a single center that reports clinical presentations, management and outcomes of blunt liver injuries based on the injury grade, hemodynamic status and management approach. The study showed a higher rate of liver injuries in young males which occurred in more than one third of patients

Table 3 Associated injuries, ISS, and blood transfusion in liver injury grades

	Grade I ($n = 74$)	Grade II ($n = 115$)	Grade III ($n = 49$)	Grade IV-V ($n = 19$)	P
Associated injuries					
Head	37 (50.0%)	50 (43.5%)	1 (2.0%)	1 (5.3%)	0.001
Chest	37 (50.0%)	60 (52.2%)	22 (44.9%)	12 (63.2%)	0.45
Pelvis	7 (9.5%)	26 (22.6%)	9 (18.4%)	5 (26.3%)	0.15
Injury severity score ≥ 16	43 (58.1%)	51 (44.3%)	27 (55.1%)	–	0.74
Glasgow coma scale ≤8	18 (24.3%)	24 (20.9%)	5 (10.2%)	1 (5.3%)	0.16
Blood transfusion	19 (25.7%)	32 (27.8%)	9 (18.4%)	10 (52.6%)	0.04
Hospital mortality	9 (12.2%)	9 (7.8%)	2 (4.1%)	0 (0.0%)	0.35

Table 4 AAST and WSES classification

Liver injury Severity	AAST		WSES (stable)		WSES (grade IV)
	Grade	n	Grade	n	n
Mild	I-II	189	I	176	13
Moderate	III	49	II	48	1
Severe[a]	IV-V	19	III	14	5

[a]Only 1 case had Grade V, *AAST* American Association for Surgery of Trauma, *WSES* World Society of Emergency Surgery classification

with blunt trauma. Conservative treatment was the option of treatment in more than a three-quarter of cases.

The mechanism of liver injury differs geographically due to socio-demographic and community factors [21, 22]. In the state of Qatar, the rate of blunt poly-trauma associated hepatic injury is high secondary to the increase in the trend of motor vehicles crashes over the recent decades [23].

Earlier studies on blunt hepatic trauma showed an association with extra-abdominal injuries involving chest and head regions as well as fractures of the long bones and pelvis [11].

It has been well established that around 80% of patients with liver injuries can be successfully managed non-operatively [22]. However, this approach could fail in up to 25% of cases due to re-bleeding, bile leak, liver necrosis or secondary sepsis. Our study demonstrated that the vast majority of patients were successfully treated conservatively. Consistent with our findings, an earlier study from Kuwait showed an 80% success rate of NOM in patients who sustained blunt liver trauma and only 4 patients (4%) failed NOM. A recent study from Albania reported a similar rate of successful conservative

Table 5 Injury characteristics and outcome in operative and non-operative management

	Non-operative ($n = 198$)	Operative ($n = 59$)	P
Age; mean±SD	31±12	32±16	0.74
Gender (male)	83.5%	86.4%	0.70
Glasgow coma scale < 8	37 (18.7%)	11 (19.3%)	0.91
Injury severity score	17(4–59)	17(5–50)	0.13
Systolic blood pressure < 90 mmHg	15 (7.6%)	7 (12.3%)	0.27
Injury severity score	18.9 ± 11.0	22.0 ± 12.4	0.11
Splenic injury	19 (9.6%)	9 (15.3%)	0.22
Kidney injury	13 (6.6%)	6 (10.2%)	0.35
Pelvic injury	34 (17.2%)	13 (22.0%)	0.39
Liver grade (I-III) AAST	190 (96.0%)	48 (81.4%)	0.001
Liver grade (IV-V) AAST	8 (4.0%)	11 (18.6%)	
FAST	52(29.5%)	29(53.7%)	0.001
CT Abdomen	137(69.2%)	40(67.8%)	0.84
WSES classification			0.03 for all
I	147(74%)	27(46%)	
II	43(22%)	7 (12%)	
III	8 (4%)	6 (10%)	
IV	–	19(32%)	
Medications			
Tranexamic acid	4(3.1%)	1(2.8%)	0.91
Factor VII	10(7.8%)	12(28.6%)	0.001
Fibrinogen	19(14.5%)	17(38.6%)	0.001
Inotropes	19(15.2%)	14(40%)	0.001
Blood transfusion	36 (18.2%)	34 (57.6%)	0.001
Hospital length of stay; median and range	7 (1–323)	13.5 (1–277)	0.23
TICU stay (days);median and range	3(1–41)	7(1–39)	0.01
Hospital mortality	13 (6.6%)	7 (12.1%)	0.17

management (83%) [3]. Another study from Turkey [24] included 300 patients (63% stable and 37% unstable), of them 192 patients treated conservatively and 108 received surgery. In this study, 13% died and the main determinants of mortality were hemodynamic instability on admission and type and grade of liver injury [24].

In our study, conservative treatment failed in six patients mainly due to delayed bleeding from hepatic hematoma, associated splenic rupture or small bowel injury. These findings reflect the improvement of the NOM approach as compared to earlier study by Bernardo et al., [14] where 60.8% of cases were treated non-operatively with a failure rate of 15%. In our series; one patient failed NOM which later successfully treated with angioembolization. Recent literature suggests that NOM in higher grade of liver injury can be considered using selective angioembolization in the absence of active bleeding. Despite the fact that angioembolization is promising adjunct for increasing the success of NOM in blunt liver injury, it could be associated with serious complications such as liver necrosis, secondary infection, liver abscess, bile leak and biloma [25].

In the present study, 23% cases underwent emergent surgery where the major indications for surgery included hemodynamic instability, acute peritonitis and associated other surgically correctable intra-abdominal injuries. Failure of NOM was related mainly to high grade liver injury. Although the failure rate was low, three cases had re-bleeding due to development of pseudoaneurysm. Current reports have suggested the rate of successful NOM to be 60–70% for high-grade liver injuries (i.e. III and above) [26].

Østerballe et al. [27] reported a 4% of pseudoaneurysm on radiological follow-up for 188 patients. The authors observed no correlation between the development of pseudoaneurysm and severity of liver injury; therefore they recommended a follow-up CT angiogram after 4–5 days to rule out such complications. As the high grade injury is the mainstay of failure, we have changed our institutional protocol to repeat the CT scan in patients with higher liver injuries grades with intravenous contrast to pick up early pseudoaneurysm development and to plan angioembolization (coiling) aiming to reduce the rate of NOM failure.

In the present study, complications related to liver injury were very few in terms of biloma in two cases and pseudoaneurysm related rebleeding in three patients. Much less to Carrillo et al. series [28]; who reported biloma of 2.8% in cases with complex blunt hepatic injuries. Bala et al. analyzed 398 patients with liver trauma and identified complications in 16 patients with high grade injury which included biloma and bile leak that was treated with drainage and endoscopic retrograde cholangiopancreatography, while three patients developed re-bleeding from pseudoaneurysm that required angioembolization [29].

Generally, in about 10–20% of severe hepatic injuries, the decision for surgery poses a difficult challenge for surgeons. Non-operative management of high grade liver injuries may carry risk of complication which can be related to the amount of blood transfusion, associated injuries, age and/or liver related complications [30]. The concept of damage control in patients with abdominal trauma is currently a valuable operative approach in unstable patients with liver injury as well as polytrauma [31].

Similar to our findings, few studies have suggested that the need for blood transfusion is lesser in patients who are managed non-operatively than those who underwent surgery [5, 21]. Notably, an earlier study from Egypt reported blood transfusion in 70.5% cases managed non-operatively [21] which is much higher than that of our study (18%). It is worthy to mention that the need of blood transfusion was not dependent on the liver injury alone.

The conservative treatment group showed no significant difference in the length of hospital stay as compared to OM group in our study which is similar to the observation from the Ghnnam et al. study [5].

In our study, the overall mortality rate was 7.8%, and most deaths accounted for significant injuries involving head or chest region and exsanguinating hemorrhage at presentation. The reported mortality rate in hepatic injury patients varies from 9 to 42%, and mostly close to 20% among the admitted patients. However, an earlier study from Saudi Arabia showed a lower rate of motility (3.5%) [5]. The observed high mortality in mild liver injury patients was mainly related to the associated head injury.

Recently, WSES classification for liver injury has been published [16], however, in our center; we still rely on the AAST for grading of solid organ injuries. According to WSES, stable patients should be treated non-operatively in grade I-III whereas WSES grade IV patients should be treated surgically without having initial CT scanning due to patients' instability. In the present study, there were 189 mild AAST cases, of them 13 patients were classified as WSES grade IV, indicating that surgical intervention was based on the patient instability due to other associated injuries. One-quarter of severe AAST cases was treated surgically and grouped as a WSES IV.

Limitations

The main limitation of the present study is the retrospective analysis of data which may limit its generalizability in addition to potential selection bias. Patients with incomplete data, prehospital or on arrival death were excluded from the current analysis which may underestimate the blunt liver injury rate. The sample size in the higher grade liver injury groups was small for reliable comparisons. The design of the study makes it difficult to carefully assess the management approach. Moreover, we lack information regarding the time to CT scan and follow-up for patients post-discharge from the hospital.

Conclusions

Blunt traumatic hepatic injuries are more common in young male population. The vast majority of hepatic injuries are mild (grade I-III) requiring conservative treatment. Therefore, non-operative management of liver injuries is a frequent approach in our practice and has been successfully considered in hemodynamic stable patient. Associated head injury could explain the high mortality in the low grade liver injuries. Major liver injuries (grades IV-V) are relatively infrequent in our cohort. All conservatively treated patients with high-grade liver injuries should be closely monitored in the intensive care unit for the indication of failure of NOM which can be treated further with the help of intervention radiology or operative management. NOM could be successful even in high graded injuries with low morbidity and mortality.

There is a role of routine repeating CT scan for high grade and the utility of angioembolization in the absence of active bleeding to decrease late failures of NOM. Introducing the new WSES classification makes clear how is important the hemodynamic status of the patients despite the lesion. However, further larger prospective and multicenter studies are needed to confirm our findings.

Acknowledgements
We would like to thank all the database registry staff of the trauma section.

Funding
This research did not receive any specific grant from any funding agency in the public, commercial or not-for-profit sector.

Authors' contributions
IA: study design, data analysis and interpretation, drafting and critical review of manuscript; SA was involved in study design, data acquisition, writing manuscript and review, AE: study design, data interpretation, writing and critical review. HA&RP: data acquisition, interpretation and drafting manuscript; HAT: study design, data interpretation, writing and critical review. All authors read and approved the final manuscript.

Competing interests
The authors have no conflict of interest, no financial issues to disclose and no funding was received for this study.

Author details
[1]Department of surgery, Trauma Surgery section, Hamad General Hospital (HGH), Doha, Qatar. [2]Department of surgery, HGH, Doha, Qatar. [3]Clinical Research, Trauma & Vascular Surgery, HGH, Doha, Qatar. [4]Clinical Medicine, Weill Cornell Medical College, PO Box 3050, Doha, Qatar.

References

1. Kozar RA, Moore FA, Moore EE, et al. Western trauma association critical decisions in trauma: nonoperative Management of Adult Blunt Hepatic Trauma. J Trauma. 2009;67:1144–9.
2. Saltzherr TP, van der Vlies CH, van Lienden KP, Beenen LF, Ponsen KJ, van Gulik TM, Goslings JC. Improved outcomes in the non-operative management of liver injuries. HPB (Oxford). 2011;13(5):350–5.
3. Buci S, Torba M, Gjata A, Kajo I, Bushi G, Kagjini K. The rate of success of the conservative management of liver trauma in a developing country. World J Emerg Surg. 2017;12:24.
4. Chatoupis K, Papadopoulou G, Kaskarelis I. New technology in the management Oliver trauma. Ann Gastroenterol. 2013;26(1):41–4.
5. Ghnnam WM, Almasry HN, Ghanem MA. Non-operative management of blunt liver trauma in a level II trauma hospital in Saudi Arabia. Int J Crit Illn Inj Sci. 2013;3(2):118–23.
6. Sartorelli KH, Frumiento C, Rogers FB, et al. Non-operative management of hepatic, splenic, and renal injuries in adults with multiple injuries. J Trauma. 2000;49:56–61.
7. Richardson JD, Franklin GA, Lukan JK, et al. Evolution in the management of hepatic trauma: a 25 year perspective. Ann Surg. 2000;232:324–30.
8. Christmas AB, Wilson AK, Manning B, et al. Selective management of blunt hepatic injuries including non-operative management is a safe and effective strategy. Surgery. 2005;138:606–11.
9. Tinkoff G, Esposito T, Reed J, et al. American Association for the Surgery of Trauma organ injury scale I: spleen, liver, and kidney, validation based on the national trauma data bank. J Am Coll Surg. 2008;207:646–55.
10. Cirocchi R, Trastulli S, Pressi E, Farinella E, Avenia S, Morales Uribe CH, Botero AM, Barrera LM. Non-operative management versus operative management in high-grade blunt hepatic injury. Cochrane Database Syst Rev. 2015;8: CD010989.
11. Malhotra AK, Fabian TC, Croce MA, et al. Blunt hepatic injury: a paradigm shift from operative to non-operative management in the 1990's. Ann Surg. 2000;231:804–13.
12. Velmahos GC, Toutouzas K, Radin R, et al. High success with nonoperative management of blunt hepatic trauma: the liver is a sturdy organ. Arch Surg 2003;138:47-Y480; discussion 480–481.
13. Paddock HN, Tepas JJ 3rd, Ramenofsky ML, et al. Management of blunt pediatric hepatic and splenic injury: similar process. different outcome Am Surg. 2004;70:1068–72.
14. Bernardo CG, Fuster J, Bombuy E, Sanchez S, Ferrer J, Loera MA, Marti J, Fondevila C, Zavala E, Garcia-Valdecasas JC. Treatment of liver trauma: operative or conservative management. Gastroenterology Res. 2010;3(1):9–18.
15. Paydar S, Mahmoodi M, Jamshidi M, Niakan H, Keshavarz M, Moeenvaziri N, et al. Perihepatic packing versus primary surgical repair in patients with blunt liver trauma; an 8-year experience. Bull Emerg Trauma. 2014;2(3):103–9.
16. Coccolini F, Catena F, Moore EE, Ivatury R, Biffl W, Peitzman A, Coimbra R, Rizoli S, Kluger Y, Abu-Zidan FM, Ceresoli M, Montori G, Sartelli M, Weber D, Fraga G, Naidoo N, Moore FA, Zanini N, Ansaloni L. WSES classification and guidelines for liver trauma. World J Emerg Surg. 2016;11:50. eCollection 2016
17. Kozar RA, Feliciano DV, Moore EE, et al. Western trauma association/critical decisions in trauma: operative Management of Adult Blunt Hepatic Trauma. J Trauma. 2011;71:1–5.
18. Arumugam S, Al-Hassani A, El-Menyar A, Abdelrahman H, Parchani A, Peralta R, Zarour A, Al-Thani H. Frequency, causes and pattern of abdominal trauma: a 4-year descriptive analysis. J Emerg Trauma Shock. 2015;8(4):193–8.
19. McCrum ML, McKee J, Lai M, Staples J, Switzer N, Widder SL. ATLS adherence in the transfer of rural trauma patients to a level I facility. Injury. 2013;44(9):1241–5.
20. Homann G, Toschke C, Gassmann P, Vieth V. Accuracy of the AAST organ injury scale for CT evaluation of traumatic liver and spleen injuries. Chin J Traumatol. 2014;17(1):25–30.
21. Saleh AF, Al Sageer E, Elheny A. Management of Liver Trauma in Minia university hospital, Egypt. Indian J Surg. 2016 Dec;78(6):442–7.

22. Beardsley C, Gananadha S. An overview of liver trauma. MSJA. 2011;3:5–10. http://msja.anu.edu.au/archive/issue/04/an-overview-of-liver-trauma.php
23. Asim M, El-Menyar A, Al-Thani H, Abdelrahman H, Zarour A, Latifi R. Blunt traumatic injury in the Arab middle eastern populations. J Emerg Trauma Shock. 7(2):88–96.
24. Kaptanoglu L, Kurt N, Sikar HE. Current approach to liver traumas. Int J Surg. 2017;39:255–9.
25. Asfar S, Khoursheed M, Al-Saleh M, Alfawaz AA, Farghaly MM, Nur AM. Management of Liver Trauma in Kuwait. Med Princ Pract. 2014;23:160–6.
26. Suen K, Skandarajah AR, Knowles B, Judson R, Thomson BN. Changes in the management of liver trauma leading to reduced mortality: 15-year experience in a major trauma Centre. ANZ J Surg. 2016;86(11):894–9.
27. Østerballe L, Helgstrand F, Axelsen T, et al. Hepatic pseudoaneurysm after traumatic liver injury; is CT follow-up warranted? Journal of Trauma Management & Outcomes. 2014;8:18.
28. Carrillo EH, Wohltmann C, Richardson JD, Polk HC Jr. Evolution in the treatment of complex blunt liver injuries. Curr Probl Surg. 2001;38(1):1–60.
29. Bala M, Abu Gazalla S, Almogy G, et al. Complications of high grade liver injuries: management and outcome with focus on bile leaks. Scandinavian Journal of Trauma, Resuscitation and Emergency Medicine. 2012;20:20.
30. Ward J, Alarcon L, Peitzman AB. Management of blunt liver injury: what is new? Eur J Trauma Emerg Surg. 2015;41(3):229–37.
31. Feliciano DV. Abdominal trauma revisited. Am Surg. 2017;83(11):1193–202.

Permissions

All chapters in this book were first published in SURGERY, by BioMed Central; hereby published with permission under the Creative Commons Attribution License or equivalent. Every chapter published in this book has been scrutinized by our experts. Their significance has been extensively debated. The topics covered herein carry significant findings which will fuel the growth of the discipline. They may even be implemented as practical applications or may be referred to as a beginning point for another development.

The contributors of this book come from diverse backgrounds, making this book a truly international effort. This book will bring forth new frontiers with its revolutionizing research information and detailed analysis of the nascent developments around the world.

We would like to thank all the contributing authors for lending their expertise to make the book truly unique. They have played a crucial role in the development of this book. Without their invaluable contributions this book wouldn't have been possible. They have made vital efforts to compile up to date information on the varied aspects of this subject to make this book a valuable addition to the collection of many professionals and students.

This book was conceptualized with the vision of imparting up-to-date information and advanced data in this field. To ensure the same, a matchless editorial board was set up. Every individual on the board went through rigorous rounds of assessment to prove their worth. After which they invested a large part of their time researching and compiling the most relevant data for our readers.

The editorial board has been involved in producing this book since its inception. They have spent rigorous hours researching and exploring the diverse topics which have resulted in the successful publishing of this book. They have passed on their knowledge of decades through this book. To expedite this challenging task, the publisher supported the team at every step. A small team of assistant editors was also appointed to further simplify the editing procedure and attain best results for the readers.

Apart from the editorial board, the designing team has also invested a significant amount of their time in understanding the subject and creating the most relevant covers. They scrutinized every image to scout for the most suitable representation of the subject and create an appropriate cover for the book.

The publishing team has been an ardent support to the editorial, designing and production team. Their endless efforts to recruit the best for this project, has resulted in the accomplishment of this book. They are a veteran in the field of academics and their pool of knowledge is as vast as their experience in printing. Their expertise and guidance has proved useful at every step. Their uncompromising quality standards have made this book an exceptional effort. Their encouragement from time to time has been an inspiration for everyone.

The publisher and the editorial board hope that this book will prove to be a valuable piece of knowledge for researchers, students, practitioners and scholars across the globe.

List of Contributors

Carsten Kamphues, Sabine Engel, Roberta Bova, Michael Hippler Benscheidt, Gero Puhl, Peter Neuhaus and Daniel Seehofer
Department of General, Visceral and Transplantation Surgery, Universitätsklinikum Charité, Campus Virchow Klinikum, Humboldt-Universität, D-13353 Berlin, Germany

Timm Denecke
Department of Radiology, Universitätsklinikum Charité, Campus Virchow Klinikum, Humboldt-Universität, D-13353 Berlin, Germany

Soondoos Raashed and Khaled Alsaleh
Upper Gastrointestinal Unit, Bankstown Hospital, Sydney, Australia

Manju D Chandrasegaram and Neil D Merrett
Upper Gastrointestinal Unit, Bankstown Hospital, Sydney, Australia
Division of Surgery, School of Medicine, University of Western Sydney, Sydney, Australia

Glen Schlaphoff
Interventional and Diagnostic Radiology, Liverpool Hospital, Sydney, Australia

Hubert Scheuerlein, Falk Rauchfuss, Julia Franke, Karin Jandt, Yves Dittmar, Gudrun Trebing and Utz Settmacher
Department of General, Visceral and Vascular Surgery, University Hospital Jena, Erlanger Allee 101, 07747 Jena, Germany

Domenico Loffredo and Alberto Marvaso
Asl Na 2-Hospital A. Rizzoli of Lacco Ameno (Ischia), Naples, Italy

Sandro Ceraso
Perfusion Science, University of Naples "Federico II", Naples, Italy

Nicola Angelo Cinelli
Bioethics, Catholic University "Sacred Heart", Rome, Italy

Aldo Rocca and Bruno Amato
Department of Clinical Medicine and Surgery, University of Naples "Federico II" Naples, Naples, Italy

Mario Vitale
Department of Medicine and Surgery, University of Salerno, Baronissi (SA), Italy

Michele Rossi
Department of Radiology, Sant'Andrea Hospital, University of Rome "Sapienza", Rome, Italy

Eugenio Annibale Genovese
Department of Radiology, University of Cagliari, Cagliari, Italy

Mariapia Cinelli
Department of Public Health, University of Naples "Federico II" Naples, Naples, Italy

Domenico Risio, Rossana Percario, Margherita Legnini, Francesco Caldaralo, Alberto D'Aulerio, Roberto Cotellese, Luca Napolitano and Paolo Innocenti
Unit of General and Laparoscopic Surgery, "G. d'Annunzio" University, Via dei Vestini 31, 66100 Chieti, Italy

Domenico Angelucci and Camilla Marinelli
Unit of Pathology, "G. d'Annunzio" University, Chieti, Italy

Nuh N Rahbari, Heike Elbers, Moritz Koch, Patrick Vogler, Fabian Striebel, Peter Schemmer, Arianeb Mehrabi, Markus W Büchler and Jürgen Weitz
Department of General, Visceral and Transplant Surgery, University of Heidelberg, Germany

Thomas Bruckner
Institute of Medical Biometry and Informatics, University of Heidelberg, Germany

Yasuhiro Kihara, Hiroshi Yokomizo and Toshihiko Hirata
Division of General Surgery, Japanese Red Cross Kumamoto Hospital, Nagamineminami 2-1-1, Higashiku, Kumamoto city, Kumamoto 861-8520, Japan

Takahiro Urata
Division of Gastroenterology, Japanese Red Cross Kumamoto Hospital, Kumamoto, Japan

Michiko Nagamine
Division of Diagnostic Pathology, Japanese Red Cross Kumamoto Hospital, Kumamoto, Japan

Marcello Donati, Antonio Biondi, Francesco Basile and Salvatore Gruttadauria
Department of Surgery. General and Oncologic Surgery Unit, Vittorio-Emanuele University Hospital of Catania, via Plebiscito 628, 95122 Catania, Italy

Xin Wang and Zusen Wang
Department of Hepatobiliary and Pancreatic Surgery, Affiliated Hospital of Qingdao University, Qingdao 266000, China

Liqun Wu
Department of Hepatobiliary and Pancreatic Surgery, Affiliated Hospital of Qingdao University, Qingdao 266000, China
Jiangsu Road 16, Qingdao 266000, China

Yanming Zhou, Lupeng Wu and Bin Li
Department of Hepatobiliary and Pancreatovascular Surgery, Oncologic Center of Xiamen, First affiliated Hospital of Xiamen University, Xiamen, China

Yaqing Xiao and Hua Li
Department of Digestive Diseases, First affiliated Hospital of Xiamen University, Xiamen, China

Syed Nabeel Zafar, Muhammad Rizwan Khan, Rushna Raza and Muhammad N Khan
Dertment of Surgery, Aga Khan University, Stadium Road, Karachi - 74800, Pakistan

Mahwash Kasi, Ammar Rafiq and Omer H Jamy
Medical College, Aga Khan University, Stadium Road, Karachi -74800, Pakistan

Takahiro Kajiwara, Yutaka Midorikawa, Shintaro Yamazaki, Tokio Higaki, Hisashi Nakayama, Masamichi Moriguchi and Tadatoshi Takayama
Department of Digestive Surgery, Nihon University School of Medicine, 30-1 Oyaguchikami-cho, Itabashi-ku, Tokyo 173-8610, Japan

Shingo Tsuji
Genome Science Division, Research Center for Advanced Science and Technologies, University of Tokyo, 4-6-1 Komaba, Meguro-ku, Tokyo 153-8904, Japan

Danzi Michele, Grimaldi Luciano and Reggio Stefano
Department of Specialized Surgery - Division of Gastrointestinal Surgery Rehabilitation of Election and Emergency. "Federico II" University, Naples -Italy

Fabozzi Massimiliano
Department of General Surgery. "U. Parini" Hospital, Aosta - Italy

Danzi Roberta and Soscia Ernesto
Department of Diagnostic Imaging and Radiotherapy. "Federico II" University, Naples - Italy

Amato Bruno
Department of General, Geriatric, Oncologic Surgery and Advanced Technologies. "Federico II" University, Naples - Italy

Mostafa A Hamad
Departments of General Surgery, Faculty of Medicine, Assiut University, Assiut, Egypt

Hussein El-Amin
Departments of Medicine, Faculty of Medicine, Assiut University, Assiut, Egypt

Takehiro Noji, Takahiro Tsuchikawa, Yuma Ebihara, Toru Nakamura, Kentaro Kato, Joe Matsumoto, Eiichi Tanaka, Toshiaki Shichinohe and Satoshi Hirano
Department of Gastroenterological Surgery II, Graduate School of Medicine, Hokkaido University, N15W7, Kita-ku, Sapporo Hokkaido 060-8638, Japan

Enver Fekaj and Mehmet Maxhuni
Department of Abdominal Surgery, University Clinical Centre of Kosovo, Rrethi i Spitalit, str: p.n., Pristina 10000, Republic of Kosovo

Arben Gjata
Department of Surgery, University Clinical Centre, "Nene Tereza", Rruga Dibres 370, Tirana, Albania

Shuichi Aoki, Masamichi Mizuma, Hiroki Hayashi, Kei Nakagawa, Takanori Morikawa, Fuyuhiko Motoi, Takeshi Naitoh and Michiaki Unno
Department of Surgery, Tohoku University Graduate School of Medicine, Aobaku, Sendai, Japan

Shinichi Egawa
Division of International Cooperation for Disaster Medicine, Tohoku University, 1-1 Seiryomachi, Aobaku, Sendai 980-8574, Japan

Hiromichi Ishii, Akinori Noguchi, Tomoyuki Fukami, Riho Sugimoto, Hiroyuki Tada, Hiroki Takeshita, Seiji Umehara, Hiroyuki Izumi, Naoki Tani, Masahide Yamaguchi and Tetsuro Yamane
Department of Surgery, Matsushita Memorial Hospital, 5-55 Sotojima-cho, Moriguchi city, Osaka 570-8540, Japan

Konrad Kobryń, Rafał Paluszkiewicz, Krzysztof Dudek, Urszula Michał Korba, Piotr Remiszewski, Michał Grąt, Waldemar Patkowski and Marek Krawczyk
Department of General, Transplant and Liver Surgery, Medical University of Warsaw, Poland. Banacha Street 1a, 02-097 Warsaw, Poland

Ołdakowska-Jedynak, Joanna Raszeja-Wyszomirska and Piotr Milkiewicz
Department of Hepatology and Internal Diseases, Medical University of Warsaw, Warsaw, Poland

Sandra de Sousa, Olivier Tobler and Pouya Iranmanesh
Division of Abdominal Surgery, Geneva University Hospitals, Faculty of Medicine, Rue Gabrielle-Perret-Gentil 4, 1205, Geneva, Switzerland

Philippe Morel and Christian Toso
Division of Abdominal Surgery, Geneva University Hospitals, Faculty of Medicine, Rue Gabrielle-Perret-Gentil 4, 1205, Geneva, Switzerland
Hepato-pancreatico-biliary Center, Geneva University Hospitals, Faculty of Medicine, Geneva, Switzerland

Jean-Louis Frossard
Division of Gastro-intestinal Disease and Hepatology, Geneva University Hospitals, Faculty of Medicine, Geneva, Switzerland
Hepato-pancreatico-biliary Center, Geneva University Hospitals, Faculty of Medicine, Geneva, Switzerland

Jimme K. Wiggers, Rowan F. van Golen, Annemiek M. Dekker, Thomas M. van Gulik and Michal Heger
Department of Surgery, Surgical Laboratory, Academic Medical Center, University of Amsterdam, Amsterdam, The Netherlands

Joanne Verheij
Department of Pathology, Academic Medical Center, University of Amsterdam, Amsterdam, The Netherlands

Heng-Chih Pan
Department of Nephrology, Chang Gung Memorial Hospital, Keelung, Taiwan

Ying-Jen Chen
Division of General Internal Medicine and Geriatrics Medicine, Chang Gung Memorial Hospital, Taipei, Taiwan

Jhe-Ping Lin and Ming-Jung Tsai
Chang Gung University College of Medicine, Taoyuan, Taiwan

Chang-Chyi Jenq, Ming-Yang Chang, Ya-Chung Tian, Cheng-Chieh Hung, Ji-Tseng Fang, Chih-Wei Yang and Yung-Chang Chen
Chang Gung University College of Medicine, Taoyuan, Taiwan
Kidney Research Center, Department of Nephrology, Chang Gung Memorial Hospital, Taipei, Taiwan

Wei-Chen Lee
Chang Gung University College of Medicine, Taoyuan, Taiwan
Laboratory of Immunology, Department of General Surgery, Chang Gung Memorial Hospital, Taipei, Taiwan

Ming-Hung Tsai
Chang Gung University College of Medicine, Taoyuan, Taiwan
Division of Gastroenterology, Chang Gung Memorial Hospital, Taipei, Taiwan

Pei-Chun Fan and Chih-Hsiang Chang
Kidney Research Center, Department of Nephrology, Chang Gung Memorial Hospital, Taipei, Taiwan

Haibo Zou, Lanyun Luo, Hua Xue, Guan Wang, Xiankui Wang, Le Luo, Yutong Yao, Guangming Xiang and Xiaolun Huang
Department of Hepatobiliary Surgery, Sichuan Academy of Medical Sciences and Sichuan Provincial People's Hospital, #32, Section 2, West 1st Ring Road, Chengdu 610072, China

Daniel Pindak, Jana Pavlendova, Miroslav Tomas and Juraj Pechan
Department of Surgical Oncology, Slovak Medical University, Bratislava, Slovakia

National Cancer Institute, Klenova 1, 833 10 Bratislava 3, Slovakia

Jozef Dolnik and Robert Duchon
National Cancer Institute, Klenova 1, 833 10 Bratislava 3, Slovakia

Deniz Balci, Elvan Onur Kirimker and Arda Cetinkaya
Department of General Surgery, Ankara University School of Medicine, K4 06590 Sihhiye, Ankara, Turkey

Menekse Ozcelik and Zekeriyya Alanoglu
Department of Anesthesiology, Ankara University School of Medicine, Ankara, Turkey

Evren Ustuner and Sadik Bilgic
Department of Radiology, Ankara University School of Medicine, Ankara, Turkey

Mehmet Cakici, Bahadir Inan and Ahmet Ruchan Akar
Department of Cardiovascular Surgery, Ankara University School of Medicine, Ankara, Turkey

Ying-Yang Liao
Nutrition Department, Affiliated Tumor Hospital of Guangxi Medical University, Nanning, China

Ning-Fu Peng, Jian-Hong Zhong and Le-Qun Li
Hepatobiliary Surgery Department, Affiliated Tumor Hospital of Guangxi Medical University, Nanning 530021, Guangxi Province, China

Di Long, Peng-Cheng Yu and Sen Zhang
Colorectal Anal Surgery Department, The First Affiliated Hospital of Guangxi Medical University, Nanning 530021, China

Hans Michael Hau, Florian Thalmann, Mehmet Haluk Morgul, Undine Lange, Rudolf Ascherl, Dirk Uhlmann, Hans-Michael Tautenhahn, Georg Wiltberger and Michael Bartels
Department of Visceral, Transplantation, Vascular and Thoracic Surgery, University Hospital of Leipzig, Liebigstrasse 20, 04103 Leipzig, Germany

Moritz Schmelzle, Georgi Atanasov and Christian Benzing
Department of General, Visceral and Transplant Surgery, Campus Virchow, Charité Universitätsmedizin Berlin, Augustenburger Platz 1, Berlin, Germany

Roman Ganzer
Department of Urology, University of Leipzig, Leipzig, Germany

Christoph Lübbert
Division of Infectious Diseases and Tropical Medicine, Department of Gastroenterology and Rheumatology, Leipzig University Hospital, Leipzig, Germany

René Fahrner, Falk Rauchfuss and Utz Settmacher
University Hospital Jena, Division of General, Visceral and Vascular Surgery, Am Klinikum 1, 07740 Jena, Germany

Hubert Scheuerlein
University Hospital Jena, Division of General, Visceral and Vascular Surgery, Am Klinikum 1, 07740 Jena, Germany
St. Vincenz Hospital, Division of General and Visceral Surgery, Am Busdorf 2, 33098 Paderborn, Germany

Hesham Abd Elaziz
Department of Surgery, Theodore Bilharz Research Institute, Cairo, Egypt

Asaad F. Salama
Department of Surgery, Theodore Bilharz Research Institute, Cairo, Egypt
Department of Surgery, Al-Jahra Hospital, Jahra, Kuwait

Hisham Rizk and Wisam Jamal
Department of Surgery, Theodore Bilharz Research Institute, Cairo, Egypt
Department of Surgery, University of Jeddah, Jeddah, Kingdom of Saudi Arabia

Alaa Magdy, Magdy Basheer and Ibrahim Dawoud
Department of Surgery, Mansoura University Hospital, Gihan El Sadat St., Mansoura 35511, Dakahlia, Egypt

Mohamed E. Abd Ellatif
Department of Surgery, Mansoura University Hospital, Gihan El Sadat St., Mansoura 35511, Dakahlia, Egypt
Department of Surgery, Hafr Elbatin Central Hospital, Hafr Elbatin, Kingdom of Saudi Arabia

Ayman El Nakeeb
Gastroenterology Surgical Center, Mansoura University, Mansoura, Egypt

Guoyong Chen, Sidong Wei, Jianjun Sun, Gaofeng Tang and Jianbin Chen
Center of Hepatopancreaticobiliary Surgery, Henan Provincial People's Hospital, Zhengzhou, Henan 450003, China

Zhongwu Zou
Hubei Vocational-Technical College School of Medicine, Xiaogan 432000, China

Shaotang Zhou
Center of Hepatopancreaticobiliary Surgery and Liver transplantation, 100 Xisihuang Middle Road, Fengtai District, Beijing 100039, China

LingXiang Kong, Ming Li, Lei Li, Li Jiang, Jiayin Yang and Lvnan Yan
Department of Liver Surgery, West China Hospital of Sichuan University, Chengdu, Sichuan Province, China

Dongbin Liu, Feng Cao, Jiafeng Liu, Dahua Xu, Yuehua Wang and Fei Li
Department of General Surgery, Xuanwu Hospital, Capital Medical University, Beijing 100053, People's Republic of China

Anwar Jarrad
Hepatology, Gastroenterology and Hepatobiliary/Transplant Unit, Jordan Hospital, Amman, Jordan

Abdalla Bashir
General and Transplant Surgery, Jordan Hospital, Amman, Jordan

Aiman Obed
Hepatobiliary and Transplant Surgery, Jordan Hospital, Amman, Jordan

Oliver Beetz, Michael Klein, Florian W. R. Vondran, Felix Oldhafer, Sebastian Cammann, Jürgen Klempnauer and Moritz Kleine
Department of General, Visceral and Transplant Surgery, Medizinische Hochschule Hannover, Carl-Neuberg-Strasse 1, 30625 Hannover, Germany

Harald Schrem
Department of General, Visceral and Transplant Surgery, Medizinische Hochschule Hannover, Carl-Neuberg-Strasse 1, 30625 Hannover, Germany
Core Facility Quality Management Transplantation, Integrated Research and Treatment Center Transplantation (IFB-Tx), Hannover Medical School, Hannover, Germany

Jill Gwiasda
Core Facility Quality Management Transplantation, Integrated Research and Treatment Center Transplantation (IFB-Tx), Hannover Medical School, Hannover, Germany

Karl J. Oldhafer
Department of General, Visceral and Oncological Surgery, Asklepios Klinik Barmbek, Hamburg, Germany

Andrea Boni, Giovanni Cochetti, Michele Del Zingaro, Francesca Quadrini, Alessio Paladini, Diego Cocca and Ettore Mearini
Department of Surgical and Biomedical Sciences, Division of Urological, Andrological surgery and Minimally-invasive techniques, University of Perugia, Perugia, Italy

Stefano Ascani
Institute of Pathologic Anatomy, "Santa Maria" Hospital, Terni, Italy

Mohamad Dughayli, Sergey Shimunov, Sherry Johnson and Fadi Baidoun
Department of General Surgery, Henry Ford Wyandotte Hospital, 2333 Biddle Avenue, Wyandotte, MI 48192, USA

Bachar Halimeh
Alfaisal University, Riyadh, Saudi Arabia

Louai R. Zaidan, Elhaitham K. Ahmed and Khalil Terro
Alfaisal University, Riyadh, Saudi Arabia
Specialized Medical Center Hospital, Riyadh, Saudi Arabia

Yasser Radwan
Specialized Medical Center Hospital, Riyadh, Saudi Arabia

Ibrahim Afifi, Husham Abdelrahman, Ruben Peralta and Hassan Al-Thani
Department of surgery, Trauma Surgery section, Hamad General Hospital (HGH), Doha, Qatar

Sheraz Abayazeed
Department of surgery, HGH, Doha, Qatar

Ayman El-Menyar
Clinical Research, Trauma and Vascular Surgery, HGH, Doha, Qatar
Clinical Medicine, Weill Cornell Medical College, Doha, Qatar

Index